HAIR RESTORATION

PROCEDURES IN COSMETIC DERMATOLOGY

PROCEDURES IN COSMETIC DERMATOLOGY

HAIR RESTORATION

Murad Alam, MD, MSCI, MBA
Professor and Vice-Chair
Department of Dermatology,
Professor
Departments of Surgery, Otolaryngology, and Medical Social Sciences
Northwestern University Feinberg School of Medicine
Chicago, Illinois

Jeffrey S. Dover, MD, FRCPC, FRCP
Director
SkinCare Physicians
Chestnut Hill, Massachusetts;
Associate Clinical Professor of Dermatology
Yale University School of Medicine;
Adjunct Associate Professor of Dermatology
Brown Medical School
Providence, Rhode Island

Series Editors
Jeffrey S. Dover, MD, FRCPC, FRCP
Murad Alam, MD, MSCI, MBA

ELSEVIER

Elsevier
1600 John F. Kennedy Blvd.
Ste 1800
Philadelphia, PA 19103-2899

Content Strategist: Jessica L. McCool/Charlotta Kryhl
Content Development Specialist: Akanksha Marwah
Publishing Services Manager: Shereen Jameel
Project Manager: Beula Christopher
Design Direction: Patrick C. Ferguson

Printed in India

Last digit is the print number: 9   8   7   6   5   4   3   2   1

Procedures in Cosmetic Dermatology
Series Editors: Jeffrey S. Dover, MD, FRCPC, FRCP and
Murad Alam, MD, MSCI, MBA

Recently published volumes:

2023
Botulinum Toxin
Fifth edition
Alastair Carruthers,
MA, BM, BCh, FRCPC, FRCP(Lon),
Jean Carruthers, MD, FRCS(C), FRC(Ophth),
Jeffrey S. Dover, MD, FRCPC, FRCP,
Murad Alam, MD, MSCI, MBA, and
Omer Ibrahim, MD
ISBN 978-0-323-83116-1

2023
Lasers, Lights, and Energy Devices
Fifth edition
Elizabeth L. Tanzi, MD, FAAD, Jeffrey S. Dover, MD,
FRCPC, FRCP, and Leah K. Spring, DO, FAAD
ISBN 978-0-323-82905-2

2020
Chemical Peels
Third edition
Suzan Obagi, MD
ISBN 978-0-323-65389-3

2017
Botulinum Toxin
Fourth edition
Alastair Carruthers, MA, BM, BCh, FRCPC, FRCP(Lon) and
Jean Carruthers, MD, FRCS(C), FRC(Ophth)
ISBN 978-0-323-47659-1

2017
Soft Tissue Augmentation
Fourth edition
Alastair Carruthers, MA, BM, BCh, FRCPC, FRCP(Lon) and
Jean Carruthers, MD, FRCS(C), FRC(Ophth)
ISBN 978-0-323-47658-4

Forthcoming volumes:

2023
Soft Tissue Augmentation
Fifth edition
Jean Carruthers, MD, FRCS(C), FRC(Ophth),
Alastair Carruthers, MA, BM,
BCh, FRCPC, FRCP(Lon), Jeffrey S. Dover, MD, FRCPC, FRCP,
Murad Alam, MD, MSCI, MBA, and Omer Ibrahim, MD
ISBN 978-0-323-83075-1

2023
Advanced Lifting
First edition
Hooman Khorasani, MD and Eyal Levit, MD
ISBN 978-0-323-67326-6

2023
Cosmetic Procedures in Skin of Color
First edition
Andrew F. Alexis, MD, MPH
ISBN 978-0-323-83144-4

2024
Photodynamic Therapy
Third edition
Macrene Alexiades, MD, PhD
ISBN 978-0-443-10689-7

2024
Cosmeceuticals
Fourth edition
Zoe Diana Draelos, MD
ISBN 978-0-443-11808-1

To my mentor, Kenneth A. Arndt, a true scholar whose inquisitiveness, curiosity, enthusiasm, support, and friendship have guided me through my career.

To my father, Mark – a great teacher, listener, and role model.

And especially to my wife, Tania, for her never-ending encouragement, patience, support, love, and friendship, and for being my moral compass.

Jeffrey S. Dover

To my parents, Rahat and Rehana, my sister Nigar, and my favorite niece and nephew, Noor and Ali.

Many thanks to all our chapter contributors, who were so kind to sign on to this project.

A very special thanks to Bianca Kang, without whose organizational skills, determination, and coaxing this would never have reached completion.

Murad Alam

CONTRIBUTORS

Crystal Aguh, MD
Assistant Professor
Department of Dermatology
Johns Hopkins University School of Medicine
Baltimore, Maryland

Murad Alam, MD, MSCI, MBA
Professor and Vice-Chair
Department of Dermatology
Northwestern University Feinberg School of Medicine;
Professor
Departments of Surgery, Otolaryngology, and Medical
    Social Sciences
Northwestern University Feinberg School of Medicine
Chicago, Illinois

Katherine Almengo, BS, MS
Medical Student
Medical Education
University of Toledo College of Medicine and Life
    Sciences
Toledo, Ohio

Marc R. Avram, MD
Clinical Professor of Dermatology
Dermatology
Weill Cornell Medical School
New York, New York

Sarah Benton, MD
Resident Physician
AMITA Health Resurrection Medical Center
Chicago, Illinois

Wilma Fowler Bergfeld, MD
Senior Dermatologist
Director of Dermatopathology
Cleveland Clinic
Cleveland, Ohio

Valerie D. Callender, MD
Associate Professor
Department of Dermatology
Howard University
Washington, District of Columbia;

Medical Director
Callender Dermatology and Cosmetic Center
Glenn Dale, Maryland

Fiore Casale, MMS
Junior Specialist
Department of Dermatology
University of California, Irvine
Irvine, California

Yu-Feng Chang, MD, MS
Doctor of Medicine
Clinical Research Fellow
Department of Dermatology
Brigham and Women's Hospital
Boston, Massachusetts

Maria Colavincenzo, MD
Assistant Professor
Department of Dermatology
Northwestern University Feinberg School of Medicine
Chicago, Illinois

Jeffrey S. Dover, MD, FRCPC, FRCP
Director of SkinCare Physicians
Department of Dermatology
SkinCare Physicians
Chestnut Hill, Massachusetts;
Associate Clinical Professor of Dermatology
Department of Dermatology
Yale University School of Medicine
New Haven, Connecticut;
Adjunct Associate Professor of Dermatology
Department of Dermatology
Brown Medical School
Providence, Rhode Island

Ronda Farah, MD
Assistant Professor
Department of Dermatology
University of Minnesota
Minneapolis, Minnesota

Lynne Goldberg, MD
Professor
Dermatology and Pathology and Laboratory Medicine
Boston University School of Medicine
Boston, Massachusetts

Ciara Grayson, MD
Resident Physician
Department of Dermatology
Henry Ford Hospital
Detroit, Michigan

Nicole Heinen, BS
Student
Department of Dermatology
University of Minnesota
Minneapolis, Minnesota

Maria Hordinsky, MD
Professor, Chair, and Director of the Clinical
    Research Division
Department of Dermatology
University of Minnesota
Minneapolis, Minnesota

Omer Ibrahim, MD
Dermatologist
Chicago Cosmetic Surgery and Dermatology
Chicago, Illinois

Jared Jagdeo, MD, MS
Associate Professor
Department of Dermatology
SUNY Downstate
Brooklyn, New York

Taylor A. Jamerson, MD
Resident Physician
University of Michigan Medical School
Ann Arbor, Michigan

Negar Kahen, MD
Clinical Research Fellow
Department of Dermatology
Northwestern University Feinberg School of Medicine
Chicago, Illinois

Bianca Y. Kang, MD
Postdoctoral Research Fellow
Department of Dermatology
Northwestern University Feinberg School of Medicine
Chicago, Illinois

Shilpi Khetarpal, MD
Assistant Professor of Dermatology
Department of Dermatology
Cleveland Clinic Foundation
Cleveland, Ohio

Alana Kurtti, MD
Resident Physician
Englewood Health
Englewood, New Jersey

Kristen Lo Sicco, MD, FAAD
Associate Professor
Department of Dermatology
New York University Langone Health;
Director
New York University Skin and Cancer Unit
New York, New York

Amy McMichael, MD
Professor and Chair
Department of Dermatology
Wake Forest Baptist Medical Center
Winston-Salem, North Carolina

Natasha Mesinkovska, MD, PHD
Associate Professor
Department of Dermatology
University of California Irvine
Irvine, California

Cristina Nguyen, MD, MSBS, MHA
Clinical Dermatology Research Fellow
Department of Dermatology
University of California, Irvine
Irvine, California

Kelly O'Connor, MD
Resident Physician
Dermatologist
South Shore Skin Center
Norwell, Massachusetts

Achiamah Osei-Tutu, MD
Dermatologist
Osei-Tutu Dermatology
Brooklyn, New York

James Thomas Pathoulas, MD
Resident Physician
Gundersen Medical Foundation
La Crosse, Wisconsin

Geraldine Cheyana Ranasinghe, MD
Dermatologist
Department of Dermatology
Cleveland Clinic Foundation
Cleveland, Ohio

Ora Raymond, BA
Clinical Research Fellow
Department of Dermatology
University of Minnesota
Minneapolis, Minnesota

Claudia M. Ricotti, MD
Resident Physician
Department of Dermatology
Cleveland Clinic
Cleveland, Ohio

Neil S. Sadick, MD, FACP, FAACS, FACPh, FAAD
Clinical Professor
Department of Dermatology
Weill Medical College of Cornell University
New York, New York

Sara Salas, MD
Dermatologist, Hair Restoration Specialist, and
**   Founder**
Baja Hair Center and Baja Scar Institute
Tijuana, Mexico

Maryanne Makredes Senna, MD, FAAD
Assistant Professor
Department of Dermatology
Harvard Medical School;
Director of MGH Hair Loss Clinic
Department of Dermatology
Massachusetts General Hospital
Boston, Massachusetts

Jerry Shapiro, MD
Professor
Department of Dermatology
New York University
New York, New York

Katharina Shaw, MD
Resident Physician
Ronald O. Perelman Department of Dermatology
New York University
New York, New York

Mollly Stout, MD
Dermatologist
Medical Dermatology Associates of Chicago
Chicago, Illinois

Cynthia Truong, MD
Medical Student
Resident Physician
Kaiser Permanente
San Francisco, California

Frances Walocko, MD
Surgical and Cosmetic Dermatology Fellow
Department of Dermatology
Northwestern University Feinberg School of Medicine
Chicago, Illinois

PREFACE

When the Procedures in Cosmetic Dermatology series was envisioned almost two decades ago, injectables and laser procedures were perceived as the core elements of cosmetic practice. Since then, cosmetic dermatology has grown into a much broader category, with the relevant expertise of dermatologists being similarly vast. As a result, beyond updating and expanding existing volumes in this series, from time to time, we have added several new topics of importance. Now, it is our pleasure and privilege to introduce this text on Hair Restoration.

In patients of every ethnicity, age, and sex, hair loss can be disfiguring and upsetting. Hair loss may have a specific, well-defined, disease-associated cause that can be medically treated. More commonly, hair loss is diffuse, nonscarring, and associated with aging, genetic predisposition, hormonal changes, and other poorly understood factors. It is this latter type of diffuse, non-specific hair loss that this volume is primarily designed to address.

We believe this book fills a significant need. Historically, books on hair have considered hair diseases, their diagnoses, and medical treatments or described hair transplantation. However, the preponderance of hair loss patients do not have a highly morbid disease, nor do they want a hair transplant. Although the volume in your hand does discuss transplantation and differential diagnosis of diseases of the hair, its primary subject is noninvasive treatment of diffuse, nonscarring hair loss, including androgenetic alopecia. Here, treatment of androgenetic alopecia is not an afterthought or one of many topics, but the main focus.

The vast majority of men, and up to half of women, will encounter hair loss associated with androgenetic alopecia at some point in their lives. As one of the visible signs of aging, such hair loss touches us all. We do not need to be vain or willing to undergo risky procedures to combat or slow hair loss. Increasingly, there are simple procedures and interventions to address the problem. With the tools explained in this book, cosmetic dermatologists will be well prepared to provide the most appropriate, current, and comprehensive care for hair loss patients of all types.

Treatment of hair is part of dermatology, and dermatologists are the undisputed experts in treatment of hair problems, including hair loss. In this volume, the leaders in hair within the field of dermatology share their wisdom and help us all become better practitioners.

Murad Alam, MD, MSCI, MBA
Jeffrey S. Dover, MD, FRCPC, FRCP

SERIES PREFACE

Much has changed since the first edition of this series. Noninvasive and minimally invasive cosmetic procedures, as pioneered by dermatologists, have become increasingly adopted by physicians and well accepted by patients. Cosmetic dermatologic surgery procedures have been refined and improved. Interventions have become more effective, safer, and more tolerable with increasing benefit-to-risk ratios. Combination cosmetic regimens that include multiple types of procedures have been shown to achieve results comparable to those that are more invasive, and new devices and technologies continue to be introduced.

How best to keep up with these advances and ensure offerings are state of the art, at the cutting edge? The newest edition of the Procedures in Cosmetic Dermatology series keeps you there, and, for those starting out in the field, these texts quickly introduce you and bring you to the state of the art. Each book in this series is designed to quickly impart basic skills and advanced concepts in an easy-to-understand manner. We focus not on theory but on how-to. Our expert book editors and chapter authors will guide you through the learning process efficiently, so you can soon get back to treating patients.

In addition to expanding and updating our existing book topics, we now add with the 5th edition entirely new volumes on hair restoration and skin of color.

The authors are leading dermatologists in the field. Dermatologists' role in cosmetic medicine has continued to expand. Research has revealed that primary care physicians and the general public view dermatologists as experts in less invasive cosmetic procedures. A nationwide advanced fellowship program in cosmetic dermatologic surgery has been initiated to train the next generation of dermatologists to the highest standards.

What has not changed is physicians' need for clear, concise, and current direction on procedure techniques. Physicians need to be proficient in the latest methods for enhancing appearance and concealing the visible signs of aging.

To that end, we hope that you, our reader, find the books enjoyable and educational.

We thank our many contributors and wish you well on your journey of discovery.

Jeffrey S. Dover, MD, FRCPC, FRCP
Murad Alam, MD, MSCI, MBA

SERIES PREFACE FIRST EDITION

Although dermatologists have been procedurally inclined since the beginning of the specialty, particularly rapid change has occurred in the past quarter century. The advent of frozen section technique and the golden age of Mohs skin cancer surgery has led to the formal incorporation of surgery within the dermatology curriculum. More recently technological breakthroughs in minimally invasive procedural dermatology have offered an aging population new options for improving the appearance of damaged skin.

Procedures for rejuvenating the skin and adjacent regions are actively sought by our patients. Significantly, dermatologists have pioneered devices, technologies, and medications, which have continued to evolve at a startling pace. Numerous major advances, including virtually all cutaneous lasers and light-source-based procedures, botulinum exotoxin, soft tissue augmentation, dilute anesthesia liposuction, leg vein treatments, chemical peels, and hair transplants have been invented or developed and enhanced by dermatologists. Dermatologists understand procedures, and we have special insight into the structure, function, and working of skin. Cosmetic dermatologists have made rejuvenation accessible to risk-averse patients by emphasizing safety and reducing operative trauma. No specialty is better positioned than dermatology to lead the field of cutaneous surgery while meeting patient needs.

As dermatology grows as a specialty, an ever-increasing proportion of dermatologists will become proficient in the delivery of different procedures. Not all dermatologists will perform all procedures, and some will perform very few, but even the less procedurally directed among us must be well versed in the details to be able to guide and educate our patients. Whether you are a skilled dermatologic surgeon interested in further expanding your surgical repertoire, a complete surgical novice wishing to learn a few simple procedures, or somewhere in between, this book and this series are for you.

The volume you are holding is one of a series entitled Procedures in Cosmetic Dermatology. The purpose of each book is to serve as a practical primer on a major topic area in procedural dermatology.

If you want to make sure you find the right book for your needs, you may wish to know what this book is and what it is not. It is not a comprehensive text grounded in theoretical underpinnings. It is not exhaustively referenced. It is not designed to be a completely unbiased review of the world's literature on the subject. At the same time, it is not an overview of cosmetic procedures that describes these in generalities without providing enough specific information to actually permit someone to perform the procedures. Importantly, it is not so heavy that it can serve as a doorstop or a shelf filler. What this book and this series offer is a step-by-step, practical guide to performing cutaneous surgical procedures. Each volume in the series has been edited by a known authority in that subfield. Each editor has recruited other equally practical-minded, technically skilled, hands-on clinicians to write the constituent chapters. Most chapters have two authors to ensure that different approaches and a broad range of opinions are incorporated. On the other hand, the two authors and the editors also collectively provide a consistency of tone. A uniform template has been used within each chapter so that the reader will be easily able to navigate all the books in the series. Within every chapter, the authors succinctly tell it like they do it. The emphasis is on therapeutic technique; treatment methods are discussed with an eye to appropriate indications, adverse events, and unusual cases. Finally, this book is short and can be read in its entirety on a long plane ride. We believe that brevity paradoxically results in greater information transfer because cover-to-cover mastery is practicable.

We hope you enjoy this book and the rest of the books in the series and that you benefit from the many hours of clinical wisdom that have been distilled to produce it. Please keep it nearby, where you can reach for it when you need it.

Jeffrey S. Dover MD, FRCPC, FRCP
Murad Alam MD, MSCI, MBA
Year: 2005

ACKNOWLEDGEMENT

Thank you to Ms. Akanksha Marwah, Senior Content Development Specialist, Ms. Beula Christopher, Senior Project Manager, Ms. Jessica McCool, Content Strategist, and Ms. Lotta Kryhl, Senior Content Strategist, our wonderful staff at Elsevier whose hard work and organization made this first edition possible. Thank you also to our incredible medical illustrator, Ms. Sheila Macomber, for transforming the authors' sketches into beautiful, descriptive images.

CONTENTS

VIDEO CONTENTS

Evaluation of Hair Loss

1

Medical Workup for Hair Loss

Negar Kahen and Maria Colavincenzo

KEY POINTS

- Although most patients seeking hair restoration have androgenetic alopecia, there are several other potential etiologies of hair-loss disorders. It is important to exclude other causes of hair loss resembling androgenetic alopecia before considering cosmetic treatment.
- The comprehensive initial assessment of a patient seeking cosmetic hair restoration includes obtaining a full medical history, assessing risk factors for alopecia, performing a global and dermoscopic examination of the hair and scalp, as well as laboratory and histopathology assessments, when indicated.
- Effective tools that allow progressive assessment of response to cosmetic hair loss treatment include scalp photography and videodermoscopy.

BACKGROUND, DEFINITIONS, AND HISTORY

The search for hair loss remedies has been ongoing for centuries. Ancient Egyptians documented the use of a concoction of ibex, crocodile, and snake fat to stimulate hair growth, and the pursuit of hair-loss treatments continues to present day (level of evidence: 5).[1] Since the late twentieth century, several promising pharmaco-therapeutic and procedural modalities for cosmetic hair restoration have become available. Although most patients seeking cosmetic hair restoration have androgenetic alopecia (AGA), there are several other potential etiologies for hair-loss disorders, and it is important to exclude other causes of hair loss resembling AGA before considering these treatment options. In this chapter, we will review the differential diagnosis of hair loss and the notable history and examination findings for each diagnosis.

The Hair Cycle

On a normal scalp, each hair follicle cycles independently; at any given moment, a percentage of hairs are growing, while others are resting and/or shedding. The majority of hair follicles are in the anagen or growth phase (86%–95%), a few are in the catagen or involution phase (1%), and a minority are in the telogen or resting phase (about 10%) (level of evidence: 5).[2] The anagen phase lasts for about 2 to 8 years, followed by a catagen phase lasting 3 to 6 weeks. The cycle concludes with the telogen phase, lasting for approximately 3 to 5 months.[2] An overly simplified but easily recalled summary of typical phase durations is "3 years, 3 weeks, 3 months." During the telogen phase, the hair shaft matures and is eventually shed from the follicle, after which a new anagen phase may commence. As long as the percentages of follicles in each phase are stable, the density and total number of scalp hairs remain stable (level of evidence: 5).[3] Any disturbance of the hair cycle may contribute to hair loss. The timing of this cycle also has implications for the expected timing of treatment response, often on the order of months (Fig. 1.1).

DIFFERENTIAL DIAGNOSIS OF HAIR LOSS

Hair loss, or alopecia, is typically divided into two main categories: scarring and nonscarring. In scarring

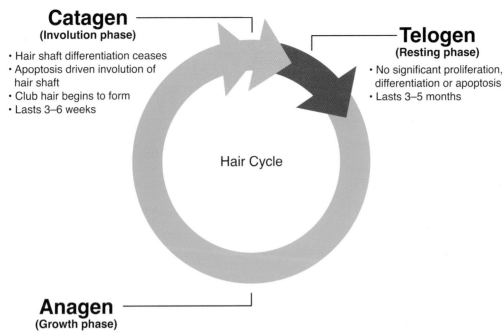

Catagen
(Involution phase)

- Hair shaft differentiation ceases
- Apoptosis driven involution of hair shaft
- Club hair begins to form
- Lasts 3–6 weeks

Telogen
(Resting phase)

- No significant proliferation, differentiation or apoptosis
- Lasts 3–5 months

Hair Cycle

Anagen
(Growth phase)

- Rapid proliferation in the hair bulb
- Hair shaft grows and differentiates
- Lasts 2–8 years

Fig. 1.1 The Hair Cycle. The scalp hair grows in cycles. During the anagen (growth) phase, the hair bulb forms and rapidly proliferates. The hair shafts are actively generated in this phase and grow to reach their maximum length and volume. During catagen (involution), the shortest of all three phases, the inferior segment of the follicle regresses and hair shaft production ceases. During the telogen (resting) phase, the hair follicle activity ceases and club hair rests loosely anchored in the hair canal. The length of each arrow shows the proportion of time the hair follicle spends in each stage.

alopecia, the hair follicle may be irreversibly destroyed and replaced by fibrous scar tissue, leading to permanent hair loss, with minimal potential for hair regrowth. Scarring alopecia is less common overall, usually found in a minority of cases in specialized hair clinics (level of evidence: 5).[4] In recent decades, however, there has been a rise in the prevalence of some scarring alopecias, for reasons that are poorly understood (level of evidence: 2b).[5] This makes the identification of any features of scarring alopecia a paramount consideration in the evaluation of patients seeking cosmetic hair restoration.

Although AGA is the most common cause of alopecia in adult patients, other nonscarring or scarring alopecia diagnoses should be considered and ruled out before pursuing cosmetic hair restoration. The most common mimickers of AGA are outlined later and will be discussed in greater detail in subsequent chapters (Fig. 1.2). In general, scarring alopecias, unlike AGA, may have symptoms, (classically itch or pain) and signs such as erythema, scaling, follicular papules, or areas of smooth follicular loss, leading to suspicion of scarring (Pearl 1.1). Other nonscarring alopecias may differ in their distribution or pattern, timing, or severity.

> **PEARL 1.1:** In general, scarring alopecias, unlike androgenetic alopecia, may have symptoms (classically itch or pain) and signs such as erythema, scaling, follicular papules, or areas of smooth follicular loss suspicious for scarring.

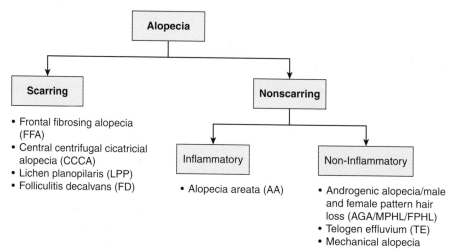

Fig. 1.2 Differential diagnosis of hair loss.

NONSCARRING ALOPECIA

Androgenetic Alopecia

AGA, also known as male pattern or female pattern hair loss (MPHL/FPHL), is a nonscarring alopecia affecting a large proportion of adults over their lifetime. AGA affects approximately 50% of men by age of 50, and 50% of women by age 60 (level of evidence: 4).[6] AGA is a genetically determined, polygenic trait. It is most prevalent in Caucasian men, who are four times more likely to develop premature balding compared with African American men.[6]

The pathophysiology of AGA involves progressive shrinkage of the hair follicles and shafts, called miniaturization (Fig. 1.3). Hairs transition over time from a normal, terminal hair to a vellus-type hair, with a potentially dramatic reduction in hair-shaft diameter. There is also a concomitant shortening of the anagen phase, resulting in shorter hair lengths. Androgen (male hormone) effects appear to drive this process over time, forming the basis for antiandrogen therapies for AGA. For reasons not yet wholly elucidated, miniaturization is typically much more prominent on the frontal and vertex scalp, with occipital sparing, leading to the typical distribution patterns seen in AGA in men and women. This difference in miniaturization over the scalp provides the basis for follicular unit transplantation, whereby nonminiaturized, typically occipital-scalp hairs are transplanted to the

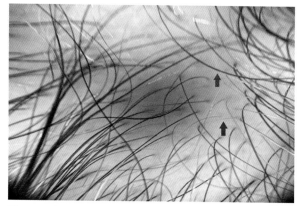

Fig. 1.3 Dermoscopic Examination of the Scalp of an Individual With Androgenetic Alopecia. Over time, hairs transition from terminal hairs *(blue arrow)* to vellus hairs *(red arrow)*.

thinned frontotemporal areas, where they retain their terminal status and may provide significant scalp coverage.

Individuals with MPHL experience varying degrees of hair loss in the bitemporal, frontal, mid-scalp, and vertex regions (Fig. 1.4). The Hamilton-Norwood scale is the leading classification system used for grading MPHL, and it has been widely reproduced for use in clinical practice (Fig. 1.5) (level of evidence: 3b).[7]

Women with FPHL typically experience diffuse hair loss in patterns described by Olsen, Ludwig, and

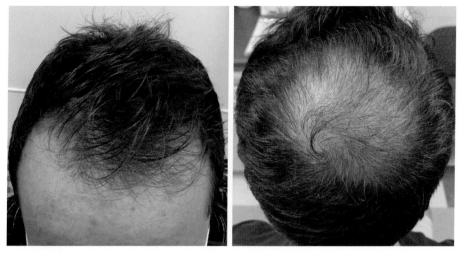

Fig. 1.4 Male Pattern Hair Loss. Bitemporal recession and thinning of the hair over the vertex are noted.

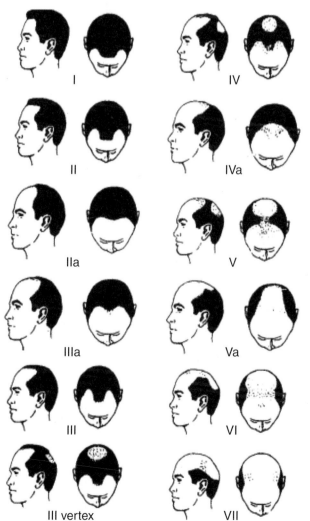

I

II

IIa

IIIa

III

III vertex

IV

IVa

V

Va

VI

VII

Fig. 1.5 Hamilton-Norwood Pattern of Hair Loss. (From Olsen EA, Weiner MS, DeLong E, Pinnell SR. Topical minoxidil in early male pattern baldness. *J Am Acad Dermatol.* 1985; 13:185-192)

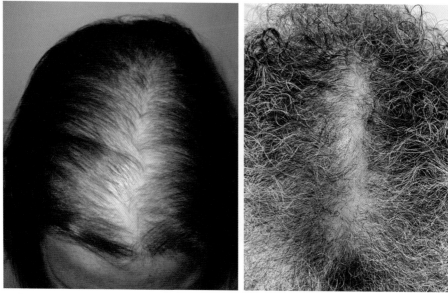

Fig. 1.6 Female Pattern Hair Loss. Women with female pattern hair loss typically experience diffuse hair loss most prominent on the crown.

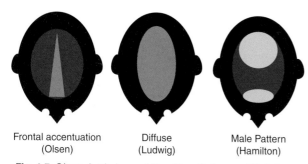

Frontal accentuation (Olsen) Diffuse (Ludwig) Male Pattern (Hamilton)

Fig. 1.7 Olsen, Ludwig, and Hamilton Patterns of Hair Loss.

PEARL 1.2: In androgenetic alopecia, miniaturization is typically prominent on the frontal and vertex scalp, with occipital sparing, leading to the distribution patterns seen in androgenetic alopecia in men and women.

Hamilton (Figs. 1.6 and 1.7) (level of evidence: 5).[8] The Olsen pattern describes accentuation of hair thinning in the anterior frontal scalp, giving the alopecic area a triangular-shaped appearance. The Ludwig pattern describes diffuse thinning of the crown region with frontal hairline preservation. Lastly, the Hamilton pattern has the classic distribution of MPHL, and an examination will reveal notable thinning in the lateral frontal part of the superior scalp and vertex (Pearl 1.2).

Telogen Effluvium

Telogen effluvium (TE) is a form of nonscarring alopecia characterized by diffuse, often acute hair shedding. Common triggering events include medical stress (e.g., severe illness, surgical procedures), emotional trauma (e.g., divorce, bankruptcy, bereavement), parturition, discontinuation of oral contraceptives, and significant weight loss or a crash diet in the months prior to hair loss (level of evidence: 5). In TE, hair loss may also be a manifestation of a general medical problem. For example, patients may present with diffuse hair loss as a symptom of thyroid disorders, anemia or iron deficiency, connective tissue disease, or as a side effect of medication (with a wide range of potentially implicated drugs). Obtaining a full medical history is essential for evaluating the potential contribution of underlying medical conditions to hair loss.

Patients with TE will often complain of increased hair shedding leading to shower drain clogging or increased hair notable on a comb/brush and pillow. They will commonly present samples of shed hair for validation (Fig. 1.8). TE and AGA frequently coexist, but the

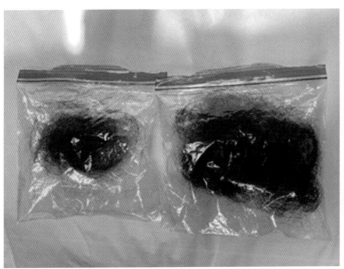 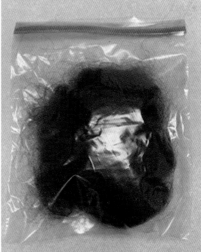

Fig. 1.8 "Hair Bag Sign." Samples of shed hair brought to a clinic by a patient with telogen effluvium.

diffuse pattern and acuity or abruptness of onset, with the primary complaint of shedding rather than increased scalp visibility, may be clues in support of the TE diagnosis.

In many cases, TE is said to "unmask" AGA, whereby patients notice their underlying MPHL/FPHL more prominently in the setting of a recent or ongoing TE episode. Thus in many cases, treatments for AGA may be instituted at the same time TE triggers are addressed (Pearl 1.3).

Alopecia Areata

Alopecia areata (AA) is a nonscarring, autoimmune, inflammatory hair-loss disorder that may affect the scalp or any hair-bearing area. Hair loss in AA can take many forms, ranging from the classic presentation, with abrupt development of well-demarcated focal patches (Fig. 1.9), to diffuse or total hair loss (alopecia totalis or universalis) (level of evidence: 5).[9] Family history of AA or related autoimmune conditions

---

> **PEARL 1.3:** Telogen effluvium and androgenetic alopecia often coexist, but the diffuse pattern, acuity, or abruptness of onset, with the primary complaint of shedding rather than increased scalp visibility, may be clues to the diagnosis of telogen effluvium.

---

can provide clues for this diagnosis. Extensive facial-hair loss (including eyebrows, eyelashes, or beard hair) should raise suspicion for this condition. Dermoscopic examination may reveal the classic "exclamation mark," or proximally tapered short hairs of active AA (Fig. 1.10).[9]

Mechanical Alopecia

The hair loss seen in this type of alopecia is caused by the exertion of excessive pulling forces, leading to mechanical damage of hair follicles. This initiates as a nonscarring process, but with chronicity, it may become scarring. Traction alopecia, related to tight hairstyles, classically causes alopecia at the fronto-temporal hairline, with a "fringe sign" of remaining short hairs at the anterior aspect (Fig. 1.11) (level of evidence: 5).[10]

Patients with trichotillomania have an abnormal urge to pull hair, which can lead to irregular patches of alopecia, often geometric in shape. Nonscalp hair (brows, lashes, pubic) is commonly affected by trichotillomania in adults.

SCARRING ALOPECIA

Lichen Planopilaris

Lichen planopilaris (LPP) is an immune mediated scarring alopecia that is more common in women

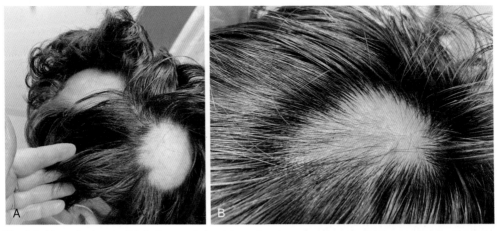

Fig. 1.9 Alopecia Areata. Well- demarcated patches of nonscarring alopecia (A). Incomplete or regrowing patches may mimic androgenetic alopecia (B).

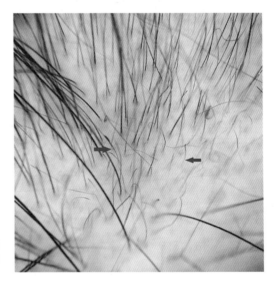

Fig. 1.10 Alopecia Areata Dermoscopic Examination. *Arrows* point to "exclamation mark hairs," or proximally tapered short hairs, a classic feature of active alopecia areata.

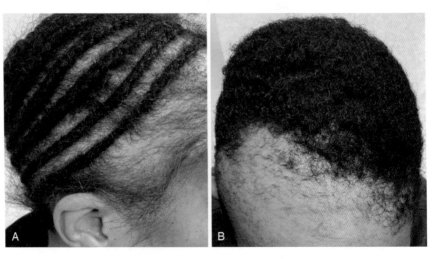

Fig. 1.11 Mechanical Alopecia. Traction alopecia (A) often presents with a "fringe sign" of thin remaining hairs anterior to alopecic patches at the anterior temporal hairline. Trichotillomania (B) may present with geometric or irregular alopecic patches.

than in men. Patients present with patchy alopecic areas, and their examination reveals follicular keratotic plugs and/or perifollicular scaling along with perifollicular erythema (Fig. 1.12) (level of evidence: 5).[11] Common presenting symptoms in the acute phase of LPP include shedding, itching, scaling, burning, and tenderness. The classic form of LPP involves the vertex, although any region of the scalp may be affected.

Frontal Fibrosing Alopecia

Frontal fibrosing alopecia (FFA) may be considered a subset of LPP with a distinct clinical pattern. FFA is a scarring alopecia characterized by progressive symmetric frontotemporal hairline recession and marked decrease or complete loss of eyebrows (Fig. 1.13) (level of evidence: 5).[12] Close examination of patients with this condition may reveal mild skin atrophy and perifollicular erythema at the

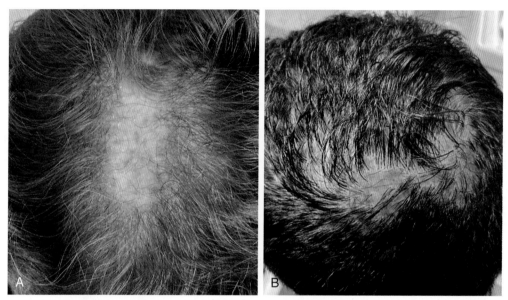

Fig. 1.12 Lichen Planopilaris. Examination reveals central scaring alopecia with scaling, erythematous perifollicular papules, and plaques (A). In darker skin types, hyperpigmentation may be more prominent than erythema (B).

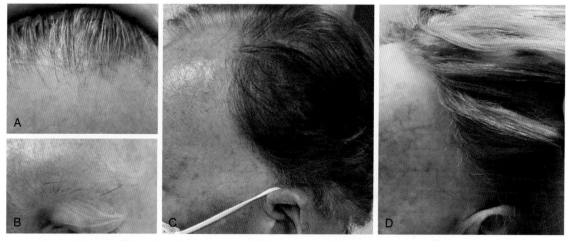

Fig. 1.13 Frontal Fibrosing Alopecia. Frontal fibrosing alopecia may be seen in male patients (A–C), but it is most commonly seen in females (D). Hairline recession and sideburn and brow loss are prominent features of this condition.

scalp margin. The classic "lonely hair sign" (level of evidence: 5)[13] refers to remaining terminal hairs at the frontal hairline margin (Fig. 1.14). This condition was initially described in postmenopausal Caucasian women but has increasingly been observed in younger women of all ethnic backgrounds and in male patients. The prevalence of FFA has increased dramatically since the 1990s, for unclear reasons (level of evidence: 4).[5] Environmental triggers (such as skin contactants) have been theorized but not proven. This condition should be considered in patients presenting with extensive eyebrow loss and in male patients with loss of beard hair (Pearl 1.4).

Central Centrifugal Cicatricial Alopecia

Central centrifugal cicatricial alopecia (CCCA) clinically presents as a patch of hair loss on the vertex or

> **PEARL 1.4:** Frontal fibrosing alopecia should be considered in patients who present with prominent loss of eyebrows or beard hair.

crown of the scalp that spreads centrifugally and spares the lateral and posterior scalp (Fig. 1.15) (level of evidence: 5).[14] This scarring alopecia is predominantly seen in women of African descent; however, it occasionally occurs in men as well. Although some have theorized that certain hair-care practices may contribute to an increased risk of developing CCCA, this relationship remains unproven. The distribution of CCCA overlaps with that of classic AGA in its prominent vertex involvement, making close inspection for any signs of inflammation or scarring a key

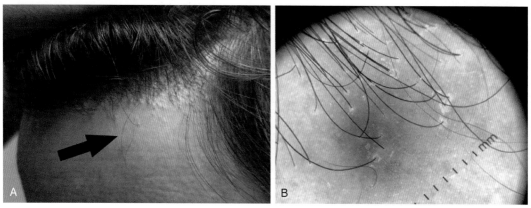

Fig. 1.14 Hairline Changes in Frontal Fibrosing Alopecia. "Lonely hair sign" (A). Dermoscopic examination reveals perifollicular scaly papules (B).

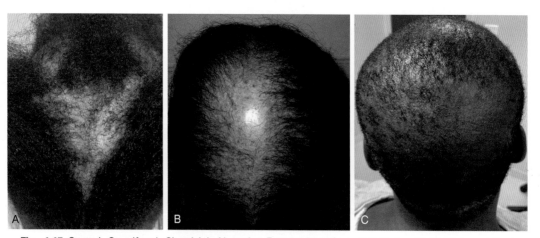

Fig. 1.15 Central Centrifugal Cicatricial Alopecia. Examination of an individual with central centrifugal cicatricial alopecia reveals smooth patches of scarring alopecia with loss of follicular ostia. Moderate (A) and severe (B) scarring alopecia of the crown to vertex in female patients are shown. Male patients (C) may also be affected.

component of the physical exam. Notably, in darker skin types, inflammation may present as hyperpigmentation rather than erythema (Pearl 1.5).

PEARL 1.5: In darker skin types, inflammation may present as hyperpigmentation rather than erythema.

Folliculitis Decalvans

Folliculitis decalvans (FD) is characterized by painful, recurrent purulent follicular exudation resulting in scarring alopecia. Examination reveals alopecic patches with follicular pustules, crusts, and tufted hairs (multiple hair shafts emerging from a single hair follicle) (Figs. 1.16 and 1.17) (level of evidence: 5).[15] This condition usually affects young adults, and its course is

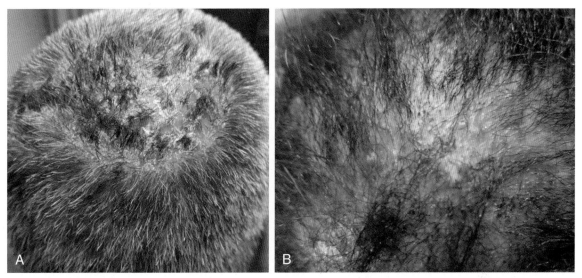

Fig. 1.16 Folliculitis Decalvans. Scarring alopecia with erythema, papules, pustules, and crusting (A). Dermatophyte infection can mimic this condition (B) and should be ruled out.

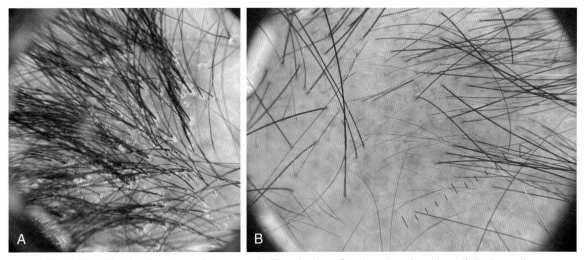

Fig. 1.17 Folliculitis Decalvans Dermoscopic Examination. Scarring alopecia with perifollicular scaling, tufted hairs and erythema on the edge of a smooth alopecic patch (A). Prominent miniaturization on the vertex of a male with androgenetic alopecia (B).

typically chronic and relapsing. Any pustules associated with alopecia on scalp examination should prompt a consideration of this entity, as well as potential infectious causes of pustules such as staphylococcal infection or dermatophytosis.

Tinea capitis, much less common among adult patients than among the pediatric population, may on occasion be mistaken for FD, as it may also present with scalp pustules and alopecia. Microscopy of scalp scrapings (especially of the broken hair shafts) and culture will reveal the infectious etiology.

INITIAL CONSULTATION AND ASSESSMENT

The main objective of initial consultation is to establish the patient's alopecia diagnosis. At this visit, a detailed history and careful examination can confirm the diagnosis of AGA and rule out other etiologies of hair loss (Table 1.1). Subsequent workup as indicated by history and examination findings can be initiated at this time (e.g., laboratory evaluation, scalp biopsy). Upon establishing the alopecia diagnosis as one amenable to cosmetic hair restoration, determining whether the patient is a suitable candidate for cosmetic hair restoration also

involves assessment of patient characteristics such as physical and emotional health. Patient education regarding available treatment modalities, potential risks and benefits, and realistic expectations in terms of efficacy and treatment timeline are important aspects of the initial consultation.

A standardized intake form addressing the following questions in steps 1 to 2 may facilitate the initial consultation assessment.

Step 1: Alopecia History

A detailed history should be obtained in patients presenting with alopecia (Table 1.2).

Step 2: Assessment of Risk Factors and Potential Contributors to Alopecia

A targeted history intake form can aid in rapidly assessing potentially relevant underlying conditions and factors affecting treatment decisions (Table 1.3).

Any potential issues identified related to mental health, such as a history of eating disorders or body dysmorphia, may affect considerations regarding the appropriateness of cosmetic hair restoration. In particular, patients with a history of body dysmorphic disorder may not be ideal candidates for cosmetic procedures

TABLE 1.1	Comparison of Clinical Features of Androgenetic Alopecia Versus Scarring Alopecias				
COMPARISON OF CLINICAL FEATURES OF ANDROGENETIC ALOPECIA VERSUS SCARRING ALOPECIAS					
	AGA	CCCA	FFA	LPP	FD
Type of alopecia	Nonscarring	Scarring	Scarring	Scarring	Scarring
Location of hair loss	Frontal, bitemporal, crown, vertex	Vertex, crown	Frontotemporal hair line, eyebrows, side-burns and beard	Commonly vertex but can occur anywhere	Vertex, occiput
Inflammation present	No	Yes, when in active phase			
Potential Symptoms	Asymptomatic	Sometimes tenderness, pruritus	Majority asymptomatic, some with tenderness, pruritus	Usually symptomatic with pruritus burning, or tenderness	Tenderness, pruritus +/− burning
Physical exam	Miniaturization	Shiny or smooth scalp, erythema or hyperpigmentation	Perifollicular erythema and follicular hyperkeratosis	Follicular keratotic plugs and/or perifollicular scaling along with perifollicular erythema	Alopecic patches with follicular pustules, crusts and tufted hairs

TABLE 1.2   Key Components of History Taking in Patients With Alopecia

Comments	Alopecia History
Seeing too much scalp is a classic complaint in AGA, while hair shedding is more common in TE/AA.	**What is your main concern for today's visit?** [ ] increased scalp visibility [ ] hair shedding [ ] hair thinning [ ] other: _____
AGA typically progresses slowly over many months to years.	**When did your hair loss begin?** _____ **Was your hair loss sudden or gradual?** [ ] sudden [ ] gradual
AGA is typically asymptomatic, while patients with scarring alopecias often present with pruritus and tenderness over the scalp.	**Are you experiencing any of the following symptoms on your scalp?** [ ] flaking [ ] itching [ ] burning [ ] pain
On occasion, the areas that look thinned to the provider are not those of concern to the patient. Therefore, it is important to establish alignment in perception of the problem. Although many postmenopausal women will note minor (not severe or patchy) brow loss and loss of body hair (e.g., not needing to shave axillae/legs), severe loss can be a clue to autoimmune diseases such as AA or FFA.	**Where have you noted hair loss (mark all that apply)?** [ ] top/front of scalp [ ] sides of scalp [ ] back of scalp [ ] arms/legs [ ] underarms [ ] groin [ ] eyebrows [ ] eyelashes [ ] mustache/beard

Evaluate for common contributors to TE. Hormonally active medications are a unique consideration in their potential effects on the hair cycle, where medication discontinuation may be a trigger for hair shedding.	**In the past 3–12 months, have you experienced any of the following?**
	[ ] hospitalization/severe medical illness/major surgery
	[ ] changes in your medications
	  [ ] started or stopped birth control pills
	  [ ] started or stopped hormone treatment
	[ ] other: _____
	[ ] severe psychological stress
	[ ] significant weight loss or weight gain

Duration of treatment, side effects of therapy, and perceived efficacy/patient satisfaction should be assessed for all medical therapies and procedures.	**What treatments/therapies have you tried in the past?** [ ] minoxidil (Rogaine) [ ] steroid injections [ ] spironolactone (Aldactone) [ ] platelet rich plasma (RPR) [ ] finasteride (Propecia) [ ] biotin [ ] LED light device/helmet [ ] hair growth supplements [ ] hair transplant procedure [ ] other: _____
AGA is a hereditary condition.	**Family History** Do you have family history of hair loss? [ ] yes [ ] no Which relative(s) were affected? _____
Reviewing any previous pathology can aid in assessment and diagnosis.	**Previous Workup** Have you seen a provider for hair loss in the past? [ ] yes [ ] no What workup has been done in the past? [ ] scalp biopsy _____ [ ] labs _____
Reviewing prior interventions can help guide future treatment planning.	**Cosmetic History** Have you had any previous cosmetic surgeries/procedures? _____ How satisfied were you with the results? _____

TABLE 1.3   Assessment of Risk Factors and Potential Contributors to Alopecia

Comments	Assessment of Risk Factors and Potential Contributors to Alopecia

Dietary restrictions and significant weight loss can be associated with hair loss.	**Nutrition**
	Are you vegan or vegetarian? [ ] yes [ ] no
	Have you experienced any of the following?
	    [ ] any recent changes in diet
	    [ ] recent weight loss or weight gain greater than 10 pounds
	    [ ] history of weight loss surgery
	    [ ] history of gastrointestinal disease

Evaluate for symptoms suggestive of hyperandrogenism, which could warrant further laboratory workup.	**Hormonal/Reproductive**
	Women:
	Have you gone through menopause [ ] yes [ ] no
	Have you recently given birth? [ ] yes [ ] no
	Are you possibly pregnant or trying to conceive? [ ] yes [ ] no
	Are your menstrual periods:
	    [ ] regular [ ] irregular [ ] no menses
	    [ ] light [ ] moderate [ ] heavy
	Do you have history of any of the following:
	    [ ] PCOS (polycystic ovarian syndrome)
	    [ ] infertility
	    [ ] unwanted facial hair or hair on chest/breasts
	    [ ] hormonal acne
	Are you currently on any of the following treatments?
	[ ] oral contraceptives
	[ ] IUD (intrauterine device)
	[ ] hormone replacement therapy
	[ ] estrogen blockers (tamoxifen, anastrozole)
	Men:
	Have you been diagnosed with:
	[ ] low libido or other sexual function disorder
	[ ] hypogonadism
	Are you currently taking:
	[ ] antiandrogens (finasteride, dutasteride)
	[ ] testosterone supplementation
	[ ] anabolic steroids

	Endocrine Do you have history of: [ ] thyroid disorder [ ] pituitary disorder [ ] delayed or abnormal puberty/development [ ] diabetes
	Heme Do you have history of: [ ] anemia/iron deficiency [ ] blood loss [ ] bleeding disorder [ ] blood thinner use

TABLE 1.3 Assessment of Risk Factors and Potential Contributors to Alopecia—cont'd	
Evaluate for anagen effluvium and assess for permanent chemotherapy-induced alopecia, defined as alopecia persisting >6mo after chemotherapy.	**Oncologic** Have you ever been diagnosed with cancer or received chemotherapy/ radiation therapy? [ ] yes [ ] no
	Autoimmune Do you have history of autoimmune disorders such as: [ ] alopecia areata [ ] vitiligo [ ] autoimmune thyroid disease [ ] inflammatory bowel disease [ ] lupus erythematous [ ] sarcoidosis [ ] other: _____
	Infectious Disease History Do you have history of: [ ] recent COVID-19 infection [ ] HIV [ ] sexually transmitted disease (including syphilis, gonorrhea, chlamydia) [ ] other infections: _____
	Cardiac Disease Do you have history of: [ ] cardiac disease (rhythm disorders, heart attack, congestive heart failure) [ ] high blood pressure
	Mental Health History Do you have history of: [ ] depression [ ] anxiety [ ] bipolar disorder [ ] eating disorder [ ] body dysmorphic disorder [ ] other:

because of abnormal fixation on hair and the inability to make objective self-assessment. Patients with a history of dissatisfaction with cosmetic procedures may present similar challenges. Alignment of patient and provider perceptions of severity is a positive factor.

Step 3: Physical Examination

The main goal of the physical examination is to establish the diagnosis of AGA and exclude other potential contributors.

A: Global Assessment

From a distance, one can evaluate for appropriateness of patient demeanor, patient mood, and global severity of alopecia. Severe nonscalp alopecia will often be evident even from a distance (e.g., alopecia universalis or severe FFA with complete brow loss).

B: Scalp Alopecia Assessment

Distribution. Does the distribution fit a typical pattern of MPHL/FPHL? Are there any focal patches of alopecia outside of these areas? Is the hair thinning even and diffuse?

Severity. Grade severity using a relevant scale, if appropriate.

Hair-pull test. Although the hair-pull test is a controversial examination technique, positive results may be a clue to TE or AA/inflammatory disorder. This test is performed by grasping roughly 40 to 60 closely grouped scalp hairs between the thumb and index fingers and gently pulling the hairs from the proximal to distal ends. The hair pulls are performed at the vertex, parietal, and occipital areas of the scalp. Broken hairs are discarded, and the remaining pulled hairs are counted. Some consider extraction of more than 10% of the hairs, or 6 to 10 hairs, as abnormal (level of evidence: 4),[16,17] although others have argued 2 or more hairs removed per pull should be characterized as abnormal (level of evidence: 4).[18]

C: Nonscalp Hair Assessment

Close examination of eyebrows, lashes, and sideburn and beard areas should be performed to assess for any signs of patchy alopecia, inflammation, or follicular scarring.

D: Nails and Other Skin Surfaces

Any signs of inflammation on the scalp suggestive of psoriasis, AA, or lichenoid process should prompt examination of nails and inquiry regarding any dermatosis affecting other skin surfaces.

E: Evaluate for Signs of Inflammation or Scarring

Does the examination reveal erythema, scale, papules, pustules, or edema?

These findings should not be seen in cases of AGA. In cases of coexisting seborrheic dermatitis, which is common, scaling and erythema may be seen along with signs of AGA. However, there should be no signs of scarring.

F: Dermoscopic Features

The dermoscopic examination is a useful technique for diagnosis and follow-up of hair and scalp disorders. Knowing the common dermoscopic features of typical hair and scalp disorders allows the clinician to distinguish between AGA and other types of scarring and nonscarring alopecias. An absence of findings suggestive of other entities in the differential diagnosis of AGA helps rule those out. With a dermatoscope, the clinician can evaluate for signs of inflammation and features suggestive of AA or scarring alopecia (such as smooth alopecic patches with an absence of follicular openings). Close examination of the frontotemporal hairline is necessary to exclude subtle cases of FFA or mechanical alopecia.

Dermoscopy enables assessment of the extent of hair-follicle miniaturization, the hallmark feature of AGA. A key distinguishing finding in AGA dermoscopic examination is hair diameter variability greater than 20% (level of evidence: 4).[19] It is helpful to compare findings in characteristically affected and unaffected areas. For example, in females, hair should be parted and examined at the vertex, mid scalp, and frontal scalp (2 cm from hairline). Clues to AGA may include lower average hair thickness in the frontal area compared with the occiput, with more than 10% of thin hairs in the frontal area (level of evidence: 4).[20]

Laboratory Workup and Additional Testing

Routine laboratory tests are useful in identifying potential underlying causes of hair loss. Commonly ordered tests include a complete blood count (CBC) to screen for anemia, iron studies (ferritin in particular), and thyroid-stimulating hormone (TSH), T3 and T4 to evaluate thyroid function.

The relationship between iron deficiency and hair loss remains controversial. Prior studies (with small sample sizes) have found associations between iron deficiency and hair loss, while others have not (level of evidence: 3b).[21-23] Iron deficiency anemia, a common cause of TE among menstruating women, should be treated with iron supplementation, and modulation of menorrhagia (where appropriate) in coordination with gynecology. The recommendation to supplement for low-normal ferritin levels, however, while widespread in practice, remains controversial.[23] Many authors believe treatment for hair loss is enhanced when iron deficiency, with or without anemia, is corrected. A common goal is ferritin values above 40 ng/mL, although there are no evidence-based targets. Iron studies may also be warranted in postmenopausal women or male patients with a history or examination findings suggestive of TE.

Some authors have suggested vitamin D deficiency may be associated with hair loss, though causality has not been established (level of evidence: 3b).[24] It is thought that vitamin D deficiency is relatively common, and many patients could benefit from supplementation. However, indications for testing and supplementation in the setting of hair loss are not firmly established (level of evidence: 3a).[25,26] It is possible that commonly identified deficiencies are not relevant to hair loss disorders.

The majority of women with FPHL do not have clinical evidence of androgen excess, such as hirsutism, severe/treatment refractory acne, or irregular menses. In women with potential signs of androgen excess, free and total testosterone and dehydroepiandrosterone sulfate (DHEAS) should be evaluated (level of evidence: 5).[27] If testosterone is greater than 200 ng/dL, or DHEAS is greater than 700 ug/dL in premenopausal or 400 ug/dL in postmenopausal women, a workup with radiographic tests to search for a tumor should be undertaken.

Other tests to evaluate hair loss should be directed by history, review of systems, and examination findings. For example, joint pains or other lupus features could suggest the need for antinuclear antibody (ANA) titer. Those with possible sexually transmitted disease exposure could necessitate syphilis serology. Though rare, diffuse nonscarring hair loss can present as the only sign of secondary syphilitic infection (level of evidence: 5).[28] Individuals presenting with galactorrhea and hair loss should be evaluated for hyperprolactinemia (level of evidence: 5).[27] Dietary restrictions or weight-loss surgery could suggest a role for serum zinc level testing. Additional investigations may be performed, depending on the clinical scenario, if there are other features revealed in a patient's history or examination that suggest potential underlying conditions.

Histopathology

In cases where there is a concern for scarring alopecia, biopsy is crucial, as it allows for early diagnosis and treatment to forestall permanent hair loss. In diagnosis of AGA, biopsy is helpful when the pattern of hair loss is not typical, or symptoms or examination findings raise suspicion of an inflammatory or scarring process. Biopsy can exclude or confirm these entities. An optimal scalp biopsy is a 4 mm punch biopsy for horizontal embedding (level of evidence: 4).[29] This is the most valuable method to reach a diagnosis of AGA, as all hair follicles can be visualized (level of evidence: 4).[30] To increase diagnostic accuracy, two specimens should be obtained. Most authors agree that selecting at least one scalp area not typically affected by AGA, such as the occipital region, may increase the chances of finding a distinct process. Because AGA preferentially affects the crown to vertex, a biopsy from this area would provide the highest yield for diagnosis of AGA (level of evidence: 5).[29]

A key histologic finding in AGA is miniaturization, the process of large, terminal follicles becoming smaller until they reach the size of vellus follicles.[30] In AGA, the total number of follicles is unchanged; however, as a result of miniaturization, there is an increase in the number of vellus hairs. In an unaffected scalp, the ratio of terminal-to-vellus hair is 7:1, and this ratio decreases in AGA. A terminal-to-vellus ratio of 3:1 is considered diagnostic of AGA (level of evidence: 4).[31] Other findings include hair-shaft diameter variation, increased fibrous tracts, and decreased follicular density in long-standing cases.[30,31] A mild peri-infundibular lymphocytic-cell infiltrate and perifollicular collagen deposition are present in 40% of cases.[31]

MONITORING AND DOCUMENTATION

Management of AGA requires long-term follow-up visits to assess and document treatment efficacy. Treatment response will allow further decision making such as adjusting treatment dose, changing therapy, or adding adjuvant treatments. Effective tools that allow progressive assessment of treatment efficacy include scalp photography and videodermoscopy.

Scalp Photography

Photography is an essential tool for tracking alopecia over time. Photography accurately captures a patient's progress and allows for objective discussion about the treatment response between the physician and the patient. Studies have also shown patients who were able to compare pre and post treatment photos had decreased alopecia-related anxiety (level of evidence: 4).[32]

The complete photographic record of a patient consists of images taken in four standard views: frontal, vertex, occipital, and both temporal areas. To reduce confounding variables, patients should be instructed to avoid use of hair products, hair prostheses, or extensions. Standardization of the photographic process and ensuring that the view, magnification, and lighting are consistent across visits is recommended. To this end, the use of a stereotactic positioning device on which the patient's chin and forehead are fixed and the given camera and flash device are mounted is suggested (level of evidence: 5).[33] Dermoscopic photos may also be helpful for tracking changes overtime in a magnified view.

Videodermoscopy

Videodermoscopy is performed using a video camera equipped with optic lenses that allow viewing at multiple magnifications and the capturing and storing of images. Similar to patient satisfaction with scalp photography, patients may appreciate the ability to view videodermoscopic images of their scalp in real time as part of their scalp assessment. Doing so may also increase patient engagement in tracking their examination progress. Some videodermoscopy devices use specialized software that allows automated and manual measurement of hair density, number of follicular units, and thickness and proportion of vellus-to-terminal hairs (level of evidence: 5).[34] These software programs introduce an objective element into the diagnostic process. However, optimization for automated calculation software is still required, as some studies have revealed errors in automatic counts in comparison to manual counts (level of evidence: 3b).[35]

FUTURE DIRECTIONS

Teledermatology is an innovative and evolving model of care delivery that has developed rapidly in tandem with technological advances, particularly in the twenty-first century. Services can be delivered through either a live-interactive or store-and-forward format, with the latter being more popular because of its lower cost and greater flexibility in coordination. Several studies report a moderate-to-high degree of diagnostic and management concordance between teledermatology and conventional in-person dermatologic visits in management of cutaneous malignancies and inflammatory skin conditions (level of evidence: 4).[36] With improvements in technology allowing patients to capture and transmit high-quality photos and video, as well as increased access to technology among patients, the use of teledermatology for assessment and management of alopecia may increase in the future. Additional research is warranted to identify the benefits and limitations of teledermatology in hair-loss disorder management.

EVIDENCE SUMMARY

- Androgenic alopecia, also known as male pattern of femal pattern hair loss, is the most common cause of hair loss worldwide, and the majority of patients seeking cosmetic hair restoration will likely carry this diagnosis. However, other nonscarring or scarring alopecia diagnoses should be considered and ruled out before pursuit of cosmetic hair restoration (strength of recommendation: A).

- Clinical clues to other diagnoses may include signs of inflammation or scarring, well-demarcated patches of alopecia, abrupt onset of hair loss, or involvement of nonscalp hair. Dermoscopic examination of the scalp of an individual with androgenic alopecia will reveal miniaturization and hair-diameter variability of greater than 20% (strength of recommendation: B).

- Scalp biopsy may aid in clarifying the type of alopecia, particularly in cases with suspected scarring. On biopsy, a terminal-to-vellus ratio of 3:1 is considered diagnostic of androgenic alopecia (strength of recommendation: B).

- In cases where other underlying medical contributors are suspected based on thorough history and examination, laboratory evaluation for conditions such as thyroid disorders, anemia, and iron deficiency should be undertaken (strength of recommendation: B).

- Photographic monitoring as part of standardized follow-up is essential for assessing a patient's response to therapy over time (strength of recommendation: B).

REFERENCES

1. Tassie GJ. Hairstyling technology and techniques used in ancient Egypt. In: Selin H, ed. *Encyclopaedia of the History of Science, Technology, and Medicine in Non-Western Cultures*. Netherlands: Springer; 2016:2155-2164.
2. Harrison S, Sinclair R. Telogen effluvium. *Clin Exp Dermatol*. 2002;27(5):389-395.
3. Malkud S. Telogen effluvium: a review. *J Clin Diagn Res*. 2015;9(9):WE01-WE03.
4. Bolduc C, Sperling LC, Shapiro J. Primary cicatricial alopecia: Lymphocytic primary cicatricial alopecias, including chronic cutaneous lupus erythematosus, lichen planopilaris, frontal fibrosing alopecia, and Graham-Little syndrome. *J Am Acad Dermatol*. 2016; 75(6):1081-1099.
5. Mirmirani P, Tosti A, Goldberg L, Whiting D, Sotoodian B. Frontal fibrosing alopecia: an emerging epidemic. *Skin Appendage Disord*. 2019;5(2):90-93.
6. Sinclair RD, Dawber RP. Androgenetic alopecia in men and women. *Clin Dermatol*. 2001;19(2):167-178.
7. Norwood OT. Male pattern baldness: classification and incidence. *South Med J*. 1975;68(11):1359-1365.
8. Olsen EA. Current and novel methods for assessing efficacy of hair growth promoters in pattern hair loss. *J Am Acad Dermatol*. 2003;48(2):253-262.
9. Wasserman D, Guzman-Sanchez DA, Scott K, McMichael A. Alopecia areata. *Int J Dermatol*. 2007;46(2):121-131.

10. Billero V, Miteva M. Traction alopecia: the root of the problem. *Clin Cosmet Investig Dermatol.* 2018;11:149-159.

11. Kang H, Alzolibani AA, Otberg N, Shapiro J. Lichen planopilaris. *Dermatol Ther.* 2008;21(4):249-256.

12. Tavakolpour S, Mahmoudi H, Abedini R, Kamyab Hesari K, Kiani A, Daneshpazhooh M. Frontal fibrosing alopecia: an update on the hypothesis of pathogenesis and treatment. *Int J Womens Dermatol.* 2019;5(2):116-123.

13. Tosti A, Miteva M, Torres F. Lonely hair: a clue to the diagnosis of frontal fibrosing alopecia. *Arch Dermatol.* 2011;147(10):1240.

14. Miteva M, Tosti A. Central centrifugal cicatricial alopecia presenting with irregular patchy alopecia on the lateral and posterior scalp. *Skin Appendage Disord.* 2015;1(1):1-5.

15. Otberg N, Kang H, Alzolibani AA, Shapiro J. Folliculitis decalvans. *Dermatol Ther.* 2008;21(4):238-244.

16. Miteva MI. Chapter 2 – Hair Pathology: The Basics. Alopecia. St. Louis, Missouri: Elsevier; 2019:23-41. 1st ed.

17. Cranwell WC, Sinclair R. Chapter 6 – Telogen Effluvium. Alopecia. St. Louis, Missouri: Elsevier; 2019:83-93. 1st ed.

18. McDonald KA, Shelley AJ, Colantonio S, Beecker J. Hair pull test: evidence-based update and revision of guidelines. *J Am Acad Dermatol.* 2017;76(3):472-477.

19. Miteva M, Tosti A. Hair and scalp dermatoscopy. *J Am Acad Dermatol.* 2012;67(5):1040-1048.

20. Rakowska A, Slowinska M, Kowalska-Oledzka E, Olszewska M, Rudnicka L. Dermoscopy in female androgenic alopecia: method standardization and diagnostic criteria. *Int J Trichology.* 2009;1(2):123-130.

21. Kantor J, Kessler LJ, Brooks DG, Cotsarelis G. Decreased serum ferritin is associated with alopecia in women. *J Invest Dermatol.* 2003;121(5):985-988.

22. Olsen EA, Reed KB, Cacchio PB, Caudill L. Iron deficiency in female pattern hair loss, chronic telogen effluvium, and control groups. *J Am Acad Dermatol.* 2010;63(6):991-999.

22. Trost LB, Bergfeld WF, Calogeras E. The diagnosis and treatment of iron deficiency and its potential relationship to hair loss. *J Am Acad Dermatol.* 2006;54(5):824-844.

24. Cheung EJ, Sink JR, English JC III. Vitamin and mineral deficiencies in patients with telogen effluvium: a retrospective cross-sectional study. *J Drugs Dermatol.* 2016;15(10):1235-1237.

25. Tamer F, Yuksel ME, Karabag Y. Serum ferritin and vitamin D levels should be evaluated in patients with diffuse hair loss prior to treatment. *Postepy Dermatol Alergol.* 2020;37(3):407-411.

26. Almohanna HM, Ahmed AA, Tsatalis JP, Tosti A. The role of vitamins and minerals in hair loss: a review. *Dermatol Ther (Heidelb).* 2019;9(1):51-70.

27. Olsen EA, Messenger AG, Shapiro J, et al. Evaluation and treatment of male and female pattern hair loss. *J Am Acad Dermatol.* 2005;52(2):301-311.

28. Piraccini BM, Broccoli A, Starace M, et al. Hair and scalp manifestations in secondary syphilis: epidemiology, clinical features and trichoscopy. *Dermatology.* 2015; 231(2):171-176.

29. Liyanage D, Sinclair R. Telogen effluvium. *Cosmetics.* 2016;3(2):13.

30. Chartier MB, Hoss DM, Grant-Kels JM. Approach to the adult female patient with diffuse nonscarring alopecia. *J Am Acad Dermatol.* 2002;47(6):809-818; quiz 818-820.

31. Stefanato CM. Histopathology of alopecia: a clinicopathological approach to diagnosis. *Histopathology.* 2010;56(1):24-38.

32. Pathoulas JT, Flanagan KE, Walker CJ, Wiss IMP, Azimi E, Senna MM. Evaluation of standardized scalp photography on patient perception of hair loss severity, anxiety, and treatment. *J Am Acad Dermatol.* 2021; 85:1640-1641. doi:10.1016/j.jaad.2020.12.059.

33. Trueb RM. Female Alopecia: Guide to Successful Management. Berlin/Heidelberg: Springer; 2013.

34. Tosti A, Asz-Sigall D, Pirmez R, eds. *Hair and Scalp Treatments: A Practical Guide.* Switzerland: Springer Nature; 2019.

35. Bilgiç Temel A, Gülkesen KH, Dicle Ö. Automated digital image analysis (TrichoScan) in male patients with androgenetic alopecia; comparison with manual marking of hairs on trichoscopic images. *Skin Res Technol.* 2018; 24(3):515-516.

36. Wang RH, Barbieri JS, Nguyen HP, et al. Clinical effectiveness and cost-effectiveness of teledermatology: where are we now, and what are the barriers to adoption? *J Am Acad Dermatol.* 2020;83(1):299-307.

2

Ethnic Differences in Hair

Ciara Grayson and Amy McMichael

KEY POINTS

- Understanding the differences in hair structure and haircare practices in African Americans compared with white, Hispanic, and Asian patients is essential when evaluating and treating hair concerns in this population.
- Structural characteristics of Afro-textured hair include a retroverted hair bulb, an S-shaped follicle, and an elliptical-shaped hair shaft.
- Hairstyles such as tight buns and ponytails, braids, dreadlocks, and weaves increase the risk of developing traction alopecia, which is present in approximately one-third of women of African descent.
- Both scarring and nonscarring alopecias can affect the skin of non-white patients. However, some types of hair loss appear to be more common in men and women of African descent, including traction alopecia, acquired trichorrhexis nodosa, seborrheic dermatitis, alopecia areata, central centrifugal cicatricial alopecia, folliculitis decalvans, acne keloidalis nuchae, and dissecting cellulitis.
- Various treatment options exist for alopecia in patients with skin of color, and the choice of treatment depends on the underlying diagnosis.
- Effective treatment options for androgenetic alopecia include topical minoxidil and low-level laser light therapy in men and women and oral 5α-reductase inhibitors in men.

INTRODUCTION

Non-white patients, specifically those of African descent, have unique hair characteristics and haircare practices. Understanding the differences seen in the hair of African Americans compared with white, Hispanic, and Asian patients is essential when evaluating and treating hair concerns in this population. Hair is classified into three types: African, Asian, and Caucasian (Fig. 2.1). Each of these differ in structure, growth rate, and density. This chapter will focus on Afro-textured hair.

The structural characteristics of Afro-textured hair include a retroverted hair bulb that resembles the shape of a golf club, an S-shaped follicle, and an elliptical-shaped hair shaft (level of evidence: 2b).[1]

The retroverted hair bulb is responsible for the curly configuration of Afro-textured hair (level of evidence: 2b).[2] One theory is that the curly nature of the hair prevents even distribution of sebum along the hair shaft, leaving the scalp oily and hair shaft prone to dryness (level of evidence: 5).[3] Additionally, Afro-textured hair is lower in density and has a slower growth rate compared with Caucasian hair (level of evidence: 5),[4] regardless of scalp region or gender (level of evidence: 2b).[5] It is important for dermatologists to understand the unique features of Afro-textured hair in addition to cultural haircare practices and hairstyles, as this may facilitate compliance with treatment and help discern practices that may negatively affect scalp disease.

African   **Asian**   **Caucasian**

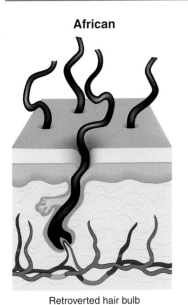   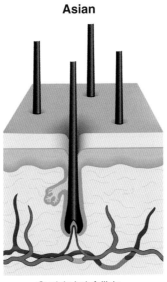   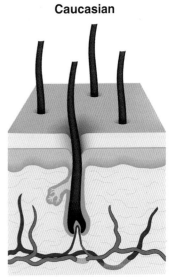

Retroverted hair bulb   Straight hair follicle   Straight and symmetrical
and S-shaped hair follicle   hair follicle

Fig. 2.1 Structure of Hair Follicles by Ethnicity. Hair is classified into three types: African, Asian, and Caucasian. (Courtesy of Sheila Macomber.)

CULTURAL DIFFERENCES IN PERSONS WITH SKIN OF COLOR

Societal beauty standards have often valued the European aesthetic, which can negatively affect Black women's perception of their own body image (level of evidence: 2b).[6] In a research study conducted by Awad et al., a cohort of black women were surveyed on body image concerns. Researchers found that hair was the most important body image domain.[6] Participants reported that their hair influenced their self-confidence.[6] Additionally, the pressure to adhere to societal and personal beauty standards led to significant sacrifices of time and money.[6] Recognition of these factors can help dermatologists understand why patients may be hesitant to change haircare practices or styles, even if recommended as part of a hair-loss treatment regimen.

Exercise also affects haircare practices. A study completed by Ahn et al. found that women of African descent modified their hairstyles to accommodate physical activity. This included wearing braids, a ponytail or bun, or the use of a scarf or hair wrap (level of evidence: 2b).[7] Additionally, 18% of these women exercised less often to avoid sweating out hairstyles.[7]

When evaluating a patient with hair loss, the place to begin is with a thorough hair-loss history. In the case of patients with Afro-textured hair, asking the right questions is paramount (Pearl 2.1). Onset and type of symptoms and the affected location of the scalp are important for all patients with hair loss, but for those with Afro-textured hair, a number of specific haircare questions must be included: use of chemical relaxers, traction-related hair styles (hair weaves, braids, locks) (level of evidence: 5),[8,9] frequency of hair washing, use of heat for straightening, and other product use. Moreover, clinicians should approach these encounters with empathy and acknowledge the significant psychosocial implications that may accompany hair loss (level of evidence: 5).[10]

PEARL 2.1: Obtaining a hair history and completing a thorough examination of the scalp are essential in diagnosing alopecia in patients with Afro-textured hair.

> **PEARL 2.2:** It is important to successfully treat inflammatory scalp disease prior to beginning any topical treatments for pattern hair loss, because the presence of inflammation can complicate treatment.

> **PEARL 2.3:** Bitemporal hair loss can be a manifestation of pattern hair loss, traction alopecia, telogen effluvium, alopecia areata, frontal fibrosing alopecia, central centrifugal cicatricial alopecia, or seborrheic dermatitis.

COMMON FORMS OF HAIR LOSS THAT AFFECT PATIENTS WITH SKIN OF COLOR

Although we will focus on androgenetic alopecia (AGA), several other forms of hair loss are important to discuss, as they may be in the differential diagnosis of AGA or complicating the treatment of AGA (Pearl 2.2).

Nonscarring Alopecias

Nonscarring alopecias are common and can be associated with hairstyles and haircare practices. With prompt diagnosis and treatment, hair regrowth is attainable. In this section, we present several nonscarring alopecias that may be seen in patients with Afro-textured hair.

Androgenetic Alopecia or Pattern Hair Loss

Androgenetic alopecia (AGA), also known as female or male pattern hair loss (FPHL/MPHL), is a common nonscarring alopecia with a characteristic pattern distribution. The population frequency and severity increase with age in both men and women. Patients typically experience slow, progressive hair loss, and associated symptoms may include pruritus and trichodynia (level of evidence: 5).[11] The prevalence of pattern hair loss is highest in Caucasian males and females compared with Asians (level of evidence: 2b).[12] There is currently no data on the prevalence of pattern hair loss in men and women of African descent.

FPHL presents as a reduction in scalp hair density, primarily in the vertex and frontal scalp. This is caused by follicular miniaturization and an increase in vellus follicles (level of evidence: 2b).[13] The vellus hair follicles have a reduced anagen cycle, leading to short, fine hair shafts (level of evidence: 5).[14] As the hairs become thinner, the central part appears wider on the frontal scalp compared with the occipital scalp (level of evidence: 5).[15] Women may present with diffuse thinning in the vertex scalp, thinning that is more prominent in the frontal scalp, resulting in a "Christmas tree pattern" (level of evidence: 5),[16] or bitemporal thinning.[14] Although bitemporal hair loss is common in FPHL, it can also be seen in traction alopecia, telogen effluvium (TE), alopecia areata (AA), frontal fibrosing alopecia

(FFA), central centrifugal cicatricial alopecia (CCCA), and seborrheic dermatitis (level of evidence: 5).[17] In FPHL, the frontal hairline is typically spared (Pearl 2.3). The etiology is likely caused by an interplay of genetics, hormones, and environmental factors. Although some women with FPHL have excessive androgen production, others have normal levels of androgens,[14] leaving the exact role of androgens in FPHL poorly understood.

MPHL presents as hair loss in the temporal, midfrontal, or vertex scalp. Dihydrotestosterone binds to androgen receptors in hair follicles, which leads to suppression of hair growth by miniaturization of hair follicles (level of evidence: 5).[18] The severity and areas of involvement are variable. Different regional patterns of hair loss are caused by differences in follicle sensitivity to dihydrotestosterone.[18]

The differential diagnosis of pattern hair loss is extensive and includes CCCA, FFA, folliculitis decalvans (FD), and, rarely, dissecting cellulitis (DC). The presence of inflammation or scarring is not consistent with pattern hair loss and should prompt consideration of another cause of alopecia. Underlying medical conditions such as eating disorders leading to malnutrition, iron deficiency, or thyroid dysfunction should also be explored, as they may result in diffuse hair loss that may appear more pronounced on the vertex scalp caused by mild underlying pattern hair loss (level of evidence: 5).[11] The goal of treatment is to prevent progression of hair loss and reverse the miniaturization process. Treatment options that have proven to be effective in randomized controlled trials include topical minoxidil and low-level laser light therapy in men and women, and oral 5α-reductase inhibitors in men (level of evidence: 1b).[19-21] Other off-label treatment options for women include oral 5α-reductase inhibitors, as well as antiandrogen therapies such as spironolactone, cyproterone acetate (outside the United States), and flutamide (level of evidence: 5).[22] In the twenty-first century, low-dose, oral minoxidil has been gaining favor for the treatment of pattern hair loss in both men and women. Scalp hair restoration may be performed for men and women with severe cases (level of evidence: 5).[23]

PEARL 2.4: Hairstyles such as tight buns and ponytails, braids, dreadlocks, and weaves increase the risk of developing traction alopecia, which is present in approximately one-third of women of African descent.

Traction Alopecia

Approximately one-third of women of African descent have traction alopecia, which clinically appears as thinning and hair loss at the frontotemporal scalp. Although it is typically believed that traction alopecia is caused by excessive tension on the hair shaft (level of evidence: 2b)[24] as a result of tight hair styling and haircare practices (level of evidence: 5),[25] it is not known if there is genetic predisposition contributing to the development of traction alopecia. Hairstyles that result in increased risk of traction alopecia include tight buns and ponytails, braids, dreadlocks, and weaves (level of evidence: 2b).[26–28] The prevalence is higher in long, relaxed hair and when styles such as braids are applied to relaxed hair (Pearl 2.4).[28] Scalp symptoms in the frontotemporal scalp, such as stinging, pain, pustules, and crusting, are the harbingers of tight hair styles and increase the likelihood of the clinical appearance of traction alopecia (level of evidence: 2b).[28,29] Clinically, perifollicular erythema is the first sign of traction alopecia (level of evidence: 2b).[30] The fringe sign, or presence of vellus hairs along the frontal or temporal scalp, is both sensitive and specific to traction alopecia.[30] Tenting of the hair follicle, which occurs when the hair is pulled so tightly that it raises the scalp, is also indicative of excessive tension.[30] Early intervention is paramount in treatment of traction alopecia, as only early stages are thought to be nonscarring; long-standing traction can be unresponsive to treatments or changes in haircare practices. Patients should be encouraged to discontinue high-risk hairstyles immediately. A discussion including gentle hair-style recommendations that can replace high-traction styles should occur. Even nocturnal hair treatments such as hair wrapping that can aggravate traction should be discussed, as they must be discontinued as well (level of evidence: 5).[31] Medical treatments include oral and topical antibiotics if there is folliculitis, and topical or intralesional corticosteroids if inflammation is present (level of evidence: 5).[32] Intralesional corticosteroids combined with topical minoxidil have shown to be effective (level of evidence: 2b),[33] as has topical minoxidil alone (level of evidence: 1a).[34] There have been reports of successful hair transplantation, punch grafting, and rotation flaps for advanced traction alopecia (level of evidence: 4).[27,35]

Acquired Trichorrhexis Nodosa

Afro-textured hair retains less moisture and is more fragile than other hair types, which increases susceptibility to breakage (level of evidence: 2b).[36,37] In acquired trichorrhexis nodosa (ATN), the hair shaft is fragile, dull, and may have visible nodes (level of evidence: 5).[38] Clinically, ATN can be identified by broken hair shafts with frayed ends of uneven lengths (level of evidence: 5).[39] Gentle tugging on the distal ends of the hair shaft (tug test) may result in breakage of small hair fragments (level of evidence: 5).[39] Topical minoxidil may cause scalp dryness, which is more commonly seen when the 5% solution is used for its increased propylene glycol content (level of evidence: 5).[40] This dryness may extend down the hair shaft, making it difficult to use topical minoxidil. Khumalo et al. found that Afro-textured hair has the same distribution of cysteine-rich proteins as white and Asian hair, suggesting physical trauma rather than trichothiodystrophy triggers the hair fragility seen in patients of African descent (level of evidence: 2b).[41] Additionally, haircare practices such as chemical relaxers, permanent hair color, drying agents such as gels and spritzes, and thermal straightening, including the use of ceramic flat irons, have been associated with an increased risk of ATN (level of evidence: 5).[4,37,39] Treatment of ATN includes screening for and treating underlying conditions such as hypothyroidism, iron deficiency, and nutritional deficiencies followed by discontinuation of haircare practices that increase risk of breakage. A healthy haircare routine that consists of moisturizing shampoo and moisturizing products used no more than once per week and the use of leave-in hair shaft conditioners to help moisturize the hair is recommended (level of evidence: 5).[42]

Seborrheic Dermatitis

Seborrheic dermatitis is a chronic inflammatory condition that affects sebaceous-rich areas such as the forehead, eyebrows, nasolabial folds, and scalp. Although the etiology is unknown, *Malassezia furfur* is likely involved in the pathogenesis (level of evidence: 5).[43] African American patients commonly seek help from dermatologists for this condition, which was the third most common diagnosis in a large database study and in the top five conditions seen in a study of patients in a skin of color clinic (level of evidence: 2b).[44,45] As the presence of inflammation can complicate the topical treatment of pattern hair loss, it is important to successfully treat seborrheic dermatitis prior to beginning any topical treatments for pattern hair loss.

Clinically, seborrheic dermatitis presents as scaly, flaky, and sometimes hypopigmented plaques. Inflammation and pruritis of the scalp can cause the patient to repetitively scratch the affected area, which may result in hair loss (level of evidence: 2b).[46] To effectively treat seborrheic dermatitis, dermatologists must be aware of the cultural differences in haircare practices of patients with skin of color. Infrequent washing and the use of hair oils and pomades, both of which commonly occur in this population, may exacerbate seborrheic dermatitis (level of evidence: 5).[47] Patients often apply these products to improve flaking and pruritus. Treatment modalities include antidandruff shampoos that contain zinc pyrithione, selenium sulfide, and tar.[47] The shampoo should be applied only to the scalp to minimize dryness along the hair shaft. Topical corticosteroids, antifungals, and calcineurin inhibitors have also proven effective (level of evidence: 5).[48] Patients with Afro-textured hair should be encouraged to wash their hair once a week or biweekly and refrain from excessive use of hair oils and pomades on the scalp.[47]

Alopecia Areata

Alopecia areata (AA) is autoimmune, inflammatory hair loss that may affect the scalp and/or body. Although the pathogenesis is not completely understood, studies have shown that cytotoxic NKD2+ T cells are necessary and sufficient to induce alopecia in mice. This work led to the understanding that IL-15 (required for the growth of natural killer cells) has been identified as a potential therapeutic target with Janus kinase (JAK) inhibitors affecting the signaling pathway of IL-15 (level of evidence: 2b).[49,50] In a study completed using the National Alopecia Areata Registry, researchers found that African Americans have higher odds of AA compared with their Caucasian counterparts (level of evidence: 3b).[51] Clinically, AA presents as a sudden onset of patchy hair loss without signs of scarring or inflammation (level of evidence: 5).[52] The extent of hair loss can vary from a small patch to complete loss of hair over the entire scalp and body. Rarely, bitemporal or vertex hair loss in AA may mimic pattern hair loss. Exclamation point hairs (short hairs that are thicker distally compared with proximally) are pathognomonic for AA (level of evidence: 5).[53] Patients are typically

asymptomatic, but some may experience itching, tingling, or dysesthesia prior to the onset of hair loss.[53] Spontaneous hair regrowth may occur with subsequent relapse. Treatment includes topical, oral, or intralesional corticosteroids, topical minoxidil, and methotrexate (level of evidence: 1b).[54,57,58]

Scarring Alopecias

Scarring or cicatricial alopecias are a result of inflammation that leads to follicular unit destruction. Once the hair follicle is no longer viable, hair loss is irreversible. This section includes details about clinical appearance and treatment options for scarring alopecias commonly seen in patients with Afro-textured hair. CCCA and FD are often in the differential diagnosis of pattern hair loss, and vertex and frontal thinning may occur in all these entities. Acne keloidalis nuchae (AKN) can interfere with donor area hair growth in patients with pattern hair loss, so this form of hair loss should be effectively treated.

Central Centrifugal Cicatricial Alopecia

Central centrifugal cicatricial alopecia (CCCA) is the most common cause of scarring hair loss in patients of African descent (level of evidence: 5).[59] It is a chronic, progressive, and inflammatory form of hair loss that begins on the vertex of the scalp and spreads centrifugally (level of evidence: 3b).[60] The prevalence has been reported to range from 2.7% to 5.6%, and the average age of presentation is 36 years (level of evidence: 2b).[41,59,61] Hair breakage in the vertex of the scalp has been reported as an early manifestation of CCCA (level of evidence: 4).[62] This may be difficult for patients to visualize and appreciate, emphasizing the importance of a thorough scalp and hair examination when patients present to the dermatologist. It is also crucial to illicit a family history of hair loss, as one study found CCCA to be inherited in an autosomal dominant fashion with partial penetrance (level of evidence: 2b).[63] Additionally, various research studies have found that haircare practices such as wearing braids with extensions, sew-in weaves, and glue-in weaves are associated with the development of CCCA (level of evidence: 3b).[63,64] A 2019 study by Malki et al. sought to identify a genetic association of CCCA (level of evidence: 3b).[65] They found that mutations in the *PADI3* gene, which is responsible for proper hair-shaft formation, are associated with CCCA. This data, combined with studies that noted an association between haircare practices and CCCA, suggest that the pathogenesis of CCCA is likely multifactorial. Clinical examination will reveal a smooth, shiny scalp with decreased or absent follicular ostia (level of evidence: 4).[60] Although this disease may be asymptomatic, some patients experience pruritis, pain, pustules, or tenderness.[25,59,62] The goal of treatment is to stop inflammation and scarring to preserve any remaining hair follicles. First, patients should be encouraged to discontinue all traumatic hair styling. Medical treatment includes the use of topical and intralesional corticosteroids, antidandruff shampoos, antimalarials, and oral and topical antibiotics (level of evidence: 5).[66] Topical minoxidil can be used to prolong the anagen phase and treat coexisting FPHL (level of evidence: 5).[67] If the inflammation has been controlled for a year, hair transplantation may be an option (level of evidence: 4).[68] However, it is important to note that presence of scarring may hinder successful hair restoration. Discussion of realistic expectations with the patient is paramount and should focus on preventing progression of disease rather than hair regrowth.

Folliculitis Decalvans

Folliculitis decalvans (FD) is a neutrophilic cicatricial alopecia that presents with alopecic patches, pustules, crusts, and tufted hairs (level of evidence: 2b).[69] The patches most commonly occur in the vertex of the scalp, and associated symptoms include pruritus, pain, and burning (level of evidence: 2b).[69,70] It predominately affects young to middle-aged African American males (level of evidence: 2b).[59,69–72] The etiology of FD is unknown. However, it is believed to be a result of an abnormal immune response to *Staphylococcus aureus* (level of evidence: 4).[69,73] Treatment aims to reduce inflammation and pustules. Oral and topical antibiotics and topical and intralesional corticosteroids have shown to be effective in disease remission (level of evidence: 5).[74] Additionally, isotretinoin and red-light photodynamic therapy have been reported to result in disease remission (Pearl 2.5).[74]

Acne Keloidalis Nuchae

Another follicular disorder that predominately affects males of African descent is acne keloidalis nuchae

(AKN). This chronic folliculitis leads to destruction of the follicles, resulting in patchy, cicatricial alopecia. The incidence is reported to be 0.5% to 13.6% in African Americans and 9.4% in Nigerians (level of evidence: 2b).[75–77] Short haircuts, shaving the scalp, and getting a haircut at the barber are believed to be inciting factors (level of evidence: 2b).[77,78] Clinically, AKN presents as fibrotic papules and pustules on the occipital scalp and posterior neck (level of evidence: 5).[77,79] Over time, the papules may coalesce to form keloidal plaques with tufted hairs (level of evidence: 5).[80] The onset of these findings is often preceded by a few hours to days of pruritis or irritation to the occipital scalp or posterior neck.[80] Aside from pruritis, other symptoms include pain and bleeding upon contact with active lesions.[80] Treatment begins with preventing exacerbating factors. Patients should be encouraged to avoid short haircuts, self-manipulation, and mechanical irritation from shirt collars and hats.[79] Medical treatment includes the use of topical and intralesional corticosteroids and topical and oral antibiotics.[79] Surgery may be considered for severe cases. There have been reports of successful treatment with excision followed by second intention healing (level of evidence: 4)[81,82] and significant improvement with long pulsed Nd:YAG laser (level of evidence: 2b).[83]

Dissecting Cellulitis

Dissecting cellulitis (DC) of the scalp is thought to be caused by abnormal follicular keratinization resulting in follicular occlusion and bacterial infection (level of evidence: 4).[84] It predominately affects African American males aged 20 to 40 years. Clinically, patients initially have folliculitis on the vertex or occipital scalp (level of evidence: 4).[85] Fluctuant nodules with abscesses and sinus tracts develop over time.[86] DC often follows a relapsing course but will eventually result in scarring alopecia and keloidal scars in the areas of chronic inflammation.[85] Oral antibiotics, isotretinoin, and corticosteroids are used to treat DC.[86] Additionally, patients treated with antitumor necrosis factor α agents, surgical excision, or Nd:YAG laser therapy reported significant improvement (level of evidence: 5).[87]

Frontal Fibrosing Alopecia

Frontal fibrosing alopecia (FFA), a variant of lichen planopilaris, is an inflammatory, cicatricial alopecia that affects the frontotemporal hairline (level of

---

PEARL 2.5: Central centrifugal cicatricial alopecia and folliculitis decalvans should be included in the differential of pattern hair loss, as they too can cause thinning in the frontal and vertex scalp.

evidence: 2b).[88] It typically affects postmenopausal women, though women of all ages have been described, as have men. It is characterized by progressive recession of the frontotemporal hairline (level of evidence: 2b).[89] Partial or complete loss of eyebrows often occurs prior to the onset of hair loss. Clinical examination will reveal frontotemporal hair loss along with perifollicular erythema and hyperkeratosis.[89] Although the etiology is not completely understood, four genes have been identified in association with FFA. The *HLA-B* gene is most strongly associated with a diagnosis of FFA (level of evidence: 3b).[90] FFA has also been associated with hormone exposure, and environmental factors (level of evidence: 3b)[91,92] in some select cases. Symptoms may include pruritis, pain, and burning.[89] Treatment aims to halt progression of the disease and includes oral 5α-reductase inhibitors, intralesional corticosteroids, and antimalarials (level of evidence: 5).[93]

FUTURE DIRECTIONS

The use of new treatment modalities for alopecia are promising. Platelet rich plasma (PRP) has a high concentration of growth factors that can act on dermal papilla cells to promote hair growth (level of evidence: 5).[94] A study assessing the effectiveness of PRP for pattern hair loss found a statistically significant increase in hair density and anagen hairs (level of evidence: 1b).[95] When PRP was compared with intralesional triamcinolone for treatment of AA, both led to significant hair regrowth compared with placebo, but patients treated with PRP had significantly increased hair regrowth compared with patients treated with intralesional triamcinolone (level of evidence: 1b).[96] There have also been reports of increase in hair density from PRP in a patient with CCCA with a mild component of FPHL and another patient with lichen planopilaris (level of evidence: 4).[97] Additionally, systemic retinoids have shown to be effective in preventing disease progression of FFA (level of evidence: 2b).[98] Several studies have demonstrated that JAK/STAT inhibitors resulted in significant scalp hair regrowth in the treatment of AA (level of evidence: 1b).[99–102] Lastly, use of topical 10% metformin resulted in visible hair growth in two patients with recalcitrant CCCA (level of evidence: 4).[103] Future research studies should include diverse patient populations and aim to better understand the pathogeneses and most efficacious treatments for nonscarring and scarring alopecias.

EVIDENCE SUMMARY

Recommendation	GRADE Strength of Recommendation	References
Low-level laser light therapy and topical minoxidil in men and women for treatment of pattern hair loss (AGA)	A	Jimenez[19]
Oral 5α-reductase inhibitors for treatment of male pattern hair loss	A	Gubelin,[20] Sato[21]
Oral Janus Kinase inhibitors for treatment of alopecia areata	B	Xing,[49] Almutairi[99]
Topical or oral corticosteroids for treatment of alopecia areata	A	Tosti,[54] Mancuso,[55] Kar[56]
Topical minoxidil for treatment of alopecia areata	C	Price,[57] expert opinion
Topical and intralesional corticosteroids, antidandruff shampoos, antimalarials, and topical and oral antibiotics for treatment of central centrifugal cicatricial alopecia	D	Expert opinion
Long pulsed Nd:YAG laser for treatment of acne keloidalis nuchae	C	Esmat[83]
Topical and intralesional corticosteroids and topical and oral antibiotics for treatment of acne keloidalis nuchae	D	Expert opinion

REFERENCES

1. Miteva M, Tosti A. 'A detective look' at hair biopsies from African-American patients. *Br J Dermatol.* 2012; 166(6):1289-1294.

2. Thibaut S, Gaillard O, Bouhanna P, Cannell DW, Bernard BA. Human hair shape is programmed from the bulb. *Br J Dermatol.* 2005;152(4):632-638.

3. Quinn CR, Quinn TM, Kelly AP. Hair care practices in African American women. *Cutis.* 2003;72(4):280-289.

4. Lewallen R, Francis S, Fisher B, et al. Hair care practices and structural evaluation of scalp and hair shaft parameters in African American and Caucasian women. *J Cosmet Dermatol.* 2015;14(3):216-223.

5. Loussouarn G. African hair growth parameters. *Br J Dermatol.* 2001;145(2):294-297.

6. Awad GH, Norwood C, Taylor DS, et al. Beauty and body image concerns among African American College Women. *J Black Psychol.* 2015;41(6):540-564.

7. Ahn CS, Suchonwanit P, Foy CG, Smith P, McMichael AJ. Hair and scalp care in African American Women who exercise. *JAMA Dermatol.* 2016;152(5):579-580.

8. Tanus A, Oliveira CC, Villarreal DJ, Sanchez FA, Dias MF. Black women's hair: the main scalp dermatoses and aesthetic practices in women of African ethnicity. *An Bras Dermatol.* 2015;90(4):450-465.

9. Haskin A, Aguh C. All hairstyles are not created equal: what the dermatologist needs to know about black hairstyling practices and the risk of traction alopecia (TA). *J Am Acad Dermatol.* 2016;75(3):606-611.

10. Marks DH, Penzi LR, Ibler E, et al. The medical and psychosocial associations of alopecia: recognizing hair loss as more than a cosmetic concern. *Am J Clin Dermatol.* 2019;20(2):195-200.

11. Blume-Peytavi U, Blumeyer A, Tosti A, et al. S1 guideline for diagnostic evaluation in androgenetic alopecia in men, women and adolescents. *Br J Dermatol.* 2011; 164(1):5-15.

12. Paik JH, Yoon JB, Sim WY, Kim BS, Kim NI. The prevalence and types of androgenetic alopecia in Korean men and women. *Br J Dermatol.* 2001;145(1):95-99.

13. Messenger AG, Sinclair R. Follicular miniaturization in female pattern hair loss: clinicopathological correlations. *Br J Dermatol.* 2006;155(5):926-930.

14. Herskovitz I, Tosti A. Female pattern hair loss. *Int J Endocrinol Metab.* 2013;11(4):e9860.

15. Price VH. Androgenetic alopecia in women. *J Investig Dermatol Symp Proc.* 2003;8(1):24-27.

16. Olsen EA. Female pattern hair loss. *J Am Acad Dermatol.* 2001;45(suppl 3):S70-S80.

17. De Souza B, Tovar-Garza A, Uwakwe L, McMichael A. Bi-temporal scalp hair loss: differential diagnosis of nonscarring and scarring conditions. *J Clin Aesthet Dermatol.* 2021;14(2):26-33.

18. Lolli F, Pallotti F, Rossi A, et al. Androgenetic alopecia: a review. *Endocrine.* 2017;57(1):9-17.

19. Jimenez JJ, Wikramanayake TC, Bergfeld W, et al. Efficacy and safety of a low-level laser device in the treatment of male and female pattern hair loss: a multicenter, randomized, sham device-controlled, double-blind study. *Am J Clin Dermatol.* 2014;15(2):115-127.

20. Gubelin Harcha W, Barboza Martínez J, Tsai TF, et al. A randomized, active- and placebo-controlled study of the efficacy and safety of different doses of dutasteride versus placebo and finasteride in the treatment of male subjects with androgenetic alopecia. *J Am Acad Dermatol.* 2014;70(3):489-498.e3.

21. Sato A, Takeda A. Evaluation of efficacy and safety of finasteride 1 mg in 3177 Japanese men with androgenetic alopecia. *J Dermatol.* 2012;39(1):27-32.

22. Atanaskova Mesinkovska N, Bergfeld WF. Hair: what is new in diagnosis and management? Female pattern hair loss update: diagnosis and treatment. *Dermatol Clin.* 2013;31(1):119-127.

23. Bunagan MJ, Banka N, Shapiro J. Hair transplantation update: procedural techniques, innovations, and applications. *Dermatol Clin.* 2013;31(1):141-153.

24. Loussouarn G, El Rawadi C, Genain G. Diversity of hair growth profiles. *Int J Dermatol.* 2005;44(suppl 1):6-9.

25. Lawson CN, Hollinger J, Sethi S, et al. Updates in the understanding and treatments of skin & hair disorders in women of color. *Int J Womens Dermatol.* 2017;3(suppl 1):S21-S37.

26. Samrao A, Chen C, Zedek D, Price VH. Traction alopecia in a ballerina: clinicopathologic features. *Arch Dermatol.* 2010;146(8):930-931.

27. Ozçelik D. Extensive traction alopecia attributable to ponytail hairstyle and its treatment with hair transplantation. *Aesthetic Plast Surg.* 2005;29(4):325-327.

28. Khumalo NP, Jessop S, Gumedze F, Ehrlich R. Hairdressing and the prevalence of scalp disease in African adults. *Br J Dermatol.* 2007;157(5):981-988.

29. Khumalo NP, Jessop S, Gumedze F, Ehrlich R. Determinants of marginal traction alopecia in African girls and women. *J Am Acad Dermatol.* 2008;59(3):432-438.

30. Samrao A, Price VH, Zedek D, Mirmirani P. The "Fringe Sign" - a useful clinical finding in traction alopecia of the marginal hair line. *Dermatol Online J.* 2011;17(11):1.

31. Samrao A, McMichael A, Mirmirani P. Nocturnal traction: techniques used for hair style maintenance while sleeping may be a risk factor for traction alopecia. *Skin Appendage Disord.* 2021;7(3):220-223.

32. Callender VD, McMichael AJ, Cohen GF. Medical and surgical therapies for alopecias in black women. *Dermatol Ther.* 2004;17(2):164-176.

33. Uwakwe LN, De Souza B, Tovar-Garza A, McMichael AJ. Intralesional triamcinolone acetonide in the treatment of traction alopecia. *J Drugs Dermatol.* 2020;19(2):128-130.

34. Sung CT, Juhasz ML, Choi FD, Mesinkovska NA. The efficacy of topical minoxidil for non-scarring alopecia: a systematic review. *J Drugs Dermatol.* 2019;18(2):155-160.

35. Earles RM. Surgical correction of traumatic alopecia marginalis or traction alopecia in black women. *J Dermatol Surg Oncol.* 1986;12(1):78-82.

36. Franbourg A, Hallegot P, Baltenneck F, Toutain C, Leroy F. Current research on ethnic hair. *J Am Acad Dermatol.* 2003;48(suppl 6):S115-S119.

37. McMichael AJ. Hair breakage in normal and weathered hair: focus on the Black patient. *J Investig Dermatol Symp Proc.* 2007;12(2):6-9.

38. Rogers M. Hair shaft abnormalities: Part I. *Australas J Dermatol.* 1995;36(4):179-186.

39. Mirmirani P. Ceramic flat irons: improper use leading to acquired trichorrhexis nodosa. *J Am Acad Dermatol.* 2010;62(1):145-147.

40. Price VH. Treatment of hair loss. *N Engl J Med.* 1999;341(13):964-973.

41. Khumalo NP, Dawber RP, Ferguson DJ. Apparent fragility of African hair is unrelated to the cystine-rich protein distribution: a cytochemical electron microscopic study. *Exp Dermatol.* 2005;14(4):311-314.

42. Haskin A, Kwatra SG, Aguh C. Breaking the cycle of hair breakage: pearls for the management of acquired trichorrhexis nodosa. *J Dermatolog Treat.* 2017;28(4):322-326.

43. Gupta AK, Batra R, Bluhm R, Boekhout T, Dawson Jr TL. Skin diseases associated with Malassezia species. *J Am Acad Dermatol.* 2004;51(5):785-798.

44. Davis SA, Narahari S, Feldman SR, Huang W, Pichardo-Geisinger RO, McMichael AJ. Top dermatologic conditions in patients of color: an analysis of nationally representative data. *J Drugs Dermatol.* 2012;11(4):466-473.

45. Alexis AF, Sergay AB, Taylor SC. Common dermatologic disorders in skin of color: a comparative practice survey. *Cutis.* 2007;80(5):387-394.

46. Osemwota O, Herbosa CM, Zhong C, Kwatra SG, Kim BS, Semenov YR. Ethnic variations in scalp pruritus and hair loss. *J Am Acad Dermatol.* 2021;84(3):792-794.

47. Taylor SC, Barbosa V, Burgess C, et al. Hair and scalp disorders in adult and pediatric patients with skin of color. *Cutis.* 2017;100(1):31-35.

48. Borda LJ, Perper M, Keri JE. Treatment of seborrheic dermatitis: a comprehensive review. *J Dermatolog Treat.* 2019;30(2):158-169.

49. Xing L, Dai Z, Jabbari A, et al. Alopecia areata is driven by cytotoxic T lymphocytes and is reversed by JAK inhibition. *Nat Med.* 2014;20(9):1043-1049.

50. Damsky W, King BA. JAK inhibitors in dermatology: the promise of a new drug class. *J Am Acad Dermatol.* 2017;76(4):736-744.

51. Lee H, Jung SJ, Patel AB, Thompson JM, Qureshi A, Cho E. Racial characteristics of alopecia areata in the United States. *J Am Acad Dermatol.* 2020;83(4):1064-1070.

52. Harries MJ, Sun J, Paus R, King Jr LE. Management of alopecia areata. *BMJ.* 2010;341:c3671.

53. Strazzulla LC, Wang EHC, Avila L, et al. Alopecia areata: disease characteristics, clinical evaluation, and new perspectives on pathogenesis. *J Am Acad Dermatol.* 2018;78(1):1-12.

54. Tosti A, Iorizzo M, Botta GL, Milani M. Efficacy and safety of a new clobetasol propionate 0.05% foam in alopecia areata: a randomized, double-blind placebo-controlled trial. *J Eur Acad Dermatol Venereol.* 2006;20(10):1243-1247.

55. Mancuso G, Balducci A, Casadio C, et al. Efficacy of betamethasone valerate foam formulation in comparison with betamethasone dipropionate lotion in the treatment of mild-to-moderate alopecia areata: a multicenter, prospective, randomized, controlled, investigator-blinded trial. *Int J Dermatol.* 2003;42(7):572-575.

56. Kar BR, Handa S, Dogra S, Kumar B. Placebo-controlled oral pulse prednisolone therapy in alopecia areata. *J Am Acad Dermatol.* 2005;52(2):287-290.

57. Price VH. Double-blind, placebo-controlled evaluation of topical minoxidil in extensive alopecia areata. *J Am Acad Dermatol.* 1987;16(3 Pt 2):730-736.

58. Strazzulla LC, Wang EHC, Avila L, et al. Alopecia areata: an appraisal of new treatment approaches and overview of current therapies. *J Am Acad Dermatol.* 2018;78(1):15-24.

59. Whiting DA, Olsen EA. Central centrifugal cicatricial alopecia. *Dermatol Ther.* 2008;21(4):268-278.

60. Sperling LC, Sau P. The follicular degeneration syndrome in black patients. 'Hot comb alopecia' revisited and revised. *Arch Dermatol.* 1992;128(1):68-74.

61. Olsen EA, Callender V, McMichael A, et al. Central hair loss in African American women: incidence and potential risk factors. *J Am Acad Dermatol.* 2011;64(2):245-252.

62. Callender VD, Wright DR, Davis EC, Sperling LC. Hair breakage as a presenting sign of early or occult central centrifugal cicatricial alopecia: clinicopathologic findings in 9 patients. *Arch Dermatol.* 2012;148(9):1047-1052.

63. Dlova NC, Jordaan FH, Sarig O, Sprecher E. Autosomal dominant inheritance of central centrifugal cicatricial alopecia in black South Africans. *J Am Acad Dermatol.* 2014;70(4):679-682.e1.

64. Gathers RC, Jankowski M, Eide M, Lim HW. Hair grooming practices and central centrifugal cicatricial alopecia. *J Am Acad Dermatol.* 2009;60(4):574-578.

65. Malki L, Sarig O, Romano MT, et al. Variant PADI3 in central centrifugal cicatricial alopecia. *N Engl J Med.* 2019;380(9):833-841.

66. Summers P, Kyei A, Bergfeld W. Central centrifugal cicatricial alopecia - an approach to diagnosis and management. *Int J Dermatol.* 2011;50(12):1457-1464.

67. Fu JM, Price VH. Approach to hair loss in women of color. *Semin Cutan Med Surg.* 2009;28(2):109-114.

68. Callender VD, Lawson CN, Onwudiwe OC. Hair transplantation in the surgical treatment of central centrifugal cicatricial alopecia. *Dermatol Surg.* 2014;40(10):1125-1131.

69. Vañó-Galván S, Molina-Ruiz AM, Fernández-Crehuet P, et al. Folliculitis decalvans: a multicentre review of 82 patients. *J Eur Acad Dermatol Venereol.* 2015;29(9):1750-1757.

70. Bunagan MJ, Banka N, Shapiro J. Retrospective review of folliculitis decalvans in 23 patients with course and treatment analysis of long-standing cases. *J Cutan Med Surg.* 2015;19(1):45-49.

71. Chandrawansa PH, Giam YC. Folliculitis decalvans–a retrospective study in a tertiary referred centre, over five years. *Singapore Med J.* 2003;44(2):84-87.

72. Tan E, Martinka M, Ball N, Shapiro J. Primary cicatricial alopecias: clinicopathology of 112 cases. *J Am Acad Dermatol.* 2004;50(1):25-32.

73. Powell JJ, Dawber RP, Gatter K. Folliculitis decalvans including tufted folliculitis: clinical, histological and therapeutic findings. *Br J Dermatol.* 1999;140(2):328-333.

74. Rambhia PH, Conic RRZ, Murad A, Atanaskova-Mesinkovska N, Piliang M, Bergfeld W. Updates in therapeutics for folliculitis decalvans: a systematic review with evidence-based analysis. *J Am Acad Dermatol.* 2019;80(3):794-801.e1.

75. Olsen EA, Bergfeld WF, Cotsarelis G, et al. Summary of North American Hair Research Society (NAHRS)-sponsored Workshop on Cicatricial Alopecia, Duke University Medical Center, February 10 and 11, 2001. *J Am Acad Dermatol.* 2003;48(1):103-110.

76. Knable Jr AL, Hanke CW, Gonin R. Prevalence of acne keloidalis nuchae in football players. *J Am Acad Dermatol.* 1997;37(4):570-574.

77. Salami T, Omeife H, Samuel S. Prevalence of acne keloidalis nuchae in Nigerians. *Int J Dermatol.* 2007;46(5):482-484.

78. East-Innis ADC, Stylianou K, Paolino A, Ho JD. Acne keloidalis nuchae: risk factors and associated disorders - a retrospective study. *Int J Dermatol.* 2017;56(8):828-832.

79. Alexis A, Heath CR, Halder RM. Folliculitis keloidalis nuchae and pseudofolliculitis barbae: are prevention and effective treatment within reach? *Dermatol Clin.* 2014;32(2):183-191.

80. Ogunbiyi A. Acne keloidalis nuchae: prevalence, impact, and management challenges. *Clin Cosmet Investig Dermatol.* 2016;9:483-489.

81. Glenn MJ, Bennett RG, Kelly AP. Acne keloidalis nuchae: treatment with excision and second-intention healing. *J Am Acad Dermatol.* 1995;33(2 Pt 1):243-246.

82. Beckett N, Lawson C, Cohen G. Electrosurgical excision of acne keloidalis nuchae with secondary intention healing. *J Clin Aesthet Dermatol.* 2011;4(1):36-39.

83. Esmat SM, Abdel Hay RM, Abu Zeid OM, Hosni HN. The efficacy of laser-assisted hair removal in the treatment of acne keloidalis nuchae; a pilot study. *Eur J Dermatol.* 2012;22(5):645-650.

84. Hoffmann E. Folliculitis et perifolliculitis capitis abscedens et suffodiens: case presentation. *Dermatol Zeitschrift.* 1908;15:122-123.

85. Scheinfeld NS. A case of dissecting cellulitis and a review of the literature. *Dermatol Online J.* 2003;9(1):8.

86. Whiting DA. Cicatricial alopecia: clinico-pathological findings and treatment. *Clin Dermatol.* 2001;19(2):211-225.

87. Thomas J, Aguh C. Approach to treatment of refractory dissecting cellulitis of the scalp: a systematic review. *J Dermatolog Treat.* 2021;32(2):144-149.

88. Kossard S, Lee MS, Wilkinson B. Postmenopausal frontal fibrosing alopecia: a frontal variant of lichen planopilaris. *J Am Acad Dermatol.* 1997;36(1):59-66.

89. Kanti V, Constantinou A, Reygagne P, Vogt A, Kottner J, Blume-Peytavi U. Frontal fibrosing alopecia: demographic and clinical characteristics of 490 cases. *J Eur Acad Dermatol Venereol.* 2019;33(10):1976-1983.

90. Tziotzios C, Petridis C, Dand N, et al. Genome-wide association study in frontal fibrosing alopecia identifies four susceptibility loci including HLA-B*07:02. *Nat Commun.* 2019;10(1):1150.

91. Moreno-Arrones OM, Saceda-Corralo D, Rodrigues-Barata AR, et al. Risk factors associated with frontal fibrosing alopecia: a multicentre case-control study. *Clin Exp Dermatol.* 2019;44(4):404-410.

92. Ramos PM, Anzai A, Duque-Estrada B, et al. Risk factors for frontal fibrosing alopecia: a case-control study in a multiracial population. *J Am Acad Dermatol.* 2021;84(3):712-718.

93. Gamret AC, Potluri VS, Krishnamurthy K, Fertig RM. Frontal fibrosing alopecia: efficacy of treatment modalities. *Int J Womens Health.* 2019;11:273-285.

94. Alves R, Grimalt R. Platelet-rich plasma and its use for cicatricial and non-cicatricial alopecias: a narrative review. *Dermatol Ther (Heidelb).* 2020;10(4):623-633.

95. Alves R, Grimalt R. Randomized placebo-controlled, double-blind, half-head study to assess the efficacy of platelet-rich plasma on the treatment of androgenetic alopecia. *Dermatol Surg.* 2016;42(4):491-497.

96. Trink A, Sorbellini E, Bezzola P, et al. A randomized, double-blind, placebo- and active-controlled, half-head study to evaluate the effects of platelet-rich plasma on alopecia areata. *Br J Dermatol*. 2013;169(3):690-694.

97. Dina Y, Aguh C. Use of platelet-rich plasma in cicatricial alopecia. *Dermatol Surg*. 2019;45(7):979-981.

98. Rakowska A, Gradzińska A, Olszewska M, Rudnicka L. Efficacy of isotretinoin and acitretin in treatment of frontal fibrosing alopecia: retrospective analysis of 54 cases. *J Drugs Dermatol*. 2017;16(10):988-992.

99. Almutairi N, Nour TM, Hussain NH. Janus kinase inhibitors for the treatment of severe alopecia areata: an open-label comparative study. *Dermatology*. 2019;235(2):130-136.

100. Liu LY, Craiglow BG, Dai F, King BA. Tofacitinib for the treatment of severe alopecia areata and variants: a study of 90 patients. *J Am Acad Dermatol*. 2017;76(1):22-28.

101. Mackay-Wiggan J, Jabbari A, Nguyen N, et al. Oral ruxolitinib induces hair regrowth in patients with moderate-to-severe alopecia areata. *JCI Insight*. 2016;1(15):e89790.

102. Jabbari A, Nguyen N, Cerise JE, et al. Treatment of an alopecia areata patient with tofacitinib results in regrowth of hair and changes in serum and skin biomarkers. *Exp Dermatol*. 2016;25(8):642-643.

103. Araoye EF, Thomas JAL, Aguh CU. Hair regrowth in 2 patients with recalcitrant central centrifugal cicatricial alopecia after use of topical metformin. *JAAD Case Rep*. 2020;6(2):106-108.

3

Diagnosis and Treatment of Scarring Alopecia

Taylor A. Jamerson, Achiamah Osei-Tutu, and Crystal Aguh

KEY POINTS

- Scarring alopecia is characterized by inflammation that leads to destruction of the pilosebaceous unit and ultimately the replacement of subcutaneous tissue with fibrous tracts. As a result, the hair loss can be disfiguring and cause significant distress in affected patients.
- Although treatment strategies for scarring alopecia center on disease subtype, the primary goal of treatment is to reduce the underlying inflammation causing the destruction of hair follicles to stop the progression of scarring and hair loss. Hair loss is often permanent and can have a significant psychological effect on patients, heightening the importance of establishing appropriate treatment expectations.
- Topical steroids, often combined with intralesional corticosteroid injections, are usually considered first-line in the treatment of scarring alopecia as a result of their demonstrated efficacy and low side-effect profile. Systemic therapies can be used for disease recalcitrant to topical and intralesional corticosteroids and are needed in most patients.
- Platelet-rich plasma is one of few treatment options for scarring alopecia that has demonstrated the potential for hair regrowth, even in patients who have failed conventional therapies.
- Surgical hair transplantation is an aesthetic treatment option that offers the unique outcome of dramatic hair restoration in scarred areas of the scalp. However, results are often variable as a result of marked fibrosis and decreased scalp vascularity in the recipient area. Caution should be taken to avoid transplantation in patients with subclinical inflammation.

BACKGROUND

Scarring or cicatricial alopecia is a diverse class of conditions of differing etiologies and clinical presentations, in most cases leading to permanent hair loss. These disorders make up approximately 7% of patients evaluated in hair-loss specialty clinics (level of evidence: 5).[1] Scarring alopecia can be primary, characterized by inflammation and destruction of the pilosebaceous unit with eventual replacement of subcutaneous tissue with fibrous tracts, or secondary as a result of trauma, cancer, radiation, or thermal burns (level of evidence: 5).[2,3] Primary cicatricial processes can be further classified into neutrophilic, lymphocytic, or mixed by the predominant inflammatory cell type seen on histology during the active phase of disease (Table 3.1) (level of evidence: 5).[4]

Unlike nonscarring alopecia where the follicular unit is preserved and treatment is centered on hair regrowth, treatment for scarring alopecia is largely aimed at reducing inflammation and preventing disease progression. Consequently, hair loss can be disfiguring and may contribute to increased psychosocial burden and decreased dermatology life quality index (DLQI) scores in patients with scarring alopecia compared with those with nonscarring alopecia (level of evidence: 1b).[5] Early

TABLE 3.1 **Classification of Primary Scarring Alopecias**		
Lymphocytic	**Neutrophilic**	**Mixed**
• Alopecia mucinosa	• Dissecting cellulitis	• Erosive pustular dermatosis
• Central centrifugal cicatricial alopecia	• Folliculitis decalvans	• Folliculitis (acne) keloidalis
• Chronic cutaneous lupus erythematosus		• Folliculitis (acne) necrotica
• Classic pseudopelade (of Brocq)		
• Lichen planopilaris		
• Classic lichen planopilaris		
• Frontal fibrosing alopecia		
• Graham-Little syndrome		

diagnosis and initiation of treatment is essential for a better prognosis in these patients.

STRUCTURAL AND FUNCTIONAL DIFFERENCES IN SCARRING ALOPECIA

The pilosebaceous unit consists of three anatomic structures: hair follicle, sebaceous gland, and arrector pili muscle (level of evidence: 5).[6] The hair follicle, an epithelial organ, can further be divided into three regions: the infundibulum (uppermost segment) extending from the insertion point of the sebaceous gland to the follicular orifice; the isthmus (middle segment) extending from the entrance of the arrector pili muscle to the insertion of the sebaceous gland; and the bulb (lowermost segment) extending from the base of the hair follicle to the arrector pili muscle.[6] Near the attachment site of the arrector pili muscle and opening of the sebaceous gland there is an area on the outer root sheath of the hair follicle called the *bulge region* where multipotent stem cells are located (level of evidence: 3a).[7,8] During the hair cycle, quiescent follicular stem cells are transiently activated in the early anagen (growth) phase

(level of evidence: 5).[9] These cells can proliferate and further differentiate to support elongation or regeneration of the hair shaft.

In nonscarring processes, while the histopathology is largely disease dependent, all conditions share the finding of an intact and healthy hair bulge region in early stages of disease, allowing the hair follicle to regenerate with sufficient treatment. Contrarily, scarring alopecia involves destructive inflammation around the infundibular, and variably isthmic, region of the hair follicle.[1] This causes damage to the follicular bulge region and leads to the loss of epithelial stem cells necessary to regenerate the hair follicle (level of evidence: 2b).[3,10] With persistent inflammation, the involved tissue becomes fibrotic, resulting in permanent hair loss. The fundamental differences between scarring and nonscarring alopecia are summarized in Table 3.2.

EVALUATION OF SCARRING ALOPECIA

Onset of scarring alopecia occurs most commonly in middle-aged adults, with only rare exceptions of familial genodermatoses developing during childhood and

TABLE 3.2 **Key Distinguishing Characteristics Between Nonscarring Alopecia and Scarring Alopecia**	
Nonscarring Alopecia	**Scarring Alopecia**
Preservation of the pilosebaceouss unit	Destruction of the pilosebaceous unit
Healthy bulge region of the hair follicle with sparing of follicular stem cells	Inflammation leads to destruction of the bulge region of the hair follicle with loss of stem cells necessary for follicular regeneration
Absence of fibrosis	Presence of fibrosis
Regeneration of the hair follicle with appropriate treatment in most cases	Permanent hair loss in scapular areas of active disease in most cases

PEARL 3.1: The threshold for a punch biopsy from two areas of the scalp, both taken from the edge of an active area of disease in patients presenting with clinical signs and symptoms concerning for a cicatricial process, should remain low, as pathology examination allows for a more definitive identification of inflammatory infiltrates.

adolescent years (level of evidence: 5).[10,11] This may be an important distinguishing clue from some nonscarring alopecias such as alopecia areata (AA), which can affect individuals at any age (level of evidence: 2a).[12] The threshold for a punch biopsy in patients presenting with clinical signs and symptoms concerning for a cicatricial process should remain low, as pathology examination allows for a more definitive identification of inflammatory infiltrates (Pearl 3.1). Often, two areas of the scalp are biopsied, both taken from the edge of an area of active inflammation to identify predominant cell types and provide possible insight on the underlying pathology (level of evidence: 5).[13] However, biopsy alone may be insufficient for making an accurate diagnosis (level of evidence: 1b).[14] A thorough patient history and clinical examination are key to establishing onset, disease course, family history, medication history, associated symptoms, and hairstyling and haircare practices. Extrascapular areas of hair growth such as the eyebrows, eyelashes, axillae, extremities, and genitalia should also be assessed, in order to establish the extent of disease involvement.

On clinical examination, there are several features that may be present to allow distinction between a cicatricial and noncicatricial process. Evidence of smooth, fibrotic alopecic patches on the scalp, follicular prominence, loss of follicular ostia, perifollicular erythema or hyperkeratosis, papules, and pustules in affected areas of the scalp are several signs that may point to a scarring process (level of evidence: 5).[15] In addition, some scarring alopecias have characteristic findings such as skin atrophy in lichen planopilaris (LPP) (level of evidence: 5)[16] and dyspigmentation in cutaneous lupus erythematosus (level of evidence: 5).[17]

This chapter will focus primarily on the most common cicatricial processes encountered by dermatologists and therefore the most important to understand: LPP, frontal fibrosing alopecia (FFA), and central centrifugal cicatricial alopecia (CCCA) (Table 3.3).

Lichen Planopilaris

Lichen planopilaris (LPP) usually presents in adult women (level of evidence: 4).[18] It is characterized clinically by perifollicular erythema and hyperkeratosis, with focal or diffuse alopecic patches involving the vertex and parietal scalp (level of evidence: 2b).[19,20] Careful examination of the face and extremities can provide additional evidence to support the diagnosis, as near total alopecia of the upper and lower extremities prior to the onset of scalp involvement has been described in several patients (level of evidence: 2b).[21] Decreased or complete loss of the eyebrows is not common in this condition, but can occur (level of evidence: 5).[22] A growing body of literature has shed light on potential disease mechanisms, including downregulation of peroxisome proliferator-activated receptor gamma (PPARG) and decreased interferon-gamma expression (level of evidence: 2b).[23,24]

TABLE 3.3 Key Characteristics of the Most Common Cicatricial Alopecias Encountered by Dermatologists: Lichen Planopilaris, Frontal Fibrosing Alopecia, and Central Centrifugal Cicatricial Alopecia	
Lichen planopilaris (LPP)	• Perifollicular erythema and hyperkeratosis • Focal or diffuse alopecic patches in the vertex or parietal scalp • Near total alopecia of the upper and lower extremities
Frontal fibrosing alopecia (FFA)	• Progressive recession of the anterior hairline, with sparing of isolated hairs • Pale, atrophic skin • Perifollicular erythema and hyperkeratosis • Decreased density or complete loss of eyebrows
Central centrifugal cicatricial alopecia (CCCA)	• Hair breakage and thinning at the scalp vertex • Associated symptoms such as tenderness, pruritis, scale, pustules or papules in the affected scalp

Frontal Fibrosing Alopecia

While histologically identical to LPP, frontal fibrosing alopecia (FFA) is considered a clinical variant as a result of its distinctive clinical presentation.[19,22] This condition primarily affects postmenopausal women between 60 and 70 years of age, but it is thought to have an earlier onset of around 40 years of age in patients of African descent (level of evidence: 2b).[25,26] Although exogenous factors such as sunscreen have been associated with disease onset, these reports have not been substantiated and remain controversial (level of evidence: 2b).[27,28] FFA characteristically presents with progressive recession of the anterior hairline, appearing as a band-like area of alopecia with sparing of isolated hairs, referred to as the "lonely hair sign" (level of evidence: 4).[29] The clinical triad of findings in FFA are (1) pale, atrophic skin, (2) perifollicular hyperkeratosis and erythema, and (3) decreased density or complete loss of the eyebrows in 70% of patients.[21,23]

Central Centrifugal Cicatricial Alopecia

Central centrifugal cicatricial alopecia (CCCA) is a scarring alopecia that predominantly affects women of African descent (level of evidence: 5).[30] CCCA presents with an insidious, centrifugal pattern of permanent hair loss beginning in the scalp vertex (level of evidence: 4).[31] In the early stages of disease, the hair loss may present as hair breakage and thinning at the crown of the scalp. This progressively expands to involve the surrounding areas with permanent hair loss. Some patients may experience symptoms secondary to inflammation of the affected scalp, including tenderness, pruritis, scale, pustules, and papules, while others have no symptoms outside of progressive hair loss.[31]

When first described in the literature, CCCA was referred to as "hot comb" alopecia as a result of the theory that disease onset was linked to hairstyling practices and then, later, to chemical relaxants (level of evidence: 2b).[32] Further studies disputed any link to hot combing or chemical relaxers, and subsequent studies suggested instead a link to extensions as these styling practices became more popular (level of evidence: 2b).[33] However, there has since been no substantial evidence to support any one hairstyling practice to the onset of CCCA, casting this hypothesis into doubt. Since a publication by Malki et al. in 2019, evidence has suggested that CCCA is an autosomal dominant condition with incomplete penetrance and is associated with variance in the *PADI3* gene in 24% of patients (level of evidence: 2b).[34] Additionally, this condition has been connected to a higher prevalence of uterine leiomyomas and type 2 diabetes, indicating potential contribution of metabolic factors in disease pathogenesis (level of evidence: 1b).[35,36]

TREATMENT APPROACHES

As stated previously, the primary goal of therapy for cicatricial alopecia is disease remission and stabilization, and this should be explicitly communicated to patients. The treatment of a primary scarring alopecia often centers on physician experience, as there is currently no gold standard approach.[16] Early initiation of treatment is key in the proper management of these conditions to slow disease progression and address symptomatology. Response to treatment is often variable, with some patients experiencing complete resolution of symptoms and control of disease progression, while others experience persistent disease despite trial of multiple therapies.[1]

Topical and Intralesional Corticosteroids

Topical potent corticosteroids, often combined with intralesional corticosteroid injections to the scalp, are generally considered a first-line therapeutic option for cicatricial alopecia.[1] The use of topical steroids has demonstrated resolution of inflammation with no evidence of disease progression after 12 weeks of therapy in some patients (level of evidence: 4).[37] Intralesional triamcinolone can be injected at a concentration of 5 to 10 mg/cc every six to eight weeks until clinical evidence of active inflammation, such as follicular prominence or perifollicular erythema, has resolved (level of evidence: 2b).[38] For patients with CCCA, assessment of disease activity is more difficult, as many women do not have overt inflammation. In these patients, a series of five to eight sessions followed by a six to nine-month treatment-free period is common.

Steroid-induced atrophy, a well-known adverse effect associated with intralesional corticosteroid injections, poses an even higher risk of occurrence in patients concurrently using potent topical steroids (level of evidence: 5).[39] Spacing out injections is essential to avoid this complication. As mentioned previously, intralesional steroid injections are generally recommended at six to eight-week intervals to reduce risk of atrophy, and potent topical corticosteroids should be used for a maximum of two-week intervals if applied daily, with a

PEARL 3.2: Intralesional steroid injections are generally recommended at six to eight-week intervals to reduce the risk of atrophy. Potent topical corticosteroids should be used for a maximum of two-week intervals if applied daily, with a one-week break in between.

one-week break in between (level of evidence: 5) (Pearl 3.2).[40] In patients who ultimately develop pale, atrophied skin at the site of injection or topical application, further injection to the area should be avoided. Steroid-induced atrophy is typically self-limited and resolves in one to two years. However, several methods have been described to improve the appearance of atrophic areas, including the use of serial saline injections, pulsed-dye laser, and fat-grafting (level of evidence: 2b).[41,42]

Systemic Therapies

Evidence of disease progression such as new areas of involvement or persistent inflammation despite topical and intralesional corticosteroids may prompt adjunctive treatment with oral agents. Most patients with scarring alopecia will require systemic therapy. Oral hydroxychloroquine has shown positive results in patients with LPP and FFA and can be considered as a second-line therapy, with effects seen three to six months after initiation.[38] In the authors' experience, patients often do well initiating oral systemic medications in addition to corticosteroid treatment. A single-center retrospective review of 40 patients with LLP and FFA found that, after 12 months, 83% of patients saw improvement in their symptoms (level of evidence: 2b).[43] Adverse reactions associated with hydroxychloroquine use are important to monitor, as this medication can cause anorexia, abdominal pain, hematologic changes, skin hyperpigmentation, and, notably, ophthalmologic damage.[38] These patients require annual monitoring by an ophthalmologist for the development of retinopathy.

In cases where symptoms persist on oral hydroxychloroquine after six months of treatment, mycophenolate mofetil and cyclosporine are immunosuppressive agents that can serve as alternative treatment options (level of evidence: 4).[44,45] Though oral corticosteroids offer quick control of inflammation, the rate of disease relapse in scarring alopecia has been reported to be as high as 80%. Thus, oral corticosteroids are generally not recommended, but can be reserved for cases of rapidly progressive, severe disease.[1,16] Oral tetracyclines such as doxycycline (100 mg twice daily), antiandrogens such as oral finasteride and dutasteride, and calcineurin inhibitors have been used in the treatment of CCCA refractory to other oral agents.[2] Finasteride and dutasteride are among the most efficacious treatments for LPP and FFA, and can be used in postmenopausal women or premenopausal women who are also on a contraceptive (level of evidence: 3a).[46] Evidence of partial hair regrowth or disease stabilization, even in severe disease, has been demonstrated in most patients (level of evidence: 2b).[47,48] Oral isotretinoin can also be used in patients with LPP and FFA to achieve disease stabilization, especially in patients with FFA who present with yellow facial papules in the early stages of disease (level of evidence: 1b).[49]

Autologous Platelet-Rich Plasma

Studied since the 1970s, primarily for applications in the stimulation of wound healing, platelet-rich plasma (PRP) has recently gained traction in its aesthetic use in dermatology for the treatment of hair loss (level of evidence: 5).[50] PRP works by enhancing cells involved in tissue regeneration such as adipose-derived stem cells and dermal fibroblasts (level of evidence: 5).[51] The proposed mechanism of PRP stimulation of hair growth is thought to involve platelet activation that leads to a cascade of reactions and ultimately the secretion of cytokines and growth factors essential in the process of wound healing (level of evidence: 5).[52] These growth factors then act on stem cells within the bulge region of the hair follicle, promoting neovascularization and follicular regeneration. In addition, beta-catenin and fibroblast growth factor-7 (FGF-7) activity has been found to be upregulated in patients after PRP treatment. The increased beta-catenin activity further induces proliferation of follicular stem cells, while upregulation of FGF-7 activity prolongs the anagen phase of the hair cycle to further stimulate growth.[52]

PRP is one of the few treatments in the literature described as an option for hair restoration in patients with cicatricial alopecia. Though PRP is primarily used as an off-label treatment for nonscarring alopecia, it has also gained attention in the literature as a feasible treatment option in cicatricial alopecia with positive results (Fig. 3.1). It has been described as a treatment option for patients who have failed conventional therapies, even producing positive results in patients with active, longstanding disease (Fig. 3.2) (level of evidence: 4).[53]

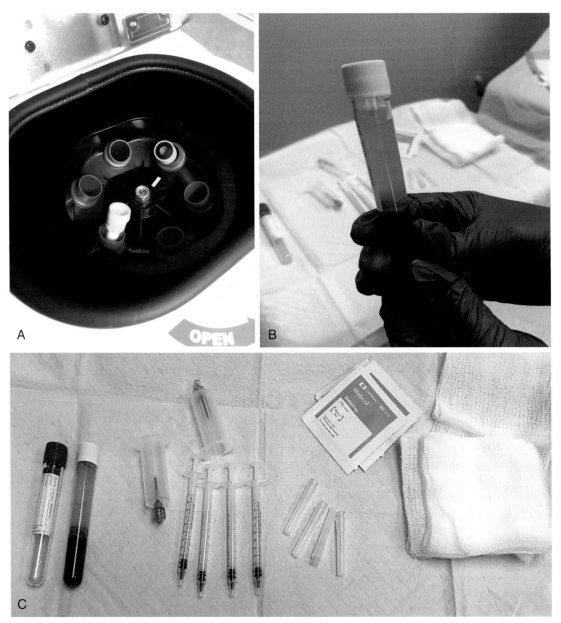

Fig. 3.1 (A) Centrifuge containing one 9 cc tube of whole blood with sodium citrate, an anticoagulant. The tube is spun at 1100 g for two 6-minute cycles with a counterbalance tube to yield 4 to 5 cc of plasma. (B) The resultant plasma after centrifugation. The bottom layer consists primarily of red blood cells. The middle layer is rich in platelets and white blood cells, and the top, gold-colored layer consists of the platelet-poor plasma. The platelet-rich plasma (PRP) is transferred to a separate tube containing a clotting cascade activator, leading to the release of growth factors. (C) Layout of the procedural materials required for a PRP session. From left to right: 0.5-M calcium chloride (clotting cascade activator), centrifuged proprietary vacutainer PRP tube, BD vacutainer luer-lok access device, BD vacutainer blood transfer device, four empty syringes, four syringe needles, alcohol wipes, and 4x4 cm gauze sponges.

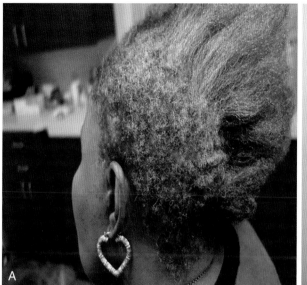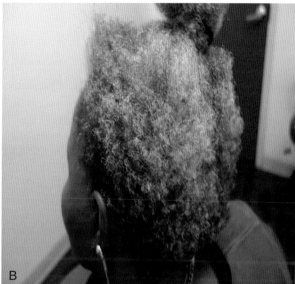

Fig. 3.2 Patient with central centrifugal cicatricial alopecia prior to platelet-rich plasma treatment (A) and 18 months after three sessions of platelet-rich plasma treatment (B).

Several case reports have been published on the use of PRP in LPP, varying from three sessions performed one month apart to four sessions administered three weeks apart (level of evidence: 4).[54] Authors noted complete regression of inflammatory symptoms such as perifollicular erythema, hyperkeratosis, and itching, evidencing potential arrest of disease progression. Only one case report describes restoration of normal follicular density across the scalp and frontal hairline in a patient with LPP after three sessions of PRP performed one month apart.[53] Lastly, resolution of symptomatology has also been described in FFA, with no evidence of progressive hair loss after five sessions of PRP at one-month intervals, in addition to improvement in perifollicular erythema, hyperkeratosis, and lichenoid papules present at the hairline (level of evidence: 4).[55] It is therefore important to manage patient expectations by providing guidance on the efficacy of PRP in slowing disease progression and improving inflammation, with possible but unlikely restoration of follicular density in affected areas of the scalp.

An important pretreatment recommendation all providers should consider prior to initiating PRP treatment is the concurrent use of topical minoxidil formulations. Topical minoxidil should not be initiated within three months of starting PRP sessions as a result of terminal hair shedding experienced by some patients at the start of topical minoxidil application (level of evidence: 2b).[56] This could potentially compromise PRP results. If patients have been on long-term topical minoxidil therapy initiated more than three months prior to the start of PRP, patients can be continued on this therapy throughout PRP sessions (Pearl 3.3).

PRP is usually a well-tolerated treatment. It has minimal side effects, with the exception of discomfort during the treatment. Patients can expect edema or erythema of the injection sites, pain, and headache immediately after treatment (level of evidence: 1b).[57] These symptoms usually resolve within hours of treatment. The use of analgesics with antiplatelet activity such as nonsteroidal anti-inflammatory drugs (NSAIDs) should be avoided to prevent counteracting the effects of treatment. A cold pack applied before and after a PRP session can be helpful in tempering pain (level of evidence: 4).[58] In addition, koebernization, or the

> **PEARL 3.3:** Topical minoxidil should not be initiated within 3 months of starting platelet-rich plasma sessions because of terminal hair shedding at the start of topical minoxidil application experienced by some patients.

> **PEARL 3.4:** Evidence of disease reactivation has been reported in patients as soon as six months after their last platelet-rich plasma session, warranting continued, longitudinal treatment with repeat platelet-rich plasma sessions.

induction of new areas of disease, is a theoretical concern with PRP treatment. However, this has yet to be reported in the literature.[54] Lastly, patients should be counseled that the results achieved with PRP sessions are not indefinite. Evidence of disease reactivation has been reported in patients as soon as six months after their last PRP session.[53] Therefore, the need for continued, longitudinal treatment with repeat PRP sessions should be expected and discussed with patients (Pearl 3.4).

Hair Transplantation

Surgical hair transplantation should be approached with caution in patients with cicatricial alopecia. Although more commonly used in patients with nonscarring alopecia, hair transplantation offers the possibility of hair growth in scarred areas of the scalp for select patients.

The consultation visit is key in establishing candidacy for surgical hair restoration. A thorough examination of the scalp is important in patients with cicatricial alopecia, as any evidence of inflammation is an absolute contraindication to hair transplantation. It is generally recommended patients undergo aggressive medical management with antiinflammatory agents and show disease stability with no clinical signs of active inflammation for at least 12 months prior to considering surgical hair restoration (level of evidence: 4).[59] A punch biopsy of the recipient site can help prevent transplantation of active areas of disease by ensuring there is no subclinical evidence of inflammation. The intended donor site should also be identified and examined at this time to ensure that an adequate number of follicular units are present (at least 40 follicular units/cm^2) (level of evidence: 5).[60]

A detailed medical and dermatologic history can aid in identification of conditions, such as seborrheic dermatitis, that can affect hair growth without treatment (level of evidence: 5).[61] Obtaining an in-depth history of hairstyling and haircare practices is also fundamental in providing early guidance to correct harmful practices

that can later compromise graft survival. This should also involve a discussion of postprocedural hairstyling plans to aid in selection of the appropriate donor harvesting technique and allow adequate time for the patient to coordinate with their hairstylist, if necessary, especially in patients of color who often have their hair routinely styled in a salon. All patients with scarring hair loss should be counseled on the possibility of disease reactivation and the lower rate of graft survival in fibrotic scalp tissue (level of evidence: 4).[62]

Once a patient has been deemed an appropriate candidate for hair transplantation, a test session is recommended to observe if the sample graft will take prior to pursuing full transplantation. This consists of harvesting five to six round, 4-mm grafts from the donor scalp and transplanting the grafts into corresponding 3.5-mm recipient sites located in the scarred, alopecic area (Fig. 3.3).[62] A window of three to six months should be allotted to monitor for proper hair growth and disease stability at the test site. Patients should be advised that hair regrowth at the grafted sites is expected to be relatively slow compared with areas of unaffected, healthy scalp (level of evidence: 2b).[63] Once graft survival and hair regrowth of the test sites has been documented, patients can then proceed with full hair transplantation (Pearl 3.5).

The best surgical technique for hair transplantation in patients with scarring alopecia depends on several factors, such as the location and extent of hair loss, expected surgical scarring, vascular supply, texture of hair, and preferred patient hairstyling (level of evidence: 5).[64] Linear strip excision (LSE) and follicular unit extraction (FUE) are the two main donor harvesting techniques used in surgical hair restoration (level of evidence: 5).[65] For patients with CCCA who have curly, textured hair, FUE is a preferred method with the use of larger grafts and larger recipient sites to decrease the risk of transection (graft failure) and offer more scalp coverage.[62] This technique involves harvesting follicular units with 0.9 to 1.25 mm punch excisions made from the safe donor area (region of the scalp expected to be spared from disease involvement in the occipital scalp) and offers less visible scarring compared with LSE (level of evidence: 2b).[66] However, FUE does require extended time to harvest donor hairs and is associated with a higher transection rate of curled follicular units.[67] The larger donor area in this procedure that requires shaving may also be a concern for female patients. LSE instead involves harvesting a 1-cm single strip from the donor

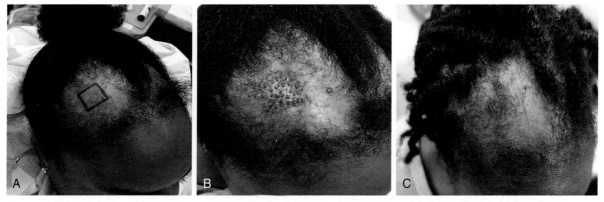

Fig. 3.3 Patient with biopsy-proven central centrifugal cicatricial alopecia with test-graft area outlined for transplantation of test grafts (A) and immediately after transplantation of test grafts in the scarred, fibrotic scalp (B). Demonstrated growth and take of test grafts in the recipient, affected scalp (C). This patient would be considered a candidate for hair transplantation.

> **PEARL 3.5:** Once a patient has been deemed an appropriate candidate for hair transplantation, a test session is recommended to observe if the sample graft will take prior to pursuing full transplantation., This consists of harvesting five to six round, 4-mm grafts from the donor scalp and transplanting the grafts into corresponding 3.5-mm recipient sites located in the scarred, alopecic area.

region above the occipital protuberance extending from helix to helix (level of evidence: 5).[67] This method is associated with lower risk of transection, but results in more visible scarring (level of evidence: 5).[67,68]

A review of 34 patients with various forms of primary scarring alopecia revealed that 76.5% of patients had moderate-to-positive results after hair transplantation (level of evidence: 3a).[69] Particularly, patients with a diagnosis of CCCA had positive outcomes, with continued hair growth and graft survival noted even two years after hair transplantation. Notably, all patients with unsatisfactory postoperative outcomes had a diagnosis of LPP or FFA. Short-term success rates of hair transplantation in LPP and FFA have been reported as 75% and 29%, respectively, at one-year follow-up (level of evidence: 3a),[70] long-term graft survival is poor secondary to disease recurrence within four years of surgical hair restoration in most patients (levels of evidence: 5; 4).[71,72]

After hair transplantation, patients are recommended to follow up in 10 to 14 days to examine the surgical sites for proper wound healing or signs of infection. As a result of marked fibrosis in the recipient area, scalp vascularity raises heightened concern.[64] The risk of graft failure, ischemia, hypoxia, infection, and necrosis are increased as a result and can compromise graft viability. After hair transplantation, the scalp should be washed daily and proper care must be given to the surgical areas to reduce risk of infection and crusting until the sites have completely healed (Fig. 3.4). In addition, topical minoxidil formulations have been used as an adjunct treatment preoperatively for at least one week, and postoperatively for a duration of five weeks, to increase blood flow at the recipient site and improve the likelihood of graft survival.[62] Oral pentoxifylline (400 mg three times daily) can also be used two weeks prior to surgical transplantation to increase oxygenation to the cicatricial areas of the scalp (level of evidence: 5).[73] Shedding of catagen hairs after FUE hair transplantation can be expected one to two weeks after the procedure (level of evidence: 5).[74] New hair follicles are expected to grow in place of these lost hairs within the next 8 to 12 months. Intraoperative PRP can reduce catagen loss of grafted hairs and may have the additional value of increasing follicular density (level of evidence: 1b).[75] After 15 months, providers should be able to assess the need for additional transplantation.

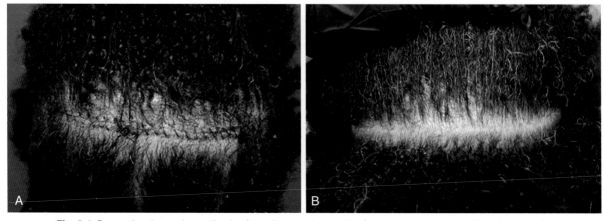

Fig. 3.4 Donor-site closure immediately after a linear strip excision for hair transplantation (A) and 12 months postprocedurally with a well-healed, concealed scar (B).

Low-Level Light Therapy

Low-level light therapy (LLLT) is an expanding technology discovered in the 1960s and has since been used in medical applications for the reduction of pain and inflammation, prevention of tissue damage, and stimulation of tissue repair and regeneration (level of evidence: 5).[76] LLLT consists of exposing tissue to low-levels of near infrared and red light at energy levels less than those used in other forms of laser therapy such as ablation (level of evidence: 5).[77]

For dermatologic use in hair loss, LLLT is currently cleared by the U.S. Food and Drug Administration (FDA) for the treatment of androgenetic alopecia (AGA) in Fitzpatrick skin types I to IV (level of evidence: 2a).[78] Though there are few studies on the use of LLLT in scarring alopecia, reports on the use of LLLT in LPP and FFA have suggested this treatment modality offers an effective, noninvasive treatment option for patients with incomplete response to topical and oral agents (level of evidence: 4).[79] Marked decrease in inflammation and increased hair thickening were observed after six months of LLLT at 246 red LED (wavelength of 630 nm and a fluence of 4 J/cm^2) for 15 minutes daily (level of evidence: 4).[80] In addition, these patients had a mean decrease of 0.87 in their lichen planopilaris activity index (LPPAI) score. Notably, one patient in a separate study was able to reduce the required dosage of oral hydroxychloroquine needed for disease management without relapse.[79] Larger cohort studies are needed to inform formal recommendations, but it is worth highlighting that no side effects have been reported in patients using LLLT for treatment of LPP or FFA.

EXPECTED OUTCOMES

Scarring alopecia typically results in permanent, irreversible hair loss. Treatment strategies differ for each subtype of cicatricial alopecia, and importantly, each patient. Spontaneous regrowth of hair is not expected, and currently there are no known methods to induce neogenesis of destroyed hair follicles. Therefore, the primary goal of treatment is to target the inflammatory cells destroying the hair follicle to slow or stop the progression of scarring and hair loss (Table 3.4).[2]

TABLE 3.4   Summary of Treatment Options for Primary Scarring Alopecia

Treatment Options for Primary Scarring Alopecia

Medical
- Topical corticosteroids
- Intralesional corticosteroids

Oral agents:
- Hydroxychloroquine
- Mycophenolate mofetil
- Cyclosporine
- Oral tetracyclines
- Antiandrogens
- Calcineurin inhibitors

Non-Invasive
- Low-level light therapy

Invasive
- Platelet-rich plasma
- Hair transplantation

Additionally, reduction of symptomatology is often achieved with treatment of the active inflammation and can serve as a clinical indication of patient response to therapies. In some cases, early initiation of treatment can result in regeneration of hair follicles that were once under inflammatory attack but have yet to fully succumb to fibrosis. This is important, as patients may experience hair regrowth in areas previously thought to represent end-stage scarring.[53] This may be evidenced by some improvement in follicular density with treatment. Every effort must be made by the treating physician to establish appropriate expectations for treatment, including likely prolonged duration of treatment, especially considering the psychological effect of scarring alopecia.

FUTURE DIRECTIONS

Some progress has been made in the identification of new therapies for scarring alopecias such as LPP and CCCA. Case reports and small retrospective analyses on the use of peroxisome proliferator-activated receptor gamma (PPARG) agonists in the treatment of LPP have described positive response (in both symptom and disease control) to oral pioglitazone, a thiazolidinedione used in the treatment of type 2 diabetes mellitus (levels of evidence: 4; 4).[81,82] Additionally, tofacitinib, a Janus Kinase inhibitor approved for the treatment of psoriasis, rheumatoid arthritis, and ulcerative colitis, has demonstrated therapeutic potential in a small sample of patients with LPP (level of evidence: 4).[83] For recalcitrant CCCA, positive outcomes have been demonstrated with topical metformin cream 10% compounded in Lipoderm, showing evidence of hair regrowth (level of evidence: 4).[84] No side effects have been reported outside of dryness and irritation at the site of application on the scalp, which improved with use of a topical moisturizer. Topical metformin it is thought to be well tolerated as a result of topical therapeutic concentrations being below the threshold of notable systemic absorption.

Though developments in the twenty-first century have advanced treatment approaches to several nonscarring alopecias, scarring alopecia continues to be largely understudied. Further research into genetic markers and disease mechanisms of scarring alopecia is needed to expand existing knowledge on pathways involved in their pathogenesis and potential targets to block the downstream effects leading to these cicatricial processes.

EVIDENCE SUMMARY

- Topical and intralesional corticosteroids are the preferred first-line treatment options for primary scarring alopecia (strength of recommendation: A).
- Autologous platelet-rich plasma is an effective treatment option that offers the potential for hair regrowth, control of inflammation, and halt of disease progression in patients with centrifugal cicatricial alopecia, lichen planopilaris, and frontal fibrosing alopecia. Topical minoxidil formulations should not be initiated within three months of beginning platelet-rich plasma sessions as a result of terminal hair shedding that can compromise platelet-rich plasma results. platelet-rich plasma is well tolerated with minimal side effects that typically resolve within hours of treatment. Results are not typically sustained beyond 6 months and repeat sessions are often needed (strength of recommendation: C).
- Surgical hair restoration is an option for patients with quiescent disease and no evidence of subclinical inflammation. The best surgical technique depends on several factors to optimize graft survival. Topical minoxidil or oral pentoxifylline can be used preoperatively to increase scalp vascularity, and intraoperative platelet-rich plasma can increase follicular density of the grafted hair follicles (strength of recommendation: B).

REFERENCES

1. Filbrandt R, Rufaut N, Jones L, Sinclair R. Primary cicatricial alopecia: diagnosis and treatment. *CMAJ*. 2013;185(18):1579-1585. doi:10.1503/cmaj.111570.
2. Harries MJ, Sinclair RD, Macdonald-Hull S, et al. Management of primary cicatricial alopecias: options for treatment. *Br J Dermatol*. 2008;159:1-22.
3. Harries MJ, Paus R. The pathogenesis of primary cicatricial alopecias. *Am J Pathol*. 2010;177:2152-2162.
4. Olsen EA, Bergfield WF, Costarelis G, et al. Summary of North American Hair Research Society (NAHRS)-sponsored workshop of cicatricial alopecia. Duke University Medical Center, February 10–11, 2001. *Am Acad Dermatol*. 2003;48:103-110.
5. Katoulis AC, Christodoulou C, Liakou AI, et al. Quality of life and psychosocial impact of scarring and non-scarring alopecia in women. *J Dtsch Dermatol Ges*. 2015;13(2):137-142. English, German. doi:10.1111/ddg.12548.
6. Martel JL, Miao JH, Badri T. Anatomy, hair follicle. In: *StatPearls*. Treasure Island (FL): StatPearls Publishing; 2021.

7. Joulai Veijouye S, Yari A, Heidari F, Sajedi N, Ghoroghi Moghani F, Nobakht M. Bulge Region as a putative hair follicle stem cells niche: a brief review. *Iran J Public Health*. 2017;46(9):1167-1175.
8. Inoue K, Aoi N, Sato T, et al. Differential expression of stem-cell-associated markers in human hair follicle epithelial cells. *Lab Invest*. 2009;89(8):844-856.
9. Woo WM, Oro AE. SnapShot: hair follicle stem cells. *Cell*. 2011;146(2):334-334.e2. doi:10.1016/j.cell.2011.07.001.
10. Harries M, Trueb RM, Tosti A, et al. How not to get scar(r)ed: pointers to the correct diagnosis in patients with suspected primary cicatricial alopecia. *Br J Dermatol*. 2009:160:482-501.
11. Ross EK, Tan E, Shapiro J. Update on primary cicatricial alopecias. *J Am Acad Dermatol*. 2005;53:1-37.
12. Villasante Fricke AC, Miteva M. Epidemiology and burden of alopecia areata: a systematic review. *Clin Cosmet Investig Dermatol*. 2015;8:397-403. doi:10.2147/CCID.S53985.
13. Shapiro J. Cicatricial alopecias. *Dermatol Ther*. 2008;21:211.
14. Mirmirani P, Willey A, Headington JT, Stenn K, McCalmont TH, Price VH. Primary cicatricial alopecia: histopathologic findings do not distinguish clinical variants. *J Am Acad Dermatol*. 2005;52:637-643.
15. Kanti V, Röwert-Huber J, Vogt A, Blume-Peytavi U. Cicatricial alopecia. *J Dtsch Dermatol Ges*. 2018;16(4):435-461.
16. Assouly P, Reygagne P. Lichen planopilaris: update on diagnosis and treatment. *Cutan Med Surg*. 2009;28(1):3-10.
17. Walling HW, Sontheimer RD. Cutaneous lupus erythematosus: issues in diagnosis and treatment. *Am J Clin Dermatol*. 2009;10:365-381.
18. Chieregato C, Zini A, Barba A, Magnanini M, Rosina P. Lichen planopilaris: report of 30 cases and review of the literature. *Int J Dermatol*. 2003;42(5):342-345.
19. Poblet E, Jimenez F, Pascual A, Pique E. Frontal fibrosing alopecia versus lichen planopilaris: a clinicopathological study. *Int J Dermatol*. 2006;45:375-380.
20. Sperling LC. Lichen planopilaris. In: *An Atlas of Hair Pathology with Clinical Correlations*. New York: Parthenon Publishing Group; 2003:101-106.
21. Dina Y, Okoye GA, Aguh C. The timing and distribution of non-scalp hair loss in patients with lichen planopilaris and frontal fibrosing alopecia: a survey-based study. *J Am Acad Dermatol*. 2018;85(2):472-473.
22. Bolduc C, Sperling LC, Shapiro J. Primary cicatricial alopecia: lymphocytic primary cicatricial alopecias, including chronic cutaneous lupus erythematosus, lichen planopilaris, frontal fibrosing alopecia, and Graham–Little syndrome. *J Am Acad Dermatol*. 2016;75:1081-1099.
23. Karnik P, Tekeste Z, McCormick TS, et al. Hair follicle stem cell-specific PPAR-gamma deletion causes scarring alopecia. *J Invest Dermatol*. 2009;129(5):1243-1257.
24. Harries MJ, Meyer K, Chaudhry I, et al. Lichen planopilaris is characterized by immune privilege collapse of the hair follicle's epithelial stem cell niche. *J Pathol*. 2013;231(2):236-247.
25. Callender VD, Reid SD, Obayan O, Mcclellan L, Sperling L. Diagnostic clues to frontal fibrosing alopecia in patients of African descent. *J Clin Aesthet Dermatol*. 2016;9(4):45-51.
26. Samrao A, Chew A-L, Price V. Frontal fibrosing alopecia: a clinical review of 36 patients. *Br J Dermatol*. 2010;163(6):1296-1300.
27. Debroy Kidambi A, Dobson K, Holmes S, et al. Frontal fibrosing alopecia in men: an association with facial moisturizers and sunscreens. *Br J Dermatol*. 2017;177:260-261.
28. Callander J, Frost J, Stone N. Ultraviolet filters in hair-care products: a possible link with frontal fibrosing alopecia and lichen planopilaris. *Clin Exp Dermatol*. 2018;43:69-70.
29. Tosti A, Miteva M, Torres F. Lonely hair: a clue to the diagnosis of frontal fibrosing alopecia. *Arch Dermatol*. 2011;147(10):1240.
30. Dlova NC, Salkey KS, Callender VD, McMichael AJ. Central centrifugal cicatricial alopecia: new insights and a call for action. *J Investig Dermatol Symp Proc*. 2017;18:S54-S56.
31. Callender VD, Wright DR, Davis EC, Sperling LC. Hair breakage as a presenting sign of early or occult central centrifugal cicatricial alopecia: clinicopathologic findings in 9 patients. *Arch Dermatol*. 2012;148:1047-1052.
32. LoPresti P, Papa CM, Kligman AM. Hot comb alopecia. *Arch Dermatol*. 1968;98(3):234-238. doi:10.1001/archderm.1968.01610150020003.
33. Gathers RC, Jankowski M, Eide M, Lim HW. Hair grooming practices and central centrifugal cicatricial alopecia. *J Am Acad Dermatol*. 2009;60(4):574-578.
34. Malki L, Sarig O, Romano MT, et al. Variant PADI3 in central centrifugal cicatricial alopecia. *N Engl J Med*. 2019;380(9):833-841.
35. Dina Y, Okoye GA, Aguh C. Association of uterine leiomyomas with central centrifugal cicatricial alopecia. *JAMA Dermatol*. 2018;154(2):213-214.
36. Coogan PF, Bethea TN, Cozier YC, et al. Association of type 2 diabetes with central-scalp hair loss in a large cohort study of African American women. *Int J Womens Dermatol*. 2019;5(4):261-266.
37. Chieregato C, Zini A, Barba A, Magnanini M, Rosina P. Lichen planopilaris: report of 30 cases and review of the literature. *Int J Dermatol*. 2003;42(5):342-345.

38. Tan E, Martinka M, Ball N, et al. Primary cicatricial alopecias: clinicopathology of 112 cases. *J Am Acad Dermatol*. 2004;50:25-32.

39. Firooz A, Tehranchi-Nia Z, Ahmed AR. Benefits and risks of intralesional corticosteroid injection in the treatment of dermatological diseases. *Clin Exp Dermatol*. 1995; 20:363-370.

40. Drake LA, Dinehart SM, Farmer ER, et al. Guidelines of care for the use of topical glucocorticosteroids. *J Am Acad Dermatol*. 1996;35(4):615-619.

41. Shumaker PR, Rao J, Goldman MP. Treatment of local, persistent cutaneous atrophy following corticosteroid injection with normal saline infiltration. *Dermatol Surg*. 2005;31:1340-1343.

42. Mansouri P, Ranibar M, Abolhasani E, Chalangari R, Martits-Chalangari R, Hejazi S. Pulsed dye laser in treatment of steroid-induced atrophy. *J Cosmet Dermatol*. 2015;14:E15-E20.

43. Chiang C, Sah D, Cho BK, Ochoa BE, Price VH. Hydroxy-chloroquine and lichen planopilaris: efficacy and intro-duction of Lichen Planopilaris Activity Index scoring system. *J Am Acad Dermatol*. 2010;62(3):387-392. doi:10.1016/j.jaad.2009.08.054.

44. Lyakhovitsky A, Amichai B, Sizopoulou C, Barzilai A. A case series of 46 patients with lichen planopilaris: demo-graphics, clinical evaluation, and treatment experience. *J Dermatolog Treat*. 2015;26(3):275-279.

45. Price VH. The medical treatment of cicatricial alopecia. *Semin Cutan Med Surg*. 2006;25:56-59.

46. Dina Y, Aguh C. An algorithmic approach to the treat-ment of frontal fibrosing alopecia: a systematic review. *J Am Acad Dermatol*. 2021;85(2):508-510.

47. Vano-Galvan S, Moina-Ruiz AM, Serrano-Falcon C. Frontal fibrosing alopecia: a multicenter review of 355 patients. *J Am Acad Dermatol*. 2014;70:670-678.

48. Donovan JC. Finasteride-mediated hair regrowth and reversal of atrophy in a patient with frontal fibrosing alopecia. *JAAD Case Rep*. 2015;1(6):353-355. doi: 10.1016/j.jdcr.2015.08.003.

49. Mahmoudi H, Rostami A, Tavakolpour S, et al. Oral isotretinoin combined with topical clobetasol 0.05% and tacrolimus 0.1% for the treatment of frontal fibrosing alopecia: a randomized controlled trial. *J Dermatolog Treat*. 2022;33(1):284-290.

50. Andia I. Platelet-rich plasma Biology. In: Alves R, Grimalt R, eds. *Clinical Indications and Treatment Protocols with Platelet-Rich Plasma in Dermatology*. Barcelona: Ediciones Mayo; 2016:3-15.

51. Sclafani AP, Azzi J. Platelet preparations for use in facial rejuvenation and wound healing: a critical review of current literature. *Aesthec Plast Surg*. 2015;39:495-505.

52. Li ZJ, Choi HI, Choi DK, et al. Autologous platelet-rich plasma: a potential therapeutic tool for promoting hair growth. *Dermatol Surg*. 2012;38(7 Pt 1):1040-1046.

53. Dina Y, Aguh C. Use of platelet-rich plasma in cicatricial alopecia. *Dermatol Surg*. 2019;45(7):979-981.

54. Svigos K, Yin L, Shaw K, et al. Use of platelet-rich plasma in lichen planopilaris and its variants: a retrospective case series demonstrating treatment tolerability without koebnerization. *J Am Acad Dermatol*. 2020;83(5):1506-1509.

55. Özcan D, Tunçer Vural A, Özen Ö. Platelet-rich plasma for treatment resistant frontal fibrosing alopecia: a case report. *Dermatol Ther*. 2019;23:e13072.

56. Sinclair RD. Female pattern hair loss: a pilot study investigating combination therapy with low-dose oral minoxidil and spironolactone. *Int J Dermatol*. 2018; 57(1):104-109.

57. Tawfik AA, Osman MAR. The effect of autologous activated platelet-rich plasma injection on female pattern hair loss: a randomized placebo-controlled study. *J Cosmet Dermatol*. 2018;17(1):47-53.

58. Alves R, Grimalt R. Platelet-rich plasma and its use for cicatricial and non-cicatricial alopecias: a narrative review. *Dermatol Ther (Heidelb)*. 2020;10:623-633.

59. Rose P, Shapiro R. Transplanting into scar tissue and areas of cicatricial alopecia. In: Unger WP, Shapiro R, eds. *Hair Transplantation*. 4th ed. New York: Marcel Dekker; 2004:606-609.

60. Olsen EA, Messenger AG, Shapiro J, et al. Evaluation and treatment of male and female pattern hair loss. *J Am Acad Dermatol*. 2005;52:301-311.

61. Kristine Bunagan MJ. Diseases of the hair and scalp in Asians that are of interest to hair surgeons. In: Pathomvanich D, Imagawa K, eds. *Practical Aspects of Hair Transplantation in Asians*. Tokyo: Springer; 2018. Available at: https://doi.org/10.1007/978-4-431-56547-5_6.

62. Callender VD, Lawson CN, Onwudiwe OC. Hair trans-plantation in the surgical treatment of central centrifugal cicatricial alopecia. *Dermatol Surg*. 2014;40:1125-1131.

63. Salanitri S, Gonçalves AJ, Helene Jr A, Lopes FH. Surgical complications in hair transplantation: a series of 533 procedures. *Aesthet Surg J*. 2009;29(1):72-76.

64. Dahdah MJ, Iorizzo M. The Role of hair restoration surgery in primary cicatricial alopecia. *Skin Appendage Disord*. 2016;2(1-2):57-60. doi:10.1159/000448104.

65. Rogers NE, Callender VD. Advances and challenges in hair restoration of curly afrocentric hair. *Dermatol Clin*. 2014;32:163-171.

66. Rassman WR, Bernstein RM, McClellan R, et al. Follicu-lar unit extraction: minimally invasive surgery in hair transplantation. *Dermatol Surg*. 2002;28:720-728.

67. Avram M, Rogers N. Contemporary hair transplantation. *Dermatol Surg.* 2009;35:1705-1719.

68. Lee TS, Minton TJ. An update on hair restoration therapy. *Curr Opin Otolaryngol Head Neck Surg.* 2009; 17:287-294.

69. Ekelem C, Pham C, Atanaskova Mesinkovska N. A systematic review of the outcome of hair transplantation in primary scarring alopecia. *Skin Appendage Disord.* 2019; 5(2):65-71.

70. Lee JA, Levy DA, Patel KG, Brennan E, Oyer SL. Hair transplantation in frontal fibrosing alopecia and lichen planopilaris: a systematic review. *Laryngoscope.* 2020;131:59-66. doi:10.1002/lary.28551https://doi:10.1002/lary.28551.

71. Nusbaum BP, Nusbaum AG. Frontal fibrosing alopecia in a man: results of follicular unit test grafting. *Dermatol Surg.* 2010;36:959-962.

72. Jiménez F, Poblet E. Is hair transplantation indicated in frontal fibrosing alopecia? The results of test grafting in three patients. *Dermatol Surg.* 2013;39(7):1115-1118. doi:10.1111/dsu.12232.

73. Rose PT, Shapiro R. Transplanting into scar tissue and areas of cicatricial alopecia. In: Unger WP, Shapiro R, eds. Hair Transplantation. 4th ed. New York: Marcel Dekker; 2004:606-610.

74. Harris JA. Follicular unit extraction. *Facial Plast Surg Clin North Am.* 2013;21(3):375-384.

75. Garg S. Outcome of intra-operative injected platelet-rich plasma therapy during follicular unit extraction hair transplant: a prospective randomised study in forty patients. *J Cutan Aesthet Surg.* 2016;9(3):157-164. doi:10.4103/0974-2077.191657.

76. Avci P, Gupta GK, Clark J, Wikonkal N, Hamblin MR. Low-level laser (light) therapy (LLLT) for treatment of hair loss. *Lasers Surg Med.* 2014;46:144-151.

77. Avci P, Gupta A, Sadasivam M, et al. Low-level laser (light) therapy (LLLT) in skin: stimulating, healing, restoring. *Semin Cutan Med Surg.* 2013;32(1):41-52.

78. Adil A, Godwin M. The effectiveness of treatments for androgenetic alopecia: a systematic review and meta-analysis. *J Am Acad Dermatol.* 2017;77(1):136-141.e5. doi:10.1016/j.jaad.2017.02.054.

79. Randolph MJ, Salhi WA, Tosti A. Lichen planopilaris and low-level light therapy: four case reports and review of the literature about low-level light therapy and lichenoid dermatosis. *Dermatol Ther (Heidelb).* 2020;10: 311-319.

80. Fonda-Pascual P, Moreno-Arrones OM, Saceda-Corralo D, et al. Effectiveness of low-level laser therapy in lichen planopilaris. *J Am Acad Dermatol.* 2018;78(5): 1020-1023.

81. Peterson EL, Gutierrez D, Brinster NK, Lo Sicco KI, Shapiro J. Response of lichen planopilaris to pioglitazone hydrochloride. *J Drugs Dermatol.* 2019;18(12):1276-1279.

82. Baibergenova A, Walsh S. Use of pioglitazone in patients with lichen planopilaris. *J Cutan Med Surg.* 2012;16(2):97-100.

83. Plante J, Eason C, Snyder A, Elston D. Tofacitinib in the treatment of lichen planopilaris: a retrospective review. *J Am Acad Dermatol.* 2020;83(5):1487-1489.

84. Araoye EF, Thomas JAL, Aguh CU. Hair regrowth in 2 patients with recalcitrant central centrifugal cicatricial alopecia after use of topical metformin. *JAAD Case Rep.* 2020;6(2):106-108. doi:10.1016/j.jdcr.2019.12.008.

Minimizing and Concealing Hair Loss

4

Nutritional Supplements

Kelly O'Connor and Lynne J. Goldberg

KEY POINTS

- There are shortcomings in U.S. Food & Drug Administration (FDA)–approved treatments for androgenetic alopecia (AGA) that are currently available.
- There is a growing body of double-blind, placebo-controlled, randomized studies that demonstrate both qualitative and quantitative benefits of nutritional supplements to combat hair thinning.

- Larger studies with longer follow-up times are needed for each individual supplement to assess optimal dosing and frequency, duration of effect, and less common adverse events.
- Nutritional supplements can lead to a variety of side effects, interactions with medications, and interference with laboratory testing.

BACKGROUND, DEFINITION, AND HISTORY

Androgenetic alopecia (AGA) is prevalent, with estimates that it affects 43% of women and 83% of men by age 60 (level of evidence: 2c).[1] Depression, anxiety (level of evidence: 2b),[2] and decreased quality of life (level of evidence: 1b)[3-5] are frequently seen in these patients. Despite AGA's prevalence and morbidity, topical minoxidil in women and men and oral finasteride in men remain the only treatments approved by the U.S. Food & Drug Administration (FDA). The side effects of irritant and allergic contact dermatitis and hypertrichosis with minoxidil (level of evidence: 1a)[6] and erectile dysfunction and decreased libido with finasteride (level of evidence: 2a)[7] may affect long-term adherence. Other treatments, such as low-level laser light, show inconsistent results, and many of the supportive studies provide low-quality evidence (level of evidence: 1a).[8]

A need for additional effective and well-tolerated therapies may account for the use of complementary and alternative medicine (CAM), which is used by an estimated 35% to 69% of dermatology patients over their lifetimes (level of evidence: 3a) (Pearl 4.1).[9] One facet of CAM is nutritional supplementation. A nutraceutical is any food substance (vitamin, mineral, proprietary blend, genetically engineered food, or herbal product) that "provides medical or health benefits, including the prevention and treatment of disease" (level of evidence: 5).[10] The FDA does not regulate nutraceuticals as it does drugs, so there are no premarket safety and efficacy studies. Therefore nutraceutical companies are not permitted to market claims that their product can diagnose, prevent, treat, or cure disease (level of evidence: 5).[11] If a company does make a "structure-function" claim (e.g., saw palmetto cures androgenic alopecia), then the product must carry a disclaimer that it was not reviewed by the FDA.[11] This may be confusing to patients, who often read about conflicting associations between nutrients and diseases reported in the

> **PEARL 4.1:** A dearth of effective and well-tolerated therapies for androgenetic alopecia may account for the use of complementary and alternative medicine.

media. A systematic review found that 75% of the risk estimates in studies claiming associations between foods and cancer had either weak or no statistical significance (level of evidence: 3a).[12] Providers must bridge this knowledge gap and offer factual advice on nutraceutical risks and benefits.

INDICATIONS AND PATIENT SELECTION

Vitamin and mineral supplementation is indicated in any patient complaining of hair loss with a documented deficiency (Pearl 4.2). Certain populations are at higher risk for deficiencies, and a thorough history of diet, lifestyle, use of supplements, and current medications should be sought in all cases (Pearl 4.3). If responses raise concern for a vitamin or mineral deficiency, then laboratory testing may be pursued to determine whether supplementation is needed.

A large population at risk for nutritional deficiency is the elderly. More than 60% of senior adults have been found to have vitamin and mineral intakes lower than the estimated requirements (level of evidence: 2c).[13] Malnourishment in this population is multifactorial, and causes include decreased sensory reception in smell and taste of foods, impaired ability to chew and swallow food, reduced nutrient absorption as a result of medications, and higher rates of dementia, depression, and social isolation (level of evidence: 5).[14]

Certain medical conditions are risk factors for nutritional deficiencies. Malabsorption in patients with pancreatic or biliary disease, Crohn's disease, celiac disease, amyloidosis, parasitic infections, scleroderma, alcohol abuse disorder, or a history of bariatric weight-loss surgery renders them at particular risk for deficiencies of fat-soluble vitamins A, D, E, and K (level of evidence: 5).[15] Patients with ongoing blood loss from menorrhagia (level of evidence: 2b),[16] inflammatory

bowel disease (level of evidence: 5),[17] or colon cancer (level of evidence: 2c)[18] are at risk for iron deficiency. Iron deficiency may also be seen in pregnant women (level of evidence: 5).[19]

Pregnancy (level of evidence: 3b),[20] lactation,[21] and alcohol use disorder (level of evidence: 5)[21] may lead to biotin deficiency, while burns, sickle cell disease, collagen vascular diseases, and chronic diarrhea can cause zinc deficiency (level of evidence: 5).[22] Lastly, patients on hemodialysis are at risk for selenium deficiency caused by its removal of selenium from the blood (level of evidence: 2b).[23]

Dietary practices have been found to be associated with specific deficiencies. Vegetarians are at higher risk for iron and zinc deficiencies, because plant-based sources of those nutrients have less bioavailability than their animal-based sources (level of evidence: 5).[24] Furthermore, phytates, such as those found in cereals, whole grain bread, and legumes, are prevalent in vegetarian diets and are known to chelate zinc, making it unavailable for absorption (level of evidence: 5).[25] Overconsumption of raw egg whites can lead to biotin deficiency, because eggs contain a protein component called avidin that binds to biotin and renders it nonfunctional (level of evidence: 5).[26]

Various medications can impair the absorption of nutrients. Proton pump inhibitors (e.g., omeprazole) decrease iron absorption by reducing the acidic environment of the stomach that is necessary to transport iron across the intestinal lumen (level of evidence: 5).[27] Diuretics, valproic acid, and penicillamine lower zinc levels (level of evidence: 5),[28,29] while isotretinoin (level of evidence: 1b)[30] and valproic acid (level of evidence: 1b)[31] lower biotin levels.

Geographic location is yet another consideration. Those with inadequate sun exposure are at risk for vitamin D deficiency (level of evidence: 5),[32] while those living in places with low selenium soil content, such as Tibet, Siberia, and parts of China, are at risk for selenium deficiency (level of evidence: 5).[33]

Guidelines for laboratory testing of vitamins and minerals have not been established. In 2014, the U.S. Preventive Services Task Force (USPSTF) reviewed the utility of screening for vitamin D deficiency and found that there was insufficient evidence to assess the pros and cons of screening asymptomatic individuals (level of evidence: 5).[34] There are currently no laboratory testing recommendations for patients with AGA. Laboratory

> **PEARL 4.2:** Vitamin and mineral supplementation is indicated in any patient reporting hair loss who has a documented deficiency.

> **PEARL 4.3:** Certain patient populations are at increased risk of vitamin and mineral deficiency.

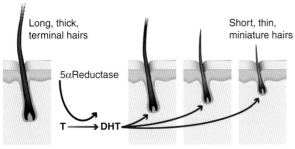

Long, thick, terminal hairs

Short, thin, miniature hairs

5αReductase

T ⟶ DHT

T = Testosterone
DHT = Dihydrotestosterone

Fig. 4.1 Miniaturization of the hair follicle is, in large, driven by dihydrotestosterone, which is catalyzed from testosterone by the enzyme 5-α-reductase. (Courtesy of Sheila Macomber.)

testing itself is not perfect. For example, biotin levels in women reporting hair loss have been shown to fluctuate up to 100% in 1 day (level of evidence: 2b).[35] Additionally, laboratory testing is not available for some ingredients of nutraceuticals, as they are not known to be essential for bodily function. Without a documented deficiency, the decision to start a nutraceutical rests on the balance between clinical trial evidence and side effect profile.

EXPECTED OUTCOMES

AGA is the result of progressive miniaturization of terminal hair follicles on the scalp (Fig. 4.1) (level of evidence: 4).[36] Miniaturization occurs as the hair follicle cycles from the anagen (growth) phase into the catagen (regression) phase, and subsequently the telogen (resting) phase (Fig. 4.2).[36] During the transition, hair shafts become thinner in diameter and hair bulbs move more superficially from the subcutis to the dermis.[36] It is hypothesized that this process is driven by a combination of hormones, stress, genetics, and environmental exposures (Fig. 4.3) (level of evidence: 5).[37] Accordingly, nutraceuticals have been studied on molecular levels for their antiandrogenic and antiinflammatory effects, which would theoretically increase the number and duration of terminal scalp hair follicles in the anagen phase.

If the treatment of AGA involves prolonging the anagen phase and reversing miniaturization, one should expect to see an increase in the percentage of hair follicles in the anagen phase, hair shaft diameter, number of terminal hairs, and hair fullness. Studies have shown this to be true with topical minoxidil, which leads to a greater proportion of hairs in the anagen phase (level of evidence: 5)[38] and increased hair counts (vellus, terminal, and total) (level of evidence: 1b).[39] Nutraceutical studies have evaluated similar endpoints to capture the reversal of miniaturization; they have included objective measures of hair-shaft diameter and hair counts (vellus, terminal, and total hairs) and subjective measures of reviewer and patient perceptions of hair fullness, thickness, and density.

Many nutraceutical studies have evaluated endpoints between 3 and 12 months of treatment. This variability may be in part caused by the lack of studies on the duration of hair regrowth in *in vivo* human hairs (level of evidence: 5).[40] Knowledge of the duration of hair follicle cycles has come from mouse xenograft models, which have shown that donor human catagen follicles will

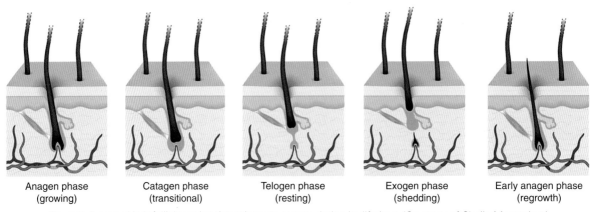

Anagen phase (growing) Catagen phase (transitional) Telogen phase (resting) Exogen phase (shedding) Early anagen phase (regrowth)

Fig. 4.2 A normal hair follicle cycles through many stages during its lifetime. (Courtesy of Sheila Macomber.)

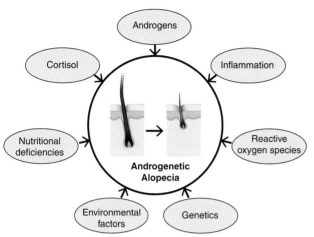

Fig. 4.3 Multiple factors contribute to the pathogenesis of androgenetic alopecia. (Courtesy of Sheila Macomber.)

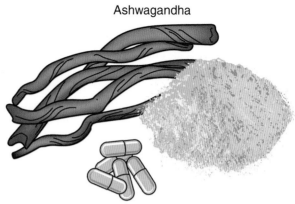

Ashwagandha

Fig. 4.4 Ashwagandha, a short perennial shrub, is a member of the nightshade family and cultivated in the drier regions of India and East Asia. (Courtesy of Sheila Macomber.)

progress to the anagen phase in recipient mice somewhere between 60 and 90 days.[40,41] Two randomized, double-blind, placebo-controlled studies on the proprietary nutraceuticals Nutrafol (level of evidence: 1b)[42] and Viviscal (level of evidence: 1b)[43] both measured results after 90 and 180 days of treatment. This is similar to prior studies on topical minoxidil, which assessed endpoints at 16 weeks (112 days)[39] and 24 weeks (168 days) (level of evidence: 1b).[44] Although it is known that discontinuation of minoxidil does not maintain treatment response (level of evidence: 1b),[45,46] studies on nutraceuticals have not assessed the duration of effects once patients stop treatment. There is a need for more studies on optimal dosing and length of nutraceutical supplementation.

TREATMENT TECHNIQUE/BEST PRACTICES (PEARL 4.4)

Ashwagandha

Ashwagandha, also known as *Withania somnifera*, is a botanical herb long thought to have a role in maintaining homeostasis by modulating the stress response (Fig. 4.4). Daily intake has been shown to significantly

> **PEARL 4.4:** Routine vitamin and mineral supplementation for all patients with androgenetic and other forms of alopecia is not advisable.

reduce circulating levels of stress hormones. An 8-week, double-blind, placebo-controlled, randomized trial demonstrated that daily intake of ashwagandha significantly reduced serum cortisol levels in healthy, stressed adults, especially at higher doses (600 mg/day > 250 mg/day) (level of evidence: 1b).[47] Study participants also reported decreased levels of stress and anxiety, and increased quality of sleep. Similar results were found in a 60-day, double-blind, placebo-controlled, randomized trial that demonstrated reduction in both serum cortisol and dehydroepiandrosterone-sulfate (DHEA-S) levels in healthy adults taking 240 mg of ashwagandha daily (level of evidence: 1b).[48] However, compared with placebo, an increase in testosterone was found in young men undergoing resistance training supplemented with 300 mg of ashwagandha twice daily (level of evidence: 1b).[49] Increased serum testosterone levels could theoretically initiate, or hasten, AGA.

Ashwagandha is an ingredient in Nutrafol, a proprietary blend of supplements that has been shown to stimulate hair growth.[42] It is unclear if ashwagandha contributes to this observed effect given that no clinical trial has evaluated the direct effect of ashwagandha on hair growth.

Biotin

Biotin is a water-soluble B-complex vitamin. It serves as a cofactor for enzymes involved in mitochondrial function of hair follicles and other metabolic functions, gene regulation, and cell signaling (level of evidence: 5).[50,51]

Biotin is often given as a supplement to patients with hair loss, because hereditary deficiency of biotin is associated with alopecia; it is also inexpensive and readily available. One retrospective cohort study found that 38% of healthy women complaining of hair loss had low levels of biotin (level of evidence: 2b);[35] however, many of these women had concurrent seborrheic dermatitis or a risk factor for biotin deficiency (e.g., inflammatory bowel disease, isotretinoin use, antibiotic treatment). Additionally, the studied population had not been diagnosed with AGA. A different study on biotin and zinc levels in male patients with AGA revealed low levels of both compared with matched controls, although biotin levels did not correlate with age or disease duration (level of evidence: 2b).[52] Furthermore, biotin levels fluctuate daily, and there are multiple compounding factors in their measurements (level of evidence: 5).[53] Although biotin has been shown to promote hair growth in biotin-deficient patients (level of evidence: 4),[54] there are no randomized, controlled trials demonstrating a beneficial effect of biotin in AGA or other types of alopecia.

Curcumin

Curcumin is the active ingredient of turmeric, a naturally occurring botanical in the ginger family (Fig. 4.5). Curcumin has been used in Ayurvedic medicine for centuries due to its anti-inflammatory effects, although it also has antioxidant, antimicrobial, antineoplastic and antiandrogenic properties (level of evidence: 5).[55] Although it can be made as an individual oral supplement, it is poorly absorbed and rapidly metabolized. The botanical piperine, which is found in black pepper, is added to commercially available supplements with curcumin to drastically increase bioavailability (level of evidence: 4).[56]

There are no clinical trials on oral curcumin for hair loss. However, a 5% topical extract has been studied with and without 5% minoxidil in comparison to placebo (level of evidence: 1b).[57] Combined therapy demonstrated statistically significant improvements in hair count, regrowth, and shedding, while treatment with topical curcumin alone did not yield significant improvements. This suggests that topical curcumin increases the penetration of topical minoxidil, which has been verified in *ex vivo* foreskin models (level of evidence: 5).[58] Although supportive evidence for curcumin alone is lacking, it may be beneficial in enhancing treatment with topical minoxidil.

Equisetum

Equisetum, or horsetail, is an herb that has long been used for its suspected anti-inflammatory, antioxidant, and antimicrobial properties (Fig. 4.6). It has been shown to inhibit 5-α-reductase *in vitro*, theoretically slowing the progression of AGA (level of evidence: 5).[59] Equisetum is believed to be effective for hair growth because of its high concentration of silicon. Physiologic concentrations of orthosilicic acid (the bioavailable form of silicon) have been shown to stimulate synthesis of type I collagen in *in vitro* human osteoblast-like cells (level of evidence: 5).[60] It is hypothesized that by activating fibroblasts, orthosilicic acid induces a favorable

Curcumin

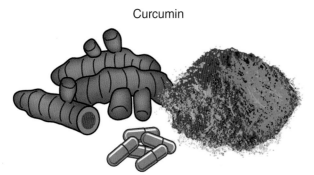

Fig. 4.5 Curcumin is the bright yellow-orange component of plants of the *Curcuma longa* species, which includes turmeric. (Courtesy of Sheila Macomber.)

Equisetum

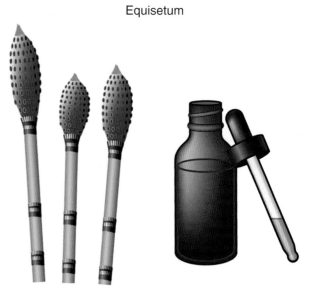

Fig. 4.6 Equisetum, commonly referred to as horsetail, is predominantly found in northern North America. (Courtesy of Sheila Macomber.)

cytokine milieu for hair growth. A double-blind, placebo-controlled, randomized trial assessed the effects of 10 mg of choline-stabilized orthosilicic acid daily in women with fine hair (level of evidence: 1b).[61] After 9 months, the treatment group had significantly thicker hair (as measured by the cross-sectional area) and a positive effect on tensile strength.[61] Although these results are promising, the supplement has not been tested on patients diagnosed with AGA.

Iron

Iron is an essential element, which means it must be obtained from the diet. It plays many crucial roles in bodily functions, including red blood cell production, oxygen transport, mitochondrial respiration, DNA replication and repair, immune function, and cell signaling (level of evidence: 5).[62] Mice with a TMPRSS6 protein (matriptase-2) mutation, which causes poor iron absorption and iron deficiency, experience a loss of body hair (level of evidence: 5).[63] It has been shown that giving these mice iron supplements can reverse the iron deficiency and restore hair growth. However, results of studies on iron and hair loss in humans are conflicting, and often AGA and telogen effluvium (TE) are not distinguished (level of evidence: 5).[64] One study on ferritin levels in women with different types of nonscarring hair loss revealed that those with AGA and alopecia areata (AA) had significantly lower levels than controls (level of evidence: 2b).[65] Another study did not find any significant decrease in ferritin levels in women with AGA compared with those with TE and controls (level of evidence: 2b).[66]

Marine Proteins

Marine proteins are a group of fish, mollusk, and marine plant species that have been isolated for the purposes of human supplementation. The first reported use of marine proteins for AGA came from a study on men in Finland comparing marine proteins mixed with equisetum (Viviscal) to a fish extract of similar composition (Fig. 4.7) (level of evidence: 1b).[67] The marine protein group demonstrated a lack of hair loss in all participants after 2 months, a significant increase in nonvellus hair counts, and less inflammation and improvement in follicular size on biopsies at 6 months. Although multiple randomized controlled trials have also shown that Viviscal leads to clinical and histologic improvement in hair growth, many have been marred by the inclusion of different types of hair loss, the lack of placebo groups, small study sizes, and follow-up times of

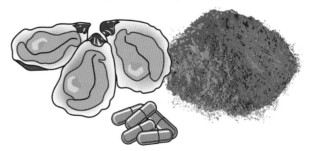

Oyster extract powder

Fig. 4.7 Oyster extract is a component of the AminoMar Marine Complex in ViviScal nutraceuticals. (Courtesy of Sheila Macomber.)

less than 4 months (level of evidence: 5, 1b, 1b).[68-70] It should be noted that Viviscal is a proprietary blend of shark cartilage, oyster powder, apple extract powder, vitamin C, L-cystine, L-methionine, and biotin, so conclusions about the efficacy of marine proteins alone cannot be made. Other proprietary supplements contain marine proteins; Nourkin has fractionated fish extract with specific lectican proteoglycans, and Nutrafol has marine collagen from cod fish scales.

Pumpkin Seed Oil

Pumpkins are members of the squash family and are native to North America (Fig 4.8). Pumpkin seed oil contains varying amounts of magnesium, potassium, calcium, sodium, selenium, iron, polyunsaturated fatty acids, tocopherols, and sterols (level of evidence: 5),[71,72] which lend antioxidant and anti-inflammatory properties. Wounded rats treated with pumpkin seed oil

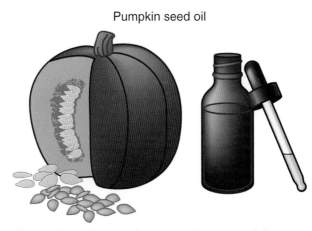

Pumpkin seed oil

Fig. 4.8 Pumpkin seed oil has antioxidant and antiinflammatory properties. (Courtesy of Sheila Macomber.)

revealed full reepithelialization with reappearance of skin appendages and well organized collagen fibers, suggesting a mechanism for hair regrowth (level of evidence: 5).[73] In a clinical study of 76 men with AGA treated with a supplement containing 400 mg of pumpkin seed oil, hair counts were significantly improved at 12 and 24 weeks compared with placebo, but hair diameters improved in both the treated and placebo groups (level of evidence: 1b).[74] However, the product used (Octa Sabal Plus) also contains mixed vegetable powder, octacosanol, corn silk, evening primrose powder, tomato powder, and red clover powder, so it is not known which ingredient, or combination of ingredients, was responsible for the observed results.

Saw Palmetto

Saw palmetto, or *Serenoa repens*, is a botanical extract made from the berries of the American dwarf tree, which can be found in the southeastern United States (Fig. 4.9) (level of evidence: 5).[75] It has been widely used in the treatment of benign prostatic hyperplasia as a result of is antiandrogenic effects. Saw palmetto is a competitive, nonselective inhibitor of 5-alpha reductase (level of evidence: 5)[76] and inhibits 50% of dihydrotestosterone from binding to nuclear androgen receptors in cultured human foreskin fibroblasts (level of evidence: 5).[77] There has been some evidence in clinical trials that saw palmetto is efficacious in treating AGA. A small pilot study showed that 200 mg of saw palmetto daily resulted in "improvement," as determined by blinded investigative staff in 6 of 10 healthy male subjects with mild-moderate AGA (60%, compared with 11% of subjects given placebo) (level of evidence: 1b).[78]

Saw palmetto

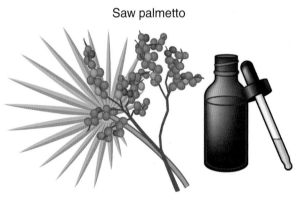

Fig. 4.9 Saw palmetto extract is from the fruit of saw palmetto, a small palm that is endemic to the southeastern United States. (Courtesy of Sheila Macomber.)

A larger study compared 320 mg of saw palmetto daily to 1 mg of finasteride daily in males with mild to moderate AGA for 24 months, finding significantly higher hair density scores for both saw palmetto (38%) and finasteride (68%) (level of evidence: 1b).[79] Additionally, saw palmetto "stabilized" AGA in 52% of cases, while 10% of the subjects continued to have progressive hair loss. The study showed that both saw palmetto and finasteride are effective treatments, but that finasteride was superior, especially for men with more severe AGA.

Another double-blind, placebo-controlled, randomized trial evaluated the efficacy of 6 months of treatment with a food supplement containing saw palmetto, L-cystine, *Equisetum* extract, zinc, and vitamins (Lambdapil) (level of evidence: 1b).[80] The treatment group saw a 23% increase in anagen to telogen ratio from baseline and a 3.7% increase in total anagen hairs (compared with a 0.8% decrease in the placebo group). Patients in the treatment group also reported statistically significant increases in hair thickness (slight to moderate) and appearance. Although this proprietary blend appears to be effective, it is unclear which ingredient, or combination of ingredients, was driving the reversal of miniaturization.

Selenium

Selenium is an essential element that is a "trace" element, meaning only small amounts are required. It acts as a cofactor for glutathione peroxidase, an enzyme involved in antioxidation, and selenium-dependent enzymes that are responsible for the conversion of inactive to active thyroxine (level of evidence: 1b).[81] It also plays a role in immune function (level of evidence: 5).[82] Animal studies have shown hair loss in rats deficient in selenium (level of evidence: 5)[83] and a selenium cofactor (level of evidence: 5).[84] Low levels of selenium were found in four children on long-term total parenteral nutrition, half of whom developed hypopigmentation of the skin and hair that resolved with intravenous supplementation over 6 to 12 months (level of evidence: 4).[85] There are no studies looking at the effects of selenium supplementation on hair growth or in populations with AGA.

Vitamin D

Vitamin D is an essential fat-soluble vitamin. Its inactive form is obtained through diet and by synthesis in the skin. It plays an important role in calcium and phosphorous metabolism and immune regulation (level of evidence: 5).[86] Ultraviolet light converts 7-dehydrocholesterol in keratinocytes to cholecalciferol, which is further metabolized in the liver and kidney to create the active form of the vitamin, 1,25-dihydroxyvitamin D (level of evidence: 5).[87] This active form functions as a steroid hormone, binding to its receptor and acting as a transcription factor.[87] In mice, the vitamin D receptor (VDR) resides intracellularly in outer root sheath of keratinocytes and mesenchymal dermal papilla cells VDRs have different levels of immunoreactivity during different stages of the hair cycle (level of evidence: 5),[88] suggesting that levels of expression change during the hair cycle. A link between vitamin D and the hair cycle is further supported by the finding of alopecia in VDR knockout mice and human genetic syndromes involving mutations in the VDR (e.g., vitamin D dependent rickets) (level of evidence: 5).[89,90] Despite this link, data on the role of vitamin D in other types of hair loss is inconclusive, as studies on TE and AGA have been small and yielded contradictory results (level of evidence: 3a).[91] No study has demonstrated that vitamin D supplementation promotes hair growth.

Vitamin E

Vitamin E is an essential fat-soluble vitamin that is composed of several compounds called tocotrienols and tocopherols (level of evidence: 5).[92] It is an antioxidant that scavenges free radicals (level of evidence: 5).[93] Because oxidative stress is important in the development of AGA (level of evidence: 5),[94] vitamin E has a potential role in treatment. A study of oral supplementation with 100 mg of vitamin E in 38 alopecia patients over 8 months resulted in a significant increase in hair counts, but no increase in hair weight (level of evidence: 1b).[95] The type of alopecia was not specified. There is little evidence that vitamin E improves hair growth in the absence of deficiency (level of evidence: 5).[96]

Zinc

Zinc is an essential trace element that functions as a cofactor for many metalloenzymes and transcription factors and plays important roles in protein synthesis, cell division, and gene regulation (level of evidence: 5).[97,98] It also has a role in the Hedgehog signaling pathway (level of evidence: 5),[99] which is involved in follicular morphogenesis. Its importance in the hair cycle is further supported by the fact that hair loss is seen in diseases of zinc deficiency. Acrodermatitis enteropathica, a rare autosomal recessive genodermatosis caused by mutation in the *SLC39A* gene that codes for a zinc-specific transporter (level of evidence: 5),[100] causes the classic triad of periorificial dermatitis, alopecia, and

diarrhea. Zinc deficiency also manifests as TE and brittle hair, which is improved with supplementation (level of evidence: 4).[101] However, the exact role of zinc in hair health is unknown. In studies of zinc levels in patients with male and female pattern hair loss, zinc levels were found to be significantly lower than in controls (level of evidence: 3b).[102,103] One study compared 50 mg of oral zinc supplementation daily, 100 mg oral calcium pantothenate supplementation daily, a combination of the two twice weekly, and topical minoxidil 2% twice daily on women with hair loss (level of evidence: 1b).[104] The greatest improvement was seen with minoxidil, but zinc supplementation showed significantly thicker hair shafts, based on dermatoscopic photographs.

PREVENTION AND MANAGEMENT OF ADVERSE EFFECTS (PEARL 4.5)

Ashwagandha

Ashwagandha capsules are well tolerated, and multiple studies reported no adverse events (level of evidence: 1b).[48,105,106] Furthermore, one of the studies compared full blood counts and lipid profiles of the placebo and treatment groups and did not find any statistically significant differences.[48]

Biotin

High levels of biotin in the serum can interfere with hormonal immunoassays that rely on biotinylated antibodies to detect the presence of an analyte (level of evidence: 5)[107] and lead to either falsely low or high results, depending on the specific assay being used. For example, thyroid-stimulating hormone (TSH) assays can yield falsely low levels in the presence of high biotin, while measurements of free T4 and T3 can be falsely elevated (level of evidence: 5).[108] Other tests that can be falsely low include those for troponin, luteinizing hormone, follicle stimulating hormone, human chorionic gonadotropin, parathyroid hormone, insulin-like growth factor 1, insulin, thyroglobulin, and C-peptide (level of evidence: 5).[109] Because of its short half-life, stopping biotin supplementation for a few days and repeating the study, or communication with the lab in

PEARL 4.5: Over supplementation can lead to side effects including, paradoxically, hair loss, effects on multiple organ systems, and interference with medical assays.

choosing an alternate assay, may be beneficial if the clinical and lab data do not correlate and a history of biotin supplementation is obtained.[107] In the case of troponin, however, falsely low values may lead to under-diagnosis of acute coronary syndrome.

Equisetum

No side effects were reported in a study of 48 women with fine hair taking 10 mg of choline-stabilized orthosilicic acid.[61] Similarly, larger studies involving daily intake of choline-stabilized orthosilicic acid (containing 3–12 mg silicon) for other medical conditions unrelated to hair did not report any side effects (level of evidence: 1b).[110,111]

Iron

Once absorbed, the body is unable to excrete excess iron; thus, it is stored in organs such as the liver, heart, and bone marrow. Systemic iron overload can ultimately lead to end organ damage (level of evidence: 5).[112] Symptoms of excess iron intake include gastrointestinal upset and pain, vomiting, and constipation, especially with doses over 20 mg/kg daily (level of evidence: 5).[113] Older studies have shown that iron supplementation can also interfere with other medications, including decreased efficacy of levothyroxine (level of evidence: 4)[114] and decreased absorption of levodopa (level of evidence: 5).[115]

Marine Proteins

People with an allergy to fish or shellfish should not ingest supplements with marine proteins, and a detailed allergy history should be obtained before use.

Saw Palmetto

Only one of the studies previously discussed reported adverse effects of nausea, constipation, and diarrhea; however, it was determined these were unlikely caused by use of the active compound.[78] One trial of 369 male patients investigated the safety and toxicity of 320, 640, and 960 mg daily (much higher than the usual pre-scribed doses) and did not observe any differences in adverse events, vital signs, laboratory test abnormalities, study withdrawal rates, or dose-response phenomena (level of evidence: 1b).[116]

Selenium

Selenium toxicity can result from excess supplementa-tion and inadvertent ingestion of foods with high levels such as chronic ingestion of Brazil nuts. Brazil nuts contain a high amount of selenium; a 1 ounce serving of six to eight nuts contains greater than 900 times the recommended daily allowance (level of evidence: 5).[117] In 2010, an error in formulation resulted in a supple-ment that contained 200 times the intended amount of selenium (level of evidence: 4).[118] According to a review, patients took this supplement for an average of 29 days, and 72% of patients with confirmed toxicity developed mild-to-severe hair loss. In addition to hair loss, other symptoms included nail changes (discoloration or brit-tleness), nausea, diarrhea, fatigue, and joint pain. A randomized study on three doses of selenium supple-mentation in a population with low selenium found that the highest dose, 300 ug/d, resulted in increased mortality after 5 years. The authors concluded that in-take over this dose should be avoided (level of evidence: 1b).[119] Death can occur from massive oral doses of sele-nium, whether accidental or intentional, and additional toxicities include renal failure, onychomadesis, and a garlic-like breath odor (level of evidence: 4).[120]

Vitamin D

Hypervitaminosis D is rare and most commonly results from accidental or uninformed intake of high-dose vitamin D supplements (level of evidence: 3a).[121] The Institute of Medicine (now the National Academy of Medicine) has defined a tolerable upper limit of vitamin D at 100 mcg (4000 IU) daily for adults, which is far below the doses reported in cases of hypervitaminosis D (frequently greater than 1000 mcg daily).[121] It does not appear that toxicity can develop from excessive sun exposure (level of evidence: 2b)[122] or by eating the rec-ommended intake of fortified foods (level of evidence: 3a).[123] Signs of intoxication from oral supplementation are a result of hypercalcemia or hyperphosphatemia, and include nausea, vomiting, abdominal pain, constipation, renal disease, headache, confusion, hypertension, bone pain, osteopenia, and osteoporosis (level of evidence: 4).[124] Populations that are more sensitive to vitamin D supplementation include those with granulomatous disorders, such as sarcoidosis and mycobacterium infec-tions (via increased 1-alpha hydroxylase activity in granulomas) and those taking hydrochlorothiazide (a calcium sparing diuretic).[121]

Vitamin E

Large, multiyear, randomized, double-blind, placebo-controlled factorial trials have demonstrated an increased risk of hemorrhagic strokes in individuals taking supplements of 400 IU of vitamin E every other day (level of evidence: 1b)[125] and 50 mg of alpha-tocopherol daily (level of evidence: 1b).[126]

Zinc

Excessive zinc supplementation can cause acute and chronic symptoms. Acute symptoms are mainly gastrointestinal, such as nausea, abdominal pain and diarrhea, and can start at doses as low as 50 mg/daily (level of evidence: 5).[127] Chronic daily ingestion leading to low copper levels has been associated with myelopathy (level of evidence: 5)[128] and sideroblastic anemia (level of evidence: 5).[129] Zinc-induced neurotoxicity may play a role in the pathogenesis of senile dementia based on molecular studies (level of evidence: 5).[130]

FUTURE DIRECTIONS

Although some nutraceuticals show promising results in small studies, larger, placebo-controlled, randomized trials in populations with a confirmed diagnosis of AGA are needed. Clinical endpoints should include a mix of objective measures (e.g., hair shaft diameter, hair density) and subjective measures (e.g., blinded reviewers, self-assessment). Objective measures give credence that nutraceuticals alter the biomechanics of a hair follicle, while subjective measures may help to ensure patient satisfaction and long-term use. Future studies should also investigate optimal dosing, length of supplementation, and effects after stopping supplementation. Many of the supplements reviewed have not been tested for longer than 6 months, so rare and chronic side effects remain unknown.

Proprietary nutraceutical blends contain a variety of ingredients. Continued improvements in techniques of purification and quantification of ingredients will lead to further clarification as to which compounds are beneficial. There is ongoing work to improve chemical assays, such as plasma-optical emission spectrometry, to measure element concentration. Furthermore, the bioavailability of individual ingredients needs further exploration to determine the best formulation for maximal absorption.

EVIDENCE SUMMARY

- Some proprietary nutraceutical blends, which contain ingredients like ashwagandha, curcumin, *equisetum*, and marine proteins, have resulted in thicker and denser hair in double-blinded, randomized, placebo-controlled clinical trials among patients reporting hair loss (strength of recommendation: B).
- Large, randomized trials of patients diagnosed with AGA are needed to assess individual ingredients, optimal dosages, and treatment lengths (strength of recommendation: C).
- Ashwagandha, curcumin, *equisetum*, marine proteins, and saw palmetto appear to have low side effect profiles, while iron, selenium, vitamin D, vitamin E, and zinc can cause notable symptoms, end stage organ damage, and decreased absorption of medications. The FDA has issued a warning that biotin supplementation may interfere with medical assays, and that patients should notify providers if they are taking biotin (strength of recommendation: B).

REFERENCES

1. Salman KE, Altunay IK, Kucukunal NA, Cerman AA. Frequency, severity and related factors of androgenetic alopecia in dermatology outpatient clinic: hospital-based cross-sectional study in Turkey. *An Bras Dermatol*. 2017; 92(1):35-40.
2. Camacho FM, García-Hernández M. Psychological features of androgenetic alopecia. *J Eur Acad Dermatol Venereol*. 2002;16(5):476-480.
3. Gupta S, Goyal I, Mahendra A. Quality of life assessment in patients with androgenetic alopecia. *Int J Trichology*. 2019;11(4):147-152.
4. Elsaie LT, Elshahid AR, Hasan HM, Soultan FAZM, Jafferany M, Elsaie ML. Cross sectional quality of life assessment in patients with androgenetic alopecia. *Dermatol Ther*. 2020;33(4):e13799.
5. Han SH, Byun JW, Lee WS, et al. Quality of life assessment in male patients with androgenetic alopecia: result of a prospective, multicenter study. *Ann Dermatol*. 2012; 24(3):311-318.
6. Suchonwanit P, Thammarucha S, Leerunyakul K. Minoxidil and its use in hair disorders: a review. *Drug Des Devel Ther*. 2019;13:2777-2786.
7. Hirshburg JM, Kelsey PA, Therrien CA, Gavino AC, Reichenberg JS. Adverse effects and safety of 5-alpha reductase inhibitors (Finasteride, Dutasteride): a systematic review. *J Clin Aesthet Dermatol*. 2016;9(7):56-62.
8. van Zuuren EJ, Fedorowicz Z, Schoones J. Interventions for female pattern hair loss. *Cochrane Database Syst Rev*. 2016;2016(5):CD007628.

9. Ernst E. The usage of complementary therapies by dermatological patients: a systematic review. *Br J Dermatol.* 2000;142(5):857-861.

10. DeFelice ST. The nutraceutical revolution: its impact on food industry R&D. *Trends Food Sci Technol.* 1995;6:59-61.

11. Center for Food Safety and Applied Nutrition. *What You Need to Know About Dietary Supplements.* Available at: https://www.fda.gov/food/dietary-supplements, November 29, 2017.

12. Schoenfeld JD, Ioannidis JP. Is everything we eat associated with cancer? A systematic cookbook review. *Am J Clin Nutr.* 2013;97:127-134.

13. Foote JA, Giuliano AR, Harris RB. Older adults need guidance to meet nutritional recommendations. *J Am Coll Nutr.* 2000;19(5):628-640.

14. Evans C. Malnutrition in the elderly: a multifactorial failure to thrive. *Perm J.* 2005;9(3):38-41.

15. Cerda JJ, Artnak EJ. Nutritional aspects of malabsorption syndromes. *Compr Ther.* 1983;9(11):35-46.

16. Napolitano M, Dolce A, Celenza G, et al. Iron-dependent erythropoiesis in women with excessive menstrual blood losses and women with normal menses. *Ann Hematol.* 2014;93:557-563.

17. Akpınar H, Çetiner M, Keshav S, Örmeci N, Törüner M. Diagnosis and treatment of iron deficiency anemia in patients with inflammatory bowel disease and gastrointestinal bleeding: iron deficiency anemia working group consensus report. *Turk J Gastroenterol.* 2017;28(2):81-87.

18. Beale AL, Penney MD, Allison MC. The prevalence of iron deficiency among patients presenting with colorectal cancer. *Colorectal Dis.* 2005;7(4):398-402.

19. Bothwell TH. Iron requirements in pregnancy and strategies to meet them. *Am J Clin Nutr.* 2000;72(suppl 1):257S-264S.

20. Perry CA, West AA, Gayle A, et al. Pregnancy and lactation alter biomarkers of biotin metabolism in women consuming a controlled diet. *J Nutr.* 2014;144(12):1977-1984.

21. Subramanya SB, Subramanian VS, Kumar JS, Hoiness R, Said HM. Inhibition of intestinal biotin absorption by chronic alcohol feeding: cellular and molecular mechanisms. *Am J Physiol Gastrointest Liver Physiol.* 2011;300(3):G494-G501.

22. Prasad AS. Clinical manifestations of zinc deficiency. *Annu Rev Nutr.* 1985;5:341-363.

23. Bogye G, Tompos G, Alfthan G. Selenium depletion in hemodialysis patients treated with polysulfone membranes. *Nephron.* 2000;84(2):119-123.

24. Hurrell R, Egli I. Iron bioavailability and dietary reference values. *Am J Clin Nutr.* 2010;91(5):1461S-1467S.

25. Hunt JR. Bioavailability of iron, zinc, and other trace minerals from vegetarian diets. *Am J Clin Nutr.* 2003;78(suppl 3):633S-639S.

26. Mock DM. Skin manifestations of biotin deficiency. *Semin Dermatol.* 1991;10(4):296-302.

27. Murray-Kolbe LE, Beard J. Iron. In: Coates PM, Betz JM, Blackman MR, et al., eds. *Encyclopedia of Dietary Supplements.* 2nd ed. London, New York: Informa Healthcare; 2010:432-438.

28. Miller SJ. Nutritional deficiency and the skin. *J Am Acad Dermatol.* 1989;21:1-30.

29. Prasad AS. Zinc deficiency. *BMJ.* 2003;326:409-410.

30. Schulpis KH, Georgala S, Papakonstantinou ED, Michas T, Karikas GA. The effect of isotretinoin on biotinidase activity. *Skin Pharmacol Appl Skin Physiol.* 1999;12(1-2):28-33.

31. Schulpis KH, Karikas GA, Tjamouranis J, Regoutas S, Tsakiris S. Low serum biotinidase activity in children with valproic acid monotherapy. *Epilepsia.* 2001;42(10):1359-1362.

32. Institute of Medicine, Food and Nutrition Board. *Dietary Reference Intakes for Calcium and Vitamin D.* Washington, DC: National Academy Press; 2010.

33. Institute of Medicine, Food and Nutrition Board. *Dietary Reference Intakes: Vitamin C, Vitamin E, Selenium, and Carotenoids.* Washington, DC: National Academy Press; 2000.

34. LeFevre ML. U.S. Preventive Services Task Force. Screening for vitamin D deficiency in adults: U.S. Preventive Services Task Force recommendation statement. *Ann Intern Med.* 2015;162(2):133-140.

35. Trüeb RM. Serum biotin levels in women complaining of hair loss. *Int J Trichology.* 2016;8(2):73-77.

36. Messenger AG, Sinclair R. Follicular miniaturization in female pattern hair loss: clinicopathological correlations. *Br J Dermatol.* 2006;155(5):926-930.

37. Farris PK, Rogers N, McMichael A, Kogan S. A novel multi-targeting approach to treating hair loss, using standardized nutraceuticals. *J Drugs Dermatol.* 2017;16(11):s141-s148.

38. Abell E. Histologic response to topically applied minoxidil in male-pattern alopecia. *Clin Dermatol.* 1988;6(4):191-194.

39. Olsen EA, Whiting D, Bergfeld W, et al. A multicenter, randomized, placebo-controlled, double-blind clinical trial of a novel formulation of 5% minoxidil topical foam versus placebo in the treatment of androgenetic alopecia in men. *J Am Acad Dermatol.* 2007;57(5):767-774.

40. Oh JW, Kloepper J, Langan EA, et al. A guide to studying human hair follicle cycling in vivo [published correction appears in J Invest Dermatol. 2016 Apr;136(4):883]. *J Invest Dermatol.* 2016;136(1):34-44.

41. Hashimoto T, Kazama T, Ito M, et al. Histologic study of the regeneration process of human hair follicles grafted onto SCID mice after bulb amputation. *J Investig Dermatol Symp Proc.* 2001;6(1):38-42.

42. Ablon G, Kogan S. A six-month, randomized, double-blind, placebo-controlled study evaluating the safety and efficacy of a nutraceutical supplement for promoting hair growth in women with self-perceived thinning hair. *J Drugs Dermatol.* 2018;17(5):558-565.

43. Ablon G, Dayan S. A randomized, double-blind, placebo-controlled, multi-center, extension trial evaluating the efficacy of a new oral supplement in women with self-perceived thinning hair. *J Clin Aesthet Dermatol.* 2015;8(12):15-21.

44. Blume-Peytavi U, Hillmann K, Dietz E, Canfield D, Garcia Bartels N. A randomized, single-blind trial of 5% minoxidil foam once daily versus 2% minoxidil solution twice daily in the treatment of androgenetic alopecia in women. *J Am Acad Dermatol.* 2011;65(6):1126-1134.e2.

45. Olsen EA, Weiner MS. Topical minoxidil in male pattern baldness: effects of discontinuation of treatment. *J Am Acad Dermatol.* 1987;17(1):97-101.

46. Price VH, Menefee E, Strauss PC. Changes in hair weight and hair count in men with androgenetic alopecia, after application of 5% and 2% topical minoxidil, placebo, or no treatment. *J Am Acad Dermatol.* 1999;41(5 Pt 1):717-721.

47. Salve J, Pate S, Debnath K, Langade D. Adaptogenic and anxiolytic effects of ashwagandha root extract in healthy adults: a double-blind, randomized, placebo-controlled clinical study. *Cureus.* 2019;11(12):e6466.

48. Lopresti AL, Smith SJ, Malvi H, Kodgule R. An investigation into the stress-relieving and pharmacological actions of an ashwagandha (Withania somnifera) extract: A randomized, double-blind, placebo-controlled study. *Medicine (Baltimore).* 2019;98(37):e17186.

49. Wankhede S, Langade D, Joshi K, Sinha SR, Bhattacharyya S. Examining the effect of Withania somnifera supplementation on muscle strength and recovery: a randomized controlled trial. *J Int Soc Sports Nutr.* 2015;12:43.

50. Almohanna HM, Ahmed AA, Tsatalis JP, Tosti A. The role of vitamins and minerals in hair loss: a review. *Dermatol Ther.* 2019;9(1):51-70.

51. Zempleni J, Hassan YI, Wijeratne SS. Biotin and biotinidase deficiency. *Expert Rev Endocrinol Metab.* 2008;3(6):715-724.

52. El-Esawy FM, Hussein MS, Ibrahim Mansour A. Serum biotin and zinc in male androgenetic alopecia. *J Cosmet Dermatol.* 2019. doi:10.1111/jocd.12865. Epub ahead of print.

53. Zempleni J, Mock DM. Biotin biochemistry and human requirements. *J Nutr Biochem.* 1999;10(3):128-138.

54. Patel DP, Swink SM, Castelo-Soccio L. A review of the use of biotin for hair loss. *Skin Appendage Disord.* 2017;3(3):166-169.

55. Fadus MC, Lau C, Bikhchandani J, Lynch HT. Curcumin: an age-old anti-inflammatory and anti-neoplastic agent. *J Tradit Complement Med.* 2016;7(3):339-346.

56. Shoba G, Joy D, Joseph T, Majeed M, Rajendran R, Srinivas PS. Influence of piperine on the pharmacokinetics of curcumin in animals and human volunteers. *Planta Med.* 1998;64(4):353-356.

57. Pumthong G, Asawanonda P, Varothai S, et al. Curcuma aeruginosa, a novel botanically derived 5α-reductase inhibitor in the treatment of male-pattern baldness: a multicenter, randomized, double-blind, placebo-controlled study. *J Dermatolog Treat.* 2012;23(5):385-392.

58. Srivilai J, Waranuch N, Tangsumranjit A, Khorana N, Ingkaninan K. Germacrone and sesquiterpene-enriched extracts from Curcuma aeruginosa Roxb. increase skin penetration of minoxidil, a hair growth promoter. *Drug Deliv Transl Res.* 2018;8(1):140-149.

59. Chaiyana W, Punyoyai C, Somwongin S, et al. Inhibition of 5α-reductase, il-6 secretion, and oxidation process of equisetum debile roxb. ex vaucher extract as functional food and nutraceuticals ingredients. *Nutrients.* 2017;9(10):1105.

60. Reffitt DM, Ogston N, Jugdaohsingh R, et al. Orthosilicic acid stimulates collagen type 1 synthesis and osteoblastic differentiation in human osteoblast-like cells in vitro. *Bone.* 2003;32(2):127-135.

61. Wickett RR, Kossmann E, Barel A, et al. Effect of oral intake of choline-stabilized orthosilicic acid on hair tensile strength and morphology in women with fine hair. *Arch Dermatol Res.* 2007;299(10):499-505.

62. Dev S, Babitt JL. Overview of iron metabolism in health and disease. *Hemodial Int.* 2017;21(suppl 1):S6-S20.

63. Du X, She E, Gelbart T, et al. The serine protease TM-PRSS6 is required to sense iron deficiency. *Science.* 2008;320(5879):1088-1092.

64. St Pierre SA, Vercellotti GM, Donovan JC, Hordinsky MK. Iron deficiency and diffuse nonscarring scalp alopecia in women: more pieces to the puzzle. *J Am Acad Dermatol.* 2010;63(6):1070-1076.

65. Kantor J, Kessler LJ, Brooks DG, Cotsarelis G. Decreased serum ferritin is associated with alopecia in women. *J Investig Dermatol.* 2003;121:985-988.

66. Olsen EA, Reed KB, Cacchio PB, Caudill L. Iron deficiency in female pattern hair loss, chronic telogen effluvium and control groups. *J Am Acad Dermatol.* 2010;63:991-999.

67. Lassus A, Eskelinen E. A comparative study of a new food supplement, viviscal, with fish extract for the treatment of hereditary androgenic alopecia in young males. *J Int Med Res.* 1992;20:445-453.

68. Hornfeldt CS, Holland M. The safety and efficacy of a sustainable marine extract for the treatment of thinning hair: a summary of new clinical research and results from a panel discussion on the problem of thinning hair and current treatments. *J Drugs Dermatol.* 2015; 14(9):s15-s22.

69. Thom E. Nourkrin: objective and subjective effects and tolerability in persons with hair loss. *J Int Med Res.* 2006;34:514-519.

70. Rizer RL, Stephens TJ, Herndon JH, Sperber BR, Murphy J, Ablon GR. A marine protein- based dietary supplement for subclinical hair thinning/loss: results of a multisite, double- blind, placebo-controlled clinical trial. *Int J Trichology.* 2015;7:156-166.

71. Martinec N, Balbino S, Dobša J, Šimunić-Mežnarić V, Legen S. Macro- and microelements in pumpkin seed oils: effect of processing, crop season, and country of origin. *Food Sci Nutr.* 2019;7(5):1634-1644.

72. Procida G, Stancher B, Cateni F, Zacchigna M. Chemical composition and functional characterisation of commercial pumpkin seed oil. *J Sci Food Agric.* 2013;93(5): 1035-1041.

73. Bardaa S, Ben Halima N, Aloui F, et al. Oil from pumpkin (Cucurbita pepo L.) seeds: evaluation of its functional properties on wound healing in rats. *Lipids Health Dis.* 2016;15:73.

74. Cho YH, Lee SY, Jeong DW, et al. Effect of pumpkin seed oil on hair growth in men with androgenetic alopecia: a randomized, double-blind, placebo-controlled trial. *Evid Based Complement Alternat Med.* 2014;2014:549721.

75. Gordon AE, Shaughnessy AF. Saw palmetto for prostate disorders. *Am Fam Physician.* 2003;67(6):1281-1283.

76. Iehlé C, Délos S, Guirou O, Tate R, Raynaud JP, Martin PM. Human prostatic steroid 5 alpha-reductase isoforms–a comparative study of selective inhibitors. *J Steroid Biochem Mol Biol.* 1995;54(5-6):273-279.

77. Sultan C, Terraza A, Devillier C, et al. Inhibition of androgen metabolism and binding by a liposterolic extract of "Serenoa repens B" in human foreskin fibroblasts. *J Steroid Biochem.* 1984;20(1):515-519.

78. Prager N, Bickett K, French N, Marcovici G. A randomized, double-blind, placebo-controlled trial to determine the effectiveness of botanically derived inhibitors of 5-alpha-reductase in the treatment of androgenetic alopecia. *J Altern Complement Med.* 2002;8(2):143-152.

79. Rossi A, Mari E, Scarno M, et al. Comparitive effectiveness of finasteride vs Serenoa repens in male androgenetic alopecia: a two-year study. *Int J Immunopathol Pharmacol.* 2012;25(4):1167-1173.

80. Narda M, Aladren S, Cestone E, Nobile V. Efficacy and safety of a food supplement containing L-cystine, Serenoa repens extract and biotin for hair loss in healthy males and females. A prospective, randomized, double-blinded, controlled clinical trial. *J Cosmo Trichol.* 2017; 3(127):2.

81. Ambroziak U, Hybsier S, Shahnazaryan U, et al. Severe selenium deficits in pregnant women irrespective of autoimmune thyroid disease in an area with marginal selenium intake. *J Trace Elem Med Biol.* 2017;44: 186-191.

82. Shreenath AP, Ameer MA, Dooley J Selenium deficiency. StatPearls. Treasure Island (FL): StatPearls Publishing; 2021. https://www.ncbi.nlm.nih.gov/books/NBK482260/.

83. Bates JM, Spate VL, Morris JS, St Germain DL, Galton VA. Effects of selenium deficiency on tissue selenium content, deiodinase activity, and thyroid hormone economy in the rat during development. *Endocrinology.* 2000;141(7):2490-2500.

84. Sengupta A, Lichti UF, Carlson BA, et al. Selenoproteins are essential for proper keratinocyte function and skin development. *PLoS One.* 2010;5(8):e12249.

85. Vinton NE, Dahlstrom KA, Strobel CT, Ament ME. Macrocytosis and pseudoalbinism: manifestations of selenium deficiency. *J Pediatr.* 1987;111(5):711-717.

86. Kriegel MA, Manson JE, Costenbader KH. Does vitamin D affect risk of developing autoimmune disease? A systematic review. *Semin Arthritis Rheum.* 2011;40(6):512-531.e8.

87. Holick MF. Sunlight and vitamin D for bone health and prevention of autoimmune diseases, cancers, and cardiovascular disease. *Am J Clin Nutr.* 2004;80(suppl 6):1678S-1688S.

88. Reichrath J, Schilli M, Kerber A, Bahmer FA, Czarnetzki BM, Paus R. Hair follicle expression of 1,25-dihydroxyvitamin D3 receptors during the murine hair cycle. *Br J Dermatol.* 1994; 131(4):477-482.

89. Xie Z, Komuves L, Yu QC, et al. Lack of the vitamin D receptor is associated with reduced epidermal differentiation and hair follicle growth. *J Invest Dermatol.* 2002; 118(1):11-16.

90. Brooks MH, Bell NH, Love L, et al. Vitamin-D-dependent rickets type II. Resistance of target organs to 1,25-dihydroxyvitamin D. *N Engl J Med.* 1978;298(18): 996-999.

91. Almohanna HM, Ahmed AA, Tsatalis JP, Tosti A. The role of vitamins and minerals in hair loss: a review. *Dermatol Ther.* 2018;9(1):51-70.

92. Traber MG. *Vitamin E. Modern Nutrition in Health and Disease.* 10th ed. Baltimore, MD: Lippincott Williams & Wilkins; 2006:396-411.

93. Serbinova E, Kagan V, Han D, Packer L. Free radical recycling and intramembrane mobility in the antioxidant properties of alpha-tocopherol and alpha-tocotrienol. *Free Radic Biol Med.* 1991;10:263-275.

94. Upton JH, Hannen RF, Bahta AW, Farjo N, Farjo B, Philpott MP. Oxidative stress-associated senescence in dermal papilla cells of men with androgenetic alopecia. *J Invest Dermatol.* 2015;135(5):1244-1252.

95. Beoy LA, Woei WJ, Hay YK. Effects of tocotrienol supplementation on hair growth in human volunteers. *Trop Life Sci Res.* 2010;21:91-99.

96. Guo EL, Katta R. Diet and hair loss: effects of nutrient deficiency and supplement use. *Dermatol Pract Concept.* 2017;7(1):1-10.

97. Ogawa Y, Kawamura T, Shimada S. Zinc and skin biology. *Arch Biochem Biophys.* 2016;611:113-119.

98. MacDonald RS. The role of zinc in growth and cell proliferation. *J Nutr.* 2000;130(suppl 5S):1500S-1508S.

99. St-Jacques B, Dassule HR, Karavanova I, et al. Sonic hedgehog signaling is essential for hair development. *Curr Biol.* 1998;8(19):1058-1068.

100. Schmitt S, Küry S, Giraud M, Dréno B, Kharfi M, Bézieau S. An update on mutations of the SLC39A4 gene in acrodermatitis enteropathica. *Hum Mut.* 2009;30:926-933.

101. Karashima T, Tsuruta D, Hamada T, et al. Oral zinc therapy for zinc deficiency-related telogen effluvium. *Dermatol Ther.* 2012;25(2):210-213.

102. El-Esawy FM, Hussein MS, Ibrahim Mansour A. Serum biotin and zinc in male androgenetic alopecia. *J Cosmet Dermatol.* 2019.

103. Dhaher SA, Yacoub AA, Jacob AA. Estimation of zinc and iron levels in the serum and hair of women with androgenetic alopecia: case-control study. *Indian J Dermatol.* 2018;63(5):369-374.

104. Siavash M, Tavakoli F, Mokhtari F. Comparing the effects of zinc sulfate, calcium pantothenate, their combination and minoxidil solution regimens on controlling hair loss in women: a randomized controlled trial. *J Res Pharm Pract.* 2017;6(2):89-93.

105. Salve J, Pate S, Debnath K, Langade D. Adaptogenic and anxiolytic effects of ashwagandha root extract in healthy adults: a double-blind, randomized, placebo-controlled clinical study. *Cureus.* 2019;11(12):e6466.

106. Wankhede S, Langade D, Joshi K, Sinha SR, Bhattacharyya S. Examining the effect of Withania somnifera supplementation on muscle strength and recovery: a randomized controlled trial. *J Int Soc Sports Nutr.* 2015;12:43.

107. Haddad RA, Giacherio K, Barkan AL. Interpretation of common endocrine laboratory tests: technical pitfalls, their mechanisms and practical considerations. *Clin Diabetes Endocrinol.* 2019;5:12.

108. Favresse J, Burlacu MC, Maiter D, Gruson D. Interferences with thyroid function immunoassays: clinical implications and detection algorithm. *Endocr Rev.* 2018;39(5):830-850. doi:10.1210/er.2018-00119.

109. Ostrowska M, Bartoszewicz Z, Bednarczuk T, Walczak K, Zgliczyński W, Glinicki P. The effect of biotin interference on the results of blood hormone assays. *Endokrynol Pol.* 2019;70(1):102-111.

110. Spector TD, Calomme MR, Anderson SH, et al. Choline-stabilized orthosilicic acid supplementation as an adjunct to calcium/vitamin D3 stimulates markers of bone formation in osteopenic females: a randomized, placebo-controlled trial. *BMC Musculoskelet Disord.* 2008;9:85.

111. Geusens P, Pavelka K, Rovensky J, et al. A 12-week randomized, double-blind, placebo-controlled multi-center study of choline-stabilized orthosilicic acid in patients with symptomatic knee osteoarthritis. *BMC Musculoskelet Disord.* 2017;18(1):2.

112. Franke GN, Kubasch AS, Cross M, Vucinic V, Platzbecker U. Iron overload and its impact on outcome of patients with hematological diseases. *Mol Aspects Med.* 2020;75:100868.

113. Aggett PJ. *Iron. Present Knowledge in Nutrition.* 10th ed. Washington, DC: Wiley-Blackwell; 2012:506-520.

114. Campbell NR, Hasinoff BB, Stalts H, Rao B, Wong NC. Ferrous sulfate reduces thyroxine efficacy in patients with hypothyroidism. *Ann Intern Med.* 1992;117:1010-1013.

115. Greene RJ, Hall AD, Hider RC. The interaction of orally administered iron with levodopa and methyldopa therapy. *J Pharm Pharmacol.* 1990;42:502-504.

116. Avins AL, Lee JY, Meyers CM, Barry MJ. Safety and toxicity of saw palmetto in the CAMUS trial. *J Urol.* 2013;189(4):1415-1420.

117. Office of Dietary Supplements. *Selenium.* NIH Office of Dietary Supplements https://ods.od.nih.gov/factsheets/Selenium-HealthProfessional/, March 26, 2021. Accessed April 3, 2021.

118. MacFarquhar JK, Broussard DL, Melstrom P, et al. Acute selenium toxicity associated with a dietary supplement. *Arch Intern Med.* 2010;170(3):256-261.

119. Rayman MP, Winther KH, Pastor-Barriuso R, et al. Effect of long term selenium supplementation on mortality: Results from a multiple-dose, randomized controlled trial. *Free Radical Biol Med.* 2018;127:46-54.

120. Hadrup N, Ravn-Haren G. Acute human toxicity and mortality after selenium ingestion: a review. *J Trace Elements Med Biol.* 2020;58:126453.

121. Hathcock JN, Shao A, Vieth R, Heaney R. Risk assessment for vitamin D. *Am J Clin Nutr.* 2007;85(1):6-18.

122. Barger-Lux MJ, Heaney RP. Effects of above average summer sun exposure on serum 25-hydroxyvitamin D and calcium absorption. *J Clin Endocrinol Metab.* 2002;87(11):4952-4956.

123. Calvo MS, Whiting SJ, Barton CN. Vitamin D fortification in the United States and Canada: current status and data needs. *Am J Clin Nutr*. 2004;80(suppl 6): 1710S-1716S.

124. Galior K, Grebe S, Singh R. Development of vitamin d toxicity from overcorrection of vitamin d deficiency: a review of case reports. *Nutrients*. 2018;10(8):953.

125. Sesso HD, Buring JE, Christen WG, et al. Vitamins E and C in the prevention of cardiovascular disease in men: the Physicians' Health Study II randomized controlled trial. *JAMA*. 2008;300(18):2123-2133.

126. The alpha-tocopherol, beta-carotene lung cancer prevention study: design, methods, participant characteristics, and compliance. The ATBC Cancer Prevention Study Group. *Ann Epidemiol*. 1994;4(1):1-10.

127. Institute of Medicine (US) Panel on Micronutrients. Dietary Reference Intakes for Vitamin A, Vitamin K, Arsenic, Boron, Chromium, Copper, Iodine, Iron, Manganese, Molybdenum, Nickel, Silicon, Vanadium, and Zinc. Washington (DC): National Academies Press (US); 2001.

128. Draine J, Simmons M. A case of copper deficiency myeloneuropathy precipitated by zinc ingestion and bariatric surgery. *S D Med*. 2020;73(4):178-180.

129. Sheqwara J, Alkhatib Y. Sideroblastic anemia secondary to zinc toxicity. *Blood*. 2013;122(3):311.

130. Mizuno D, Kawahara M. The molecular mechanisms of zinc neurotoxicity and the pathogenesis of vascular type senile dementia. *Int J Mol Sci*. 2013;14: 22067-22081.

5

Hair Cosmetics, Styling, and Processing

Ora Raymond, Nicole Heinen, Maria Hordinsky, Neil Sadick, and Ronda Farah

KEY POINTS

- Hair cosmetics, styling, and processing play key roles in counseling patients with hair loss.
- Hair and scalp health must be maintained for medical and aesthetic reasons. This includes regular shampooing, conditioning, and limiting unnecessary heat styling and processing.
- Direct-to-consumer hair cosmetics are available to create the illusion of volume or camouflage hair loss, but their use comes with some risk.

- Literature on hair cosmetics has few randomized sham-controlled trials, and most research in this area is driven by the beauty industry. Additional collaboration between clinicians and the beauty industry is needed.

BACKGROUND, DEFINITIONS, AND HISTORY

The desire for healthy hair is evolutionary, as the cosmetic appearance of hair is a primary indicator of youth (level of evidence: 5).[1-3] Hair is considered the healthiest when it lacks damage, whether self-inflicted or environmental. In 2016, the US beauty industry had an estimated revenue of 62.46 billion US dollars (level of evidence: 5).[4] The leading worldwide cosmetic manufacturer in 2019 was L'Oreal, with worldwide headquarters located in France; the company made approximately 33.4 billion US dollars that year (level of evidence: 5).[5] In 2018, the global haircare industry was valued at 87.9 billion US dollars.[4] In addition to improving hair appearance in the general population, hair cosmetics, styling, and processing have a role in altering the appearance of the hair and scalp in a way that those with hair loss value. For example, patients with androgenetic alopecia (AGA) may turn to the beauty industry for products to minimize and conceal hair loss.

Therefore, a firm knowledge base of hair cosmetics is essential for the assessment and treatment of these patients. In this chapter, we will review the fundamentals of healthy scalp and hair follicle maintenance, styling techniques, and hair processing options. Furthermore, we will emphasize their utility in the treatment of patients with AGA.

INDICATIONS AND PATIENT SELECTION

Within the United States in 2021, routine hair and scalp hygiene and styling products were readily available and routinely used in the general population. However, a thorough understanding of hair cosmetics, styling, and processing requires individuals to also understand the concept of weathering. Weathering is a hair shaft process that results in hair damage from root to tip and includes decreased shine, elasticity, and, ultimately, breakage (level of evidence: 5) (Pearl 5.1).[6,7] There are two types of weathering: natural and accelerated. In the process of natural weathering, the cuticle is worn away

> **PEARL 5.1:** Weathering is a process that results in damage to the hair shaft and may include decreased shine, elasticity, and breakage.

over time from hair brushing, combing, or other physical haircare maintenance techniques. Accelerated weathering includes damage to the hair's cuticle and cortex proteins (Fig. 5.1).[3,7] Those with long hair often demonstrate more severe weathering caused by repetitive injury of the hair shaft over time (level of evidence: 5).[8] Processes that weaken hair fiber integrity and contribute to accelerated weathering include heat styling and chemical processing such as bleaching and permanent waving (level of evidence: 5).[3,9] Processes such as straightening, bleaching, and perming alter the protein structures of hair, causing irreversible damage (level of evidence: 5).[10,11] Other environmental factors in weathering include prolonged exposure to sunlight, resulting in loss of tensile strength, color changes, embrittlement, and split ends (level of evidence: 5).[12-14] Sunlight exposure causes proteins and lipids to undergo degradation via a reaction between aromatic amino acid species and ultraviolet light, which produces reactive oxygen species such as hydrogen peroxide, hydroperoxides, and singlet oxygen.[3] Overall, weathering of the hair fiber is expected over time in those with and without hair and scalp disease.

In addition to the general population seeking hair cosmetics for hygiene and to managing weathering, those with hair and scalp disease may also turn to the beauty industry for solutions. Patients with excessive sweat, oil, dirt, or hair product use may find regular hair and scalp hygiene especially helpful for follicular aesthetic appearance and prevention of the development of scalp diseases such as dandruff, seborrheic dermatitis, or folliculitis. Those with hair or scalp disease such as psoriasis, atopic dermatitis, dermatomyositis, or tinea may find that perfecting a hair and scalp hygiene routine along with personalized styling is important for overall disease management. Furthermore, cosmetic products are the foundation of treatment for those with hair breakage such as trichorrhexis nodosa and trichoptilosis (Figs. 5.2 and 5.3).[15]

Those with AGA may find unique cosmetic benefits in styling and camouflaging to disguise hair thinning. In AGA, hair follicles are miniaturized, which contributes to the overall appearance of lower hair density in affected scalp regions. Additionally, it has been proposed that the disease process, which results in reduced follicular fiber diameter, allows for increased vulnerability to fracture and increased weathering of hair fibers (level of evidence: 5).[15,16] Those with early and mild androgenetic alopecia may find that the at-home beauty industry offers sufficient cosmetic and styling options. Those with more progressed AGA will likely need the help of dermatologists and professional stylists to camouflage hair loss as part of a comprehensive management plan.

Of note, patients with a history of contact dermatitis may find the hair and scalp cosmetics industry difficult to navigate given the numerous ingredients found in products. Routine patch testing or patch testing within a tertiary care center may be required to finesse product selection (level of evidence: 5).[17] When managing patients with alopecia, physicians must recognize that hair cosmetics, processing, and styling options are unique to

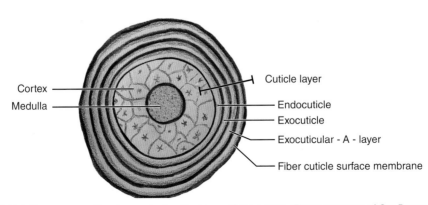

Fig. 5.1 Hair-fiber cross section demonstrating the layers of the cuticle. (Figure courtesy of Ora Raymond, BA.)

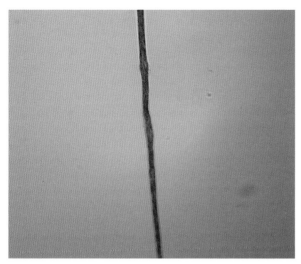

Fig. 5.2 Trichorrhexis nodosa in a female of African descent with nonbleached hair. (Figure courtesy of Ronda Farah, MD.)

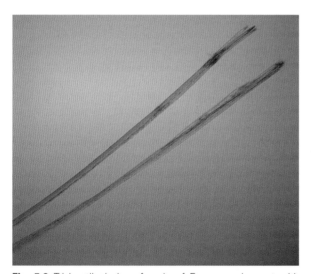

Fig. 5.3 Trichoptilosis in a female of European descent with bleached hair. (Figure courtesy of Ronda Farah, MD.)

each patient as product choices can be affected by hair and scalp disease, hair type, and social determinants of health.

EXPECTED OUTCOMES

Immediate desired changes in cosmetic appearance can be achieved with topical camouflaging agents, hair dyes, conditioning, volumizers, and heat styling

PEARL 5.2: Hair growth rate varies among individuals, and the technology to change hair growth rate is lacking.

tools in those with early AGA. Within days to weeks of initiating regular cleansing and shampooing of the scalp, a noticeable aesthetic difference in scale and scalp erythema may be noted in those with concomitant seborrheic dermatitis (level of evidence: 2b).[18-20] Over years, combining medical hair growth treatment options with hair cosmetics, styling, and processing as part of a comprehensive plan can result in an improved appearance. As the hair grows over time, scalp and hair shaft health may improve, including increased shine, length, and strength, along with decreases in hair-shaft disease (e.g., bubble hair, trichorrhexis nodosa, trichoptilosis, trichoschisis). Without addressing the AGA disease process, the disease may continue to progress, and these techniques may slowly prove to be less useful. Patients may have the expectation that, with medical treatment, their hair will grow more rapidly, and results will be immediate. However, the rate of hair growth varies among individuals and can differ from scalp location and age (level of evidence: 2b) (Pearl 5.2).[21] Adjusting patient expectations with regard to expected results and timelines is fundamental to cosmetic hair counseling success.[22,23]

TREATMENT TECHNIQUE/BEST PRACTICES

Shampooing

Shampoo is a key component of every healthy haircare routine. Although shampoos can have a variety of secondary functions, they are first and foremost scalp and hair cleansing products. Shampoos commonly come in liquid formulations; however, dry and solid shampoos also exist (level of evidence: 2b).[24,25] The goal of shampooing is to remove sebum, dirt, scale, sweat, dust, and other environmental pollutants, thus helping prevent the onset of various scalp-related conditions such as seborrheic dermatitis or dandruff (Pearl 5.3).[24] Consistent scalp and hair hygiene with shampoo usage is a cornerstone to the regimen of patients with alopecia (Fig. 5.4).

> **PEARL 5.3:** The goal of shampooing is to remove sebum, dirt, scale, sweat, dust, and other pollutants.

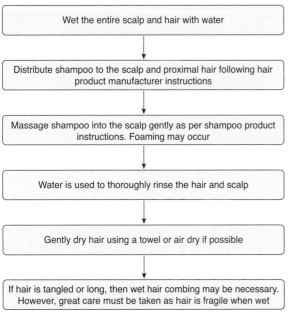

Wet the entire scalp and hair with water

↓

Distribute shampoo to the scalp and proximal hair following hair product manufacturer instructions

↓

Massage shampoo into the scalp gently as per shampoo product instructions. Foaming may occur

↓

Water is used to thoroughly rinse the hair and scalp

↓

Gently dry hair using a towel or air dry if possible

↓

If hair is tangled or long, then wet hair combing may be necessary. However, great care must be taken as hair is fragile when wet

Fig. 5.4 Recommended shampooing process.[26,27] (Figure courtesy of Ronda Farah, MD. Figure related to content from "Draelos ZD. Shampoos, conditioners, and camouflage techniques. *Dermatol Clin.* 2013;31(1):173-178." and "Teaching your child healthy hair care habits. www.aad.org. Accessed February 16, 2022. https://www.aad.org/public/everyday-care/hair-scalp-care/hair/hair-care-habits.")

Although shampoo usage is fairly ubiquitous, there can sometimes be confusion surrounding how exactly it should be used. In general, the hair should be wet, then a custom amount of shampoo should be massaged on the scalp and the proximal hair shafts (see Fig. 5.4). The shampoo should then be fully rinsed out of the hair and scalp (level of evidence: 5).[26] The amount of shampoo needed may vary between individuals and by scalp size and product type. Shampooing frequency is determined by numerous factors including hair type, hairstyle, sweat-producing activity level, and hairstyling product usage. Individuals with oily hair or fine hair may need to shampoo their hair more often than those with dry hair (level of evidence: 5).[28] Those with curly or dry hair may have more fragile hair shafts susceptible to breakage with frequent shampooing;

therefore, some patients may need to limit shampoo-based washing to approximately every 7 to 14 days (level of evidence: 5).[29,30] In the authors' experience, the presence of erythema, pruritus, flakes, or scale on the scalp or proximal hair shaft may indicate that the scalp needs to be washed more often. In general, hair should not be washed more than once a day.[28] Sometimes, patients with hair loss will shampoo their hair more often than necessary to give the appearance of more volume, as sebum can weigh down the hair. Consumers should seek shampoos labeled for their hair type.[28] For example, those that have fine hair should look with shampoo labels for "fine hair." Those with curly or dry hair should look for labels for "curly," "dry," or "very dry" hair. Those with color-treated hair or bleached hair should also look for shampoos labeled for their hair type.

In the twenty-first century, shampoo ingredients have increasingly become a topic of interest for consumers. Shampoos may contain a wide variety of ingredients: surfactants, conditioners, sequestering agents, preservatives, fragrances, specialty additives, and various other ingredients aimed at influencing the physical properties of the shampoo.[24] In general, the most important shampoo ingredients are surfactants, as they are the ingredients responsible for cleansing the hair and scalp. Surfactants reduce surface tension and can act as detergents. They are structured as amphiphilic molecules, and remove oil from the hair and scalp by attaching to water on their hydrophilic ends and oil on their lipophilic ends (level of evidence: 5).[31-33] Shampoo surfactants can be anionic, cationic, nonionic, amphoteric, or natural, and shampoos typically have more than one type of surfactant (Table 5.1).[24] Sodium laureth sulfate and amphoteric surfactants are common surfactants used in shampoos for hair loss.[26] Sodium laureth sulfate is effective at removing sebum, and is not considered to be as harsh as sodium lauryl sulfate, another anionic surfactant.[24] Sodium laureth sulfate and amphoteric surfactants are beneficial to patients with hair loss because they are gentle, but patients and dermatologists alike should be aware that cocamidopropyl betaine, an amphoteric surfactant, is a common allergen (Fig. 5.5) (level of evidence: 5).[17,34]

Shampoo components that may be beneficial for patients with hair loss are pH-adjusting acids and conditioning agents. Glycolic acid and other pH-adjusting acids are added to shampoos to neutralize the basic detergents and avoid breakage. Conditioning shampoo

TABLE 5.1 Comparison of Shampoo Surfactants[26]

Surfactant	Chemical Properties	Cleansing Ability	Examples
Anionic	Polar group is negatively charged	Deep cleansing	Sodium laureth sulfate, sodium lauryl sulfate
Cationic	Polar group is positively charged	Little sebum removal potential	Ammonioesters
Nonionic	No polar group	Mild cleansing, often used as secondary surfactant	Polyoxyethylene fatty alcohols, polyoxyethylene sorbitol esters and alkanolamides
Amphoteric	Two polar groups, one positively charged and one negatively charged	Act as anionic surfactants at high pHs and cationic surfactants at low pHs	Cocamidopropyl betaine, sodium lauriminodipropionate

From: Draelos ZD. Shampoos, conditioners, and camouflage techniques. *Dermatol Clin.* 2013;31(1):173-178.

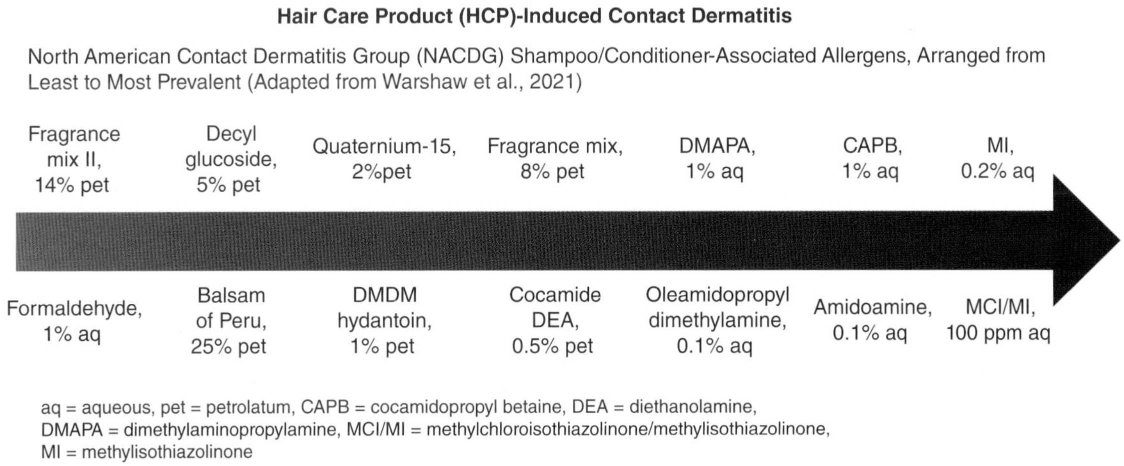

Hair Care Product (HCP)-Induced Contact Dermatitis

North American Contact Dermatitis Group (NACDG) Shampoo/Conditioner-Associated Allergens, Arranged from Least to Most Prevalent (Adapted from Warshaw et al., 2021)

Fragrance mix II, 14% pet   Decyl glucoside, 5% pet   Quaternium-15, 2%pet   Fragrance mix, 8% pet   DMAPA, 1% aq   CAPB, 1% aq   MI, 0.2% aq

Formaldehyde, 1% aq   Balsam of Peru, 25% pet   DMDM hydantoin, 1% pet   Cocamide DEA, 0.5% pet   Oleamidopropyl dimethylamine, 0.1% aq   Amidoamine, 0.1% aq   MCI/MI, 100 ppm aq

aq = aqueous, pet = petrolatum, CAPB = cocamidopropyl betaine, DEA = diethanolamine, DMAPA = dimethylaminopropylamine, MCI/MI = methylchloroisothiazolinone/methylisothiazolinone, MI = methylisothiazolinone

Fig. 5.5 North American Contact Dermatitis Group (NACDG) shampoo/conditioner-associated allergens, arranged from fewest to most haircare product reactions (in dark red). A total of 4,263 positive reactions to NACDG allergens were identified.[17] (Figure related to content from "Warshaw EM, Buonomo M, DeKoven JG, et al. Importance of supplemental patch testing beyond a screening series for patients with dermatitis. *JAMA Dermatology.* 2021;157(12):1456.")

agents, also known as 2-in-1 shampoos, often contain glycerin or dimethicone and may help with moisturizing the follicle and improving the aesthetic appearance in a patient with alopecia.[26,31,32] However, some patients may require more aggressive conditioning to avoid hair breakage.

Another category of shampoos is sulfate-free shampoos. Sulfates, particularly sodium lauryl sulfate, can be quite drying, and individuals with dry hair might not prefer them for this reason. Sulfate-free shampoos are formulated without anionic surfactants and instead

contain milder surfactants (level of evidence: 2b).[35] Despite the popularity of these shampoos, not much is known about their relative effectiveness (level of evidence: 2b).[36]

Medicated shampoos are also available to patients with specific scalp concerns such as dandruff. Dandruff, or scalp flaking, is thought to be caused by *Malassezia* yeast (level of evidence: 2b).[37] Zinc pyrithione is an antimicrobial agent commonly used in antidandruff shampoos; it functions by breaking down iron-sulfur proteins that are essential for microbe survival and improving the condition of the stratum corneum (level of evidence: 2b).[38-41] Ketoconazole is another antimicrobial agent used in antidandruff shampoos (level of evidence: 2b).[42-45] Draelos et al. performed a double-blind cross over study to compare the effectiveness and tolerability of 1% zinc pyrithione conditioning shampoo and 2% ketoconazole shampoo in women with dandruff. In terms of overall response, the majority of participants preferred the former.[19] However, a different prospective study reported that 2% ketoconazole shampoo was more effective at eliminating dandruff compared with 1% zinc pyrithione shampoo (level of evidence: 2b).[46] Selenium sulfide is another common antidandruff ingredient. In one study, it was found to be as effective as 2% ketoconazole shampoo in reducing dandruff (level of evidence: 2b).[47]

Conditioning

Conditioning agents help replace some of the moisture lost from cleansing, making the hair more manageable and aesthetically pleasing. Examples of conditioning agents are dimethicone and glycerin. Conditioners are hair products that should be applied to the ends of the hair and the length of the hair shaft, avoiding the scalp.[28] In general, the goal of conditioning is to increase the aesthetic and physical quality of the hair (Pearl 5.4). Conditioners typically contain cationic detergents, polymers, emollients, and other ingredients aimed at influencing the physical properties of the conditioner. Cationic detergents are ineffective at removing sebum, but their positive charge allows them to adhere to the negatively charged hair, which neutralizes the hair and thus reduces static.[34] Polymers can flatten the cuticle, resulting in more shine and less friction (level of evidence: 5).[34,48] Conditioners can also contain added proteins, which can temporarily increase the strength and thickness of hair.[26] There are different types of conditioners on the market, including instant, deep, and leave-in conditioners. Instant conditioners are the most common and are typically left in the hair for 5 minutes after shampooing, and are then washed out. Deep conditioners typically have a cream consistency and are left in the hair for approximately 1 to 30 minutes. In

contrast, leave-in conditioners are not meant to be washed out of the hair (level of evidence: 5).[34,49]

Use of conditioners can reduce hair breakage and thus reduce further hair loss. It is therefore recommended that patients with hair loss use conditioners (level of evidence: 5).[50] Conditioners with dimethicone are recommended to patients with hair loss because they are effective at conditioning the hair while not weighing it down.[34,50] Patients with hair loss may also benefit from conditioners with added proteins because, as mentioned, they can temporarily increase the strength and thickness of the hair. Additionally, such patients may benefit from deep conditioning treatments and leave-in conditioners. Leave-in conditioners can also temporarily increase the thickness of the hair.[26]

Hairstyling Techniques for Concealment

Different styling techniques and products can be used to conceal hair loss. These techniques may be used at any stage of hair loss, although some techniques may provide more satisfactory results in the earlier stages. In male AGA, thinning and recession may progress until a receding hairline, starting at the temples, meets the balding at the vertex (level of evidence: 5).[51] In female patients, patterned hair loss may begin with a widening central part width, which may extend into an ovular, then Christmas tree like pattern, ultimately resulting in circular balding at the mid scalp (level of evidence: 5).[52] Although the frontal hairline may be preserved, thinning at the frontal-temporal hairline is also possible in women.

In regard to hairstyles, one route for concealing hair loss is maintaining hair in its natural state and growing it longer, if possible, to increase volume and provide better natural coverage. This may reduce damage caused by tight hairstyles, artificial hairpieces, and chemical processing techniques (level of evidence: 5).[53,54] Another method to minimize the appearance of balding at the frontal anterior and mid scalp regions is the comb-over technique (Fig. 5.6). For a comb-over to be successful, the individual's hair must be grown out enough to cover the location of concern. Then, a side hair part can be created, and hair can be combed over to conceal the balding area. This method may minimize the appearance of balding at the frontal anterior and mid scalp regions. In general, it may be beneficial to choose a hairstyle that allows for more regular washing to maintain scalp health and help promote new hair growth.

PEARL 5.4: Conditioners function to improve aesthetic appearance and physical quality and reduce hair breakage.

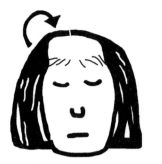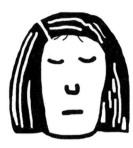

Fig. 5.6 Use of the comb-over technique to camouflage hair loss. A side part is created, then hair is "combed over" the top of the head to conceal hair loss. (Figure courtesy of Ora Raymond, BA.)

Patients may use hairstyles with braids, bandanas, and hats. However, one must be cautious of tight hairstyles, as even chronic loose tension styles can result in hair loss, thereby adding a secondary hair disease process. Strategically placed braids, locks, and extensions can be used to reduce the appearance of hair loss. However, traction alopecia, traction folliculitis, and acquired trichorrhexis nodosa have been associated with these hairstyles. Traction alopecia is commonly diagnosed in women of African descent, though it can occur in all ethnicities (level of evidence: 2b).[55] Sports that require tight hairstyles or braids, such as ballet, gymnastics, and figure skating, may cause patients to be at increased risk for traction type hair styles and should be noted by the clinician as possible secondary causes of hair loss (level of evidence: 4).[56] Limiting tight hairstyles as much as possible and encouraging low-tension styles most days of the week is optimal. Hairpieces may also increase the risk of contact dermatitis, particularly from synthetic hair and glue used in extensions.[53,54]

When styling hair, attention should be given to limit accelerated weathering. In general, hair is porous and absorbs water. Sinclair notes that damaged hair is even more porous and swells to a greater degree.[57] It is possible to extend wet hair to 30% of its original length without altering its structure permanently, although stretching hair to 80% or more induces irreversible damage and fracture (level of evidence: 5).[57,58] Draelos and Sinclair concluded that brittle or damaged hair is more likely to break when it is combed wet or towel-dried.[19,57] To minimize hair damage and prevent further thinning, fingers can be used to detangle hair when it is wet, then a wide-toothed comb can be used. Once the hair is dry, a hairbrush can be used to further detangle the hair, but its involvement should be minimized to prevent additional physical damage.[26]

Regular haircuts or trims are recommended to prevent trichoptilosis, or split ends, mediated damage, and associated hair loss.[59] Blunt or tapered distal hair fiber ends are considered to be healthier than frayed or split ends.[57] As split ends progress, cuticular disruption and the exposure of the cortex progressively weaken the hair fiber and can give a frayed "paintbrush" appearance and cause hair loss from the distal end of the fiber (level of evidence: 5).[9,59]

Heat styling at home or in a salon has long been a consumer staple within the styling industry. Although heat styling may offer a method to increase the appearance of hair volume, there are also associated risks to hair health. Different types of heat styling include straightening, curling, and blow-drying. When using a hairdryer, one must be cautious to not overheat the hair, causing a bubble-hair effect, resulting in irreversible damage.[9] Lee et al. found that, as blow dryer temperature increased, the magnitude of hair damage also increased (level of evidence: 5).[60] Various curling-iron models reach temperatures that exceed 100°C (level of evidence: 5).[61] These high temperatures can cause irreversible damage. Both curling and straightening irons are known to cause both mechanical and heat damage. Heat protectants typically contain dimethicone or cyclomethicone. Dimethicone is silicone-based and forms a protective barrier around the hair shaft (level of evidence: 5).[62] Cyclomethicone is found in some heat protectants and may also have conditioning properties (level of evidence: 5).[63]

Styling products such as gels, creams, mousses, or hairsprays may create the appearance of volume and help hold hair in place over less densely covered areas. Styling gels or mousses are usually most effective at maintaining hairstyles when applied to slightly damp, but not drenched, hair. Styling gels hold hairstyles in place more firmly than mousses.[26] In the experience of the authors, using the least amount of product necessary to achieve the desired cosmetic results is best, as product accumulation on the scalp may cause contact or irritant dermatitis, follicular plugging, and folliculitis. Patients with dermatitis, erythema, burning, or tingling following product application should be evaluated by a board-certified dermatologist for possible patch testing.[17] An additional technique for creating the illusion of volume is using a mousse or styling gel at the hair fiber's base when the hair is damp, then using a blow-dryer and brushing the hair away from the scalp simultaneously to increase the appearance of hair volume that will stay in place.[26]

Concealing pigmented powders, creams, lotions, and sprays can be used to camouflage hair loss (level of evidence: 2b).[64] Moreover, one popular method involves sprinkling synthetic or real keratin fibers onto the less densely covered areas of the scalp. These added keratin fibers are positively charged and bond to the negatively charged native hair fibers (level of evidence: 5).[65] Sade et al. recommends daily application of concealing agents and suggests the products be removed with shampoo regularly.[64] In AGA, these methods may prove most effective for diffuse thinning at the vertex and temples for men and at the frontal anterior, temples, mid scalp, and part width for women. However, it is important to note that applying these cosmetics to bald areas will look less natural compared with an application at thinning areas with some hair density present. Long-term studies detailing the effects of topical keratin concealers on hair and scalp disease are lacking. Clinicians should be aware that concealing powders may include talc as an ingredient. It is possible for talc products to be contaminated with asbestos (level of evidence: 2b).[66] Asbestos inhalation after cosmetic use of talc has been discussed in the literature (level of evidence: 4) (Pearl 5.5).[67-69] Therefore, it may behoove clinicians to avoid recommendations of talc-containing concealers.

Processing: Chemical Straightening/ Relaxing, Chemical Curling, Chemical Antifrizz

Chemical treatments such as permanent waving, relaxing, straightening, and hair smoothing are commonly used to achieve a desired aesthetic appearance (level of evidence: 2b).[49,70] Permanent waving and chemical relaxing both change the shape of the hair through breaking and reforming disulfide bonds.[49] Alkaline reducing agents are responsible for breaking the disulfide bonds.

PEARL 5.5: Clinicians should consider avoiding hair loss products containing talc, given the possibility of contamination with asbestos.

The alkalinity is necessary for opening the cuticle and thus allowing the reducing agent to break disulfide bonds in the cortex. In permanent waving treatments, the alkaline reducing agent formulation is applied to washed hair in curlers, whereas in chemical relaxing treatments, the formulation is just applied to washed hair. In both cases, the formulation is washed out after a period of time, then the hair is treated with an oxidizing agent, which acts to reform the disulfide bonds in their new positions.[49] Both permanent waving and chemical relaxing can damage the hair (level of evidence: 5).[71]

Patients may also be interested in Brazilian hair treatments such as the Brazilian keratin treatment and blowouts. Makers of keratin treatments have made claims such as reduced frizz, stronger hair, and smoother hair. The technique typically involves washing the hair, applying hydrolyzed keratin and formaldehyde, and then blow drying and straightening the hair.[70] The treatment may be left in the hair for 2 to 3 days before being washed out. Hydrolyzed keratin in these treatments may be derived from sheep's wool, horns, or hoofs.[62] The formaldehyde acts to link the added hydrolyzed keratin to the existing keratin in the hair. It is conceivable that some patients with hair loss might be drawn to this treatment for its hair-strengthening claims. However, strong evidence that Brazilian keratin treatments increase hair strength is lacking, and repetitive treatment may be harmful.[70] Another hair smoothing treatment is the Brazilian Blowout™ (North Hollywood, California, United States). One key difference between the Brazilian Blowout™ and Brazilian keratin treatments is that the Brazilian Blowout™ solution is washed out of the hair before the client leaves the salon (level of evidence: 5).[70,72]

One of the key concerns of these treatment options is the presence of formaldehyde. Formaldehyde is commonly present in Brazilian keratin treatments, and methylene glycol, a formaldehyde derivative, is listed as an ingredient in the Brazilian Blowout™ Acai Professional Smoothing Solution (level of evidence: 5).[70,73] Patients who are interested in these treatments should be aware that formaldehyde is a known irritant, allergen, and possible carcinogen.[17,70] Occupational concerns among stylists have also been raised (level of evidence: 2b).[74] The FDA alerted consumers to risks of formaldehyde exposure, including eye irritation, headaches, dizziness, throat issues, cough, chest pain, nausea, rash, and vomiting (level of evidence: 5).[75] Of note, the

International Agency for Research on Cancer (IARC) classifies formaldehyde as a human carcinogen (level of evidence: 5).[76] Long-term studies are needed to truly determine the incidence and if any long-term safety concerns exist for stylists and consumers.

Hair Dyeing

Hair coloring or "dyeing" remains a common at-home or salon practice for various age groups in the United States. There are a variety of different hair dye options, depending on how long an individual wants their color to last and what color they would like to achieve: temporary, semipermanent, demi-permanent, or permanent.[71]

The least damaging form of hair dye is temporary dye.[71] Temporary dyes are typically anionic and of high molecular weight. As such, they are not able to move past the cuticle into the cortex. Temporary dyes do not remove the color from the hair and simply sit atop the hair, so individuals with dark hair will not be able to significantly alter their hair color using this method (level of evidence: 5).[77] Patients may find them helpful to remove the yellowing of gray hair or make gray hair appear more platinum.[71,77]

Semipermanent dyes typically last between 3 to 10 shampooings (level of evidence: 5).[71,77,78] Unlike temporary dyes, semipermanent dyes are typically cationic, which attracts them to the negatively charged hair. They also have a lower molecular weight than temporary dyes, which helps them move past the cuticle. They may cover gray, add highlights, or improve hair tone.[71] Demi-permanent dyes represent an intermediary between semipermanent and permanent dyes. They contain semipermanent dyes, oxidation dye precursors, oxidizing agents, and alkalizing ingredients. These dyes last between 10 to 20 shampooings.[71,78]

Permanent dyes are the most lasting, color versatile, and popular form of hair dye. These dyes are not shampooed out of the hair and are able to alter an individual's hair color in countless ways. They employ alkalizing agents to open the cuticle along with oxidation dye precursors, oxidizing agents, and coupling bases.[78] Dermatologists and patients should be aware that p-phenylenediamine, a commonly used oxidation dye precursor, is a common allergen.[17,78]

Bleaching is the permanent lightening of the hair.[71] It typically involves applying an alkaline oxidizing agent formulation to the hair. The alkalinity is necessary to open the cuticle so that the oxidizing agent can oxidize the melanin inside (level of evidence: 5).[78,79] Patients and dermatologists should be aware that bleaching is damaging to the hair.[71] If a patient still chooses to bleach their hair, they can take certain steps to minimize damage and breakage, including limiting lightening to a color close to natural hair color.[50,71]

PREVENTION AND MANAGEMENT OF ADVERSE EVENTS

The use of hair cosmetic products, heat styling, and chemical processing all have the potential to cause adverse events. Cosmetic products applied to the scalp have the potential to cause follicular plugging, contact dermatitis, or seborrheic dermatitis. When using a new product that will be applied to the scalp or hair, it is advisable for patients with hair loss to do a "use" test, in which the patient applies the product to a clean portion of skin on their forearm twice daily for 7 to 10 days. The product should be used as it is labeled, rinsed off, and removed as directed. After cosmetic product application, the area should be monitored for signs of dermatitis such as redness, irritation, or pruritus. If any of these adverse events occur, the patient should immediately remove the product, wash the area with soap and water, and avoid the product until evaluated by a physician. The chance of promoting follicular plugging or seborrheic dermatitis can be limited by not applying cosmetic products directly to the scalp and/or ensuring they are rinsed as directed.

Heat styling such as blow drying, straightening, or curling can cause burns on the scalp, forehead, neck, and ears along with irreversible damage to the hair shaft such as bubble hair. Limiting or eliminating the use of heat styling products is recommended. Chemical processing including straightening, bleaching, and perming can cause chemical burns, damage to the hair cuticle, trichoptilosis, and hair loss (Fig. 5.7A and B). Discontinuing chemical processing is suggested for patients experiencing hair loss in addition to intense conditioning and deep conditioning (Boldac 2001).

Additionally, cosmetic ingredients, such as parabens, have been the subject of controversy for purported negative health effects. Parabens act as preservatives in many cosmetics and have the potential to cause scalp irritation.[29] There has been concern that parabens may be carcinogenic through alteration of endocrine

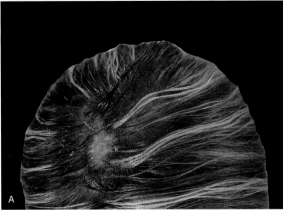

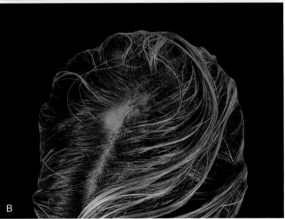

Fig. 5.7 Skin ulceration with fibrinous debris centrally and early scar formation at the periphery after chemical burn that occurred after bleaching (A). Final appearance of scar, several weeks post chemical burn. Permanent hair loss with loss of follicular ostia is noted (B). (Figure courtesy of Ronda Farah, MD.)

activity, and some have suggested a link to breast cancer in mice (level of evidence: 5).[80] The medical literature provides little evidence for these claims, and studies are lacking in humans (level of evidence: 5).[81] Nonetheless, the resulting controversy has led to the production of many paraben-free products. It has been suggested that product developers may be using preservative substitutes with higher levels of allergenicity as substitutes (level of evidence: 5).[82] For example, DMDM hydantoin, quaternium-15, methylisothiazolinone, and methylchloroisothiazolinone are frequently used as preservatives and are common allergens.[17,34] Another

example includes cocamidopropyl betaine used in shampoo products, which is a common amphoteric surfactant and has known allergen potential.[17,34] Regardless, if contact dermatitis is diagnosed, patch testing is recommended to prevent future reactions and identify a safety list for the patient.

Good physician-patient communication and education can prevent and limit the occurrence of adverse events. This communication and education may involve the patient's hairstylist. A patient-physician relationship allowing for repetitive visits and review of haircare products throughout the visit process is imperative. Patients should be counseled that hair disease is complex and that product changes may be necessary over the treatment course. Additionally, while dermatologists may recommend products, patients may not find them aesthetically suitable for their hair. Therefore, a constant line of communication on hair cosmetics at each visit is imperative for success. The hair cosmetics industry and ingredient lists are complicated, not just for clinicians, but also for consumers. Thorough understanding of hair cosmetics is imperative for the success of the patient treatment plan. Dermatologists have a unique education that makes them particularly well suited to engage in and advocate within the hair cosmetic industry on behalf of patients with hair loss and the general population.

FUTURE DIRECTIONS

The hair cosmetic styling and processing industry is rapidly changing. Integrating hair cosmetics, styling, and processing counseling into the hair patient visit is fundamental, as the aesthetic industry continues to grow within hair as it has in skincare. More styling options that are less damaging to the hair shaft are needed. Research has demonstrated that many patients with hair loss have allergies and sensitivities to haircare products. In the future, additional options for styling gels, mousse products, and conditioners with fewer potential allergens would benefit this population. Physicians must take these nuances into account when managing patients with hair and scalp disorders. Communication with the stylist and patient is of utmost importance. Furthermore, many over-the-counter cosmetic haircare products are not FDA-approved. Additional restrictions and safety measures may be warranted given the unknown long-term health effects of cosmetic hair treatments. On a national level, increased effort to share cosmetic product information with patients is needed as consumers navigate the overwhelming cosmetics industry. The cosmetic hair literature focuses on styling, processing, and hair cosmetic usage and is not filled robustly with randomized controlled trials. In fact, most of the options available do not require FDA approval. The majority of research in this area is driven by the beauty industry and studied on a healthy scalp. More collaboration between the medical world and the beauty industry is needed to truly move this field forward within the population of patients with hair loss.

EVIDENCE SUMMARY

- Overall, maintaining a healthy scalp and good hair-care practices are imperative to the clinical counseling of patients with alopecia. This includes shampooing and conditioning, along with limited heat styling and processing (strength of recommendation: A).
- Creating the illusion of volume, using topical camouflaging agents, and alternate hair styles are options for patients with hair loss (strength of recommendation: C).
- Risks of hair cosmetics include hair breakage, contact dermatitis, folliculitis, and traction alopecia (strength of recommendation: B).
- Clinicians managing AGA should have a firm understanding of hair cosmetics (strength of recommendation: C).

REFERENCES

1. Galvin D. *The World of Hair Colour: The Art and Techniques of Modern Hair Colour*. United Kingdom: Macmillan; 1977.
2. Marsh JM, Gray J, Tosti A. *Healthy Hair*. Switzerland: Springer International Publishing; 2015.
3. Gray J. Human Hair. In: McMichael AJ, Hordinsky MK, eds. *Hair and Scalp Disorders: Medical, Surgical, and Cosmetic Treatments*. 2nd ed. London: CRC Press; 2018:59-71.
4. Ridder M. *"Size of the Global Hair Care Market from 2012 to 2025 (in Billion U.S. Dollars)."* Statista https://www.statista.com/statistics/254608/global-hair-care-market-size/, March 8, 2022.
5. Ridder M. *"Revenue of the Leading 10 Beauty Manufacturers Worldwide in 2020."* Statista https://www.statista.com/statistics/243871/revenue-of-the-leading-10-beauty-manufacturers-worldwide/, March 8, 2022.
6. Ahluwalia J, Fabi SG. The psychological and aesthetic impact of age-related hair changes in females. *J Cosmet Dermatol*. 2019;18(4):1161–1169. doi:10.1111/jocd.12960.
7. Osório F, Tosti A. Hair weathering, part 2: clinical features, diagnosis, prevention, and treatment. *J Cosmet Dermatol*. 2011;24(12):555-559.
8. Gummer CL. Hair shaft effects from cosmetics and styling. *Exp Dermatol*. 1999;8(4):317.
9. Dawber R. Cosmetic and medical causes of hair weathering. *J Cosmet Dermatol*. 2002;1(4):196-201.
10. Bloch LD, Goshiyama AM, Dario MF, et al. Chemical and physical treatments damage Caucasian and Afro-ethnic hair fibre: analytical and image assays. *J Eur Acad Dermatol Venereol*. 2019;33(11):2158-2167.
11. Grosvenor AJ, Deb-Choudhury S, Middlewood PG, et al. The physical and chemical disruption of human hair after bleaching - studies by transmission electron microscopy and redox proteomics. *Int J Cosmet Sci*. 2018; 40(6):536-548.
12. Nogueira ACS, Dicelio LE, Joekes I. About photo-damage of human hair. *Photochem Photobiol Sci*. 2006; 5(2):165-169.
13. Pande CM, Jachowicz J. Hair photodamage - measurement and prevention. *J Soc Cosmet Chem*. 1993;44(2):109-122.
14. Ratnapandian S, Warner SB, Kamath YK. Photodegradation of human hair. *J Cosmet Sci*. 1998;49(5):309-320.
15. Sinclair R, Patel M, Dawson TL, et al. Hair loss in women: medical and cosmetic approaches to increase scalp hair fullness. *Br J Dermatol*. 2011;165:12-18.
16. Dinh QQ, Sinclair R. Female pattern hair loss: current treatment concepts. *Clin Interv Aging*. 2007;2(2):189-199.
17. Warshaw EM, Buonomo M, DeKoven JG, et al. Importance of supplemental patch testing beyond a screening series for patients with dermatitis. *JAMA Dermatol*. 2021; 157(12):1456.
18. Berger RS, Fu JL, Smiles KA, et al. The effects of minoxidil, 1% pyrithione zinc and a combination of both on hair density: a randomized controlled trial. *Br J Dermatol*. 2003;149(2):354-362.
19. Draelos ZD, Kenneally DC, Hodges LT, Billhimer W, Copas M, Margraf C. A comparison of hair quality and cosmetic acceptance following the use of two anti-dandruff shampoos. *J Investig Dermatology Symp Proc*. 2005;10(3):201-204.
20. Barak-Shinar D, Green LJ. Scalp seborrheic dermatitis and dandruff therapy using a herbal and zinc pyrithione-based therapy of shampoo and scalp lotion. *J Clin Aesthet Dermatol*. 2018;11(1):26-31.
21. Van Neste D. Thickness, medullation and growth rate of female scalp hair are subject to significant variation according to pigmentation and scalp location during ageing. *Eur J Dermatol*. 2004;14(1):28-32.

22. Cash TF. The psychological effects of androgenetic alopecia in men. *J Am Acad Dermatol.* 1992;26(6):926-931.

23. Cash TF, Price VH, Savin RC. Psychological effects of androgenetic alopecia on women: comparisons with balding men and with female control subjects. *J Am Acad Dermatol.* 1993;29(4):568-575.

24. Draelos ZD. Essentials of hair care often neglected: hair cleansing. *Int J Trichology.* 2010;2(1):24-29.

25. Gubitosa J, Rizzi V, Fini P, Cosma P. Hair care cosmetics: from traditional shampoo to solid clay and herbal shampoo, a review. *Cosmetics.* 2019;6(1):13.

26. Draelos ZD. Shampoos, conditioners, and camouflage techniques. *Dermatol Clin.* 2013;31(1):173-178.

27. American Academy of Dermatology. *Tips for Healthy Hair.* AAD. https://www.aad.org/public/everyday-care/hair-scalp-care/hair/healthy-hair-tips. Accessed June 17, 2021.

28. Cline A, Uwakwe LN, McMichael AJ. No sulfates, no parabens, and the "no-poo" method: a new patient perspective on common shampoo ingredients. *Cutis.* 2018;101(1):22-26.

29. American Academy of Dermatology. *African American Hair: Tips for Everyday Care.* AAD https://www.aad.org/public/diseases/hair-loss/hair-care/african-american. Accessed July 1, 2021.

30. Bouillon C. Shampoos and hair conditioners. *Clin Dermatol.* 1988;6(3):83-92.

31. Powers DH. Shampoos. In: Balsam MS, Gershon SD, Reiger MM, Sagarin E, Strianse SJ, eds. *Cosmetics Science and Technology.* 2nd ed. New York: Wiley-Interscience; 1972:73-116.

32. Im SH. Shampoo compositions. Human health handbooks no 1. 2012:434-447.

33. D'Souza P, Rathi SK. Shampoo and conditioners: what a dermatologist should know? *Indian J Dermatol.* 2015;60(3):248-254.

34. Gavazzoni Dias MF, Pichler J, Adriano A, Cecato P, de Almeida A. The shampoo pH can affect the hair: myth or reality? *Int J Trichology.* 2014;6(3):95.

35. Douglas A, Onalaja AA, Taylor SC. Hair care products used by women of African descent: review of ingredients. *Cutis.* 2020;105(4):183-188.

36. Gupta AK, Batra R, Bluhm R, Boekhout T, Dawson TL. Skin diseases associated with Malassezia species. *J Am Acad Dermatol.* 2004;51(5):785-798.

37. Reeder NL, Kaplan J, Xu J, et al. Zinc pyrithione inhibits yeast growth through copper influx and inactivation of iron-sulfur proteins. *Antimicrob Agents Chemother.* 2011;55(12):5753.

38. Reeder NL, Xu J, Youngquist RS, Schwartz JR, Rust RC, Saunders CW. The antifungal mechanism of action of zinc pyrithione. *Br J Dermatol.* 2011;165(suppl 2):9-12.

39. Warner RR, Schwartz JR, Boissy Y, Dawson TL. Dandruff has an altered stratum corneum ultrastructure that is improved with zinc pyrithione shampoo. *J Am Acad Dermatol.* 2001;45(6):897-903.

40. Marks R, Pearse AD, Walker AP. The effects of a shampoo containing zinc pyrithione on the control of dandruff. *Br J Dermatol.* 1985;112(4):415-422.

41. Trüeb RM. Shampoos: ingredients, efficacy and adverse effects. *J Dtsch Dermatol Ges.* 2007;5(5):356-365.

42. Peter RU, Richarz-Barthauer U. Successful treatment and prophylaxis of scalp seborrhoeic dermatitis and dandruff with 2% ketoconazole shampoo: results of a multicentre, double-blind, placebo-controlled trial. *Br J Dermatol.* 1995;132(3):441-445.

43. Faergemann J. Treatment of seborrhoeic dermatitis of the scalp with ketoconazole shampoo. A double-blind study. *Acta Derm Venereol.* 1990;70(2):171-172.

44. Brown M, Evans TW, Poyner T, Tooley PJH. The role of ketoconazole 2% shampoo in the treatment and prophylactic management of dandruff. *J Dermatolog Treat.* 1990;1(4):177-179.

45. Piérard-Franchimont C, Goffin V, Decroix J, Piérard GE. A multicenter randomized trial of ketoconazole 2% and zinc pyrithione 1% shampoos in severe dandruff and seborrheic dermatitis. *Skin Pharmacol Physiol.* 2002;15(6):434-441.

46. Danby FW, Maddin WS, Margesson LJ, Rosenthal D. A randomized, double-blind, placebo-controlled trial of ketoconazole 2% shampoo versus selenium sulfide 2.5% shampoo in the treatment of moderate to severe dandruff. *J Am Acad Dermatol.* 1993;29(6):1008-1012.

47. Draelos ZD. The biology of hair care. *Dermatol Clin.* 2000;18(4):651-658.

48. Bolduc C, Shapiro J. Hair care products: waving, straightening, conditioning, and coloring. *Clin Dermatol.* 2001;19(4):431-436.

49. Draelos ZD. *Hair Loss Due to Cosmetic Practices.* Accessed June 17, 2021. https://www.zoedraelos.com/articles/hair/.

50. Hamilton JB. Patterned loss of hair in man: types and incidence. *Ann N Y Acad Sci.* 1951;53(3):708-728.

51. Ludwig E. Classification of the types of androgenetic alopecia (common baldness) occurring in the female sex. *Br J Dermatol.* 1977;97:247-254.

52. Tanus A, Oliveira CC, Villarreal DJ, Sanchez FA, Dias MF. Black women's hair: the main scalp dermatoses and aesthetic practices in women of African ethnicity. *An Bras Dermatol.* 2015;90(4):450-465.

53. Callender VD, McMichael AJ, Cohen GF. Medical and surgical therapies for alopecias in black women. *Dermatol Ther.* 2004;17(2):164-176.

54. Loussouarn G, El Rawadi C, Genain G. Diversity of hair growth profiles. *Int J Dermatol.* 2005;44(suppl 1):6-9.

55. Samrao A, Chen C, Zedek D, Price VH. Traction alopecia in a ballerina: clinicopathologic features. *Arch Dermatol.* 2010;146(8):918-935.

56. Sinclair RD. Healthy hair: what is it? *J Investig Dermatol Symp Proc.* 2007;12(2):2-5.

57. Dawber R. Hair: its structure and response to cosmetic preparations. *Clin Dermatol.* 1996;14(1):105-112.

58. Draelos ZD. Hair care and dyeing. *Curr Probl Dermatol.* 2015;47:121-127.

59. Lee Y, Kim YD, Hyun HJ, Pi LQ, Jin X, Lee WS. Hair shaft damage from heat and drying time of hair dryer. *Ann Dermatol.* 2011;23(4):455-462.

60. Gummer CL. Bubble hair: a cosmetic abnormality caused by brief, focal heating of damp hair fibres. *Br J Dermatol.* 1994;131(6):901-903.

61. Gavazzoni Dias MF. Hair cosmetics: an overview. *Int J Trichology.* 2015;7(1):2-15.

62. Mariwalla K. *Cosmeceutical Compendium.* Chicago: American Society for Dermatologic Surgery; 2018.

63. Saed S, Ibrahim O, Bergfeld WF. Hair camouflage: a comprehensive review. *Int J Womens Dermatol.* 2017;3(suppl 1):S75-S80.

64. Donovan JC, Shapiro RL, Shapiro P, Zupan M, Pierre-Louis M, Hordinsky M. A review of scalp camouflaging agents and prostheses for individuals with hair loss. *Dermatol Online J.* 2012;18(8):1.

65. Steffen JE, Tran T, Yimam M, et al. Serous ovarian cancer caused by exposure to asbestos and fibrous talc in cosmetic talc powders–a case series. *J Occup Environ Med.* 2020;62(2):e65-e77.

66. Gordon RE, Fitzgerald S, Millette J. Asbestos in commercial cosmetic talcum powder as a cause of mesothelioma in women. *Int J Occup Environ Health.* 2014;20(4):318-332.

67. Tran TH, Steffen JE, Clancy KM, Bird T, Egilman DS. Talc, asbestos, and epidemiology: corporate influence and scientific incognizance. *Epidemiology.* 2019;30(6):783-788.

68. Center for Food Safety and Applied Nutrition. *Cosmetic Ingredients.* U.S. Food and Drug Administration. Available at: https://www.fda.gov/cosmetics/cosmetic-products-ingredients/cosmetic-ingredients. Accessed October 19, 2021.

69. Weathersby C, Mcmichael A. Brazilian keratin hair treatment: a review. *J Cosmet Dermatol.* 2013;12(2):144-148.

70. Draelos ZD. Chapter 6: Nonmedicated grooming products and beauty treatments. In: McMichael AJ, Hordinsky MK, eds. *Hair and Scalp Disorders: Medical, Surgical, and Cosmetic Treatments.* London: CRC Press; 2018:59-71. 2nd ed.

71. *Brazilian Blowout AÇAI Professional Smoothing Solution Brazilian Blowout Professional Smoothing Treatment Summary Sheet Textured Hair.* Accessed July 21, 2021 http://brazilianblowout.com/literature/BB_TREATMENT_SUMMARY_AA.pdf.

72. *Brazilian Blowout AÇAI Professional Smoothing Solution Brazilian Blowout Açai Professional Smoothing Solution 1.5 Product Uses & Restrictions: Professional Use Only.* Accessed July 21, 2021 https://www.brazilianblowout.com/literature/bb-msds.pdf.

73. Aglan MA, Mansour GN. Hair straightening products and the risk of occupational formaldehyde exposure in hairstylists. *Drug Chem Toxicol.* 2020;43(5):488-495.

74. Nutrition C for FS and A. *Hair-Smoothing Products that Release Formaldehyde When Heated.* FDA https://www.fda.gov/cosmetics/cosmetic-products/hair-smoothing-products-release-formaldehyde-when-heated. Published online. Accessed March 8, 2022.

75. International Agency for Research on Cancer. *IARC Monographs on the evaluation of carcinogenic risks to humans volume 88 (2006): Formaldehyde, 2-Butoxyethanol and 1-tert-Butoxypropan-2-ol.* http://monographs.iarc.fr/ENG/Monographs/vol88/index.php, June 2004.

76. França SA Da, Dario MF, Esteves VB, Baby AR, Velasco MVR. Types of hair dye and their mechanisms of action. *Cosmet.* 2015;2(2):110-126.

77. George NM, Potlapati A. Hair colouring: what a dermatologist should know? *Int J Res Dermatol.* 2021;7(3):496-502.

78. Smith RAW, Garrett B, Naqvi KR, et al. Mechanistic insights into the bleaching of melanin by alkaline hydrogen peroxide. *Free Radic Biol Med.* 2017;108:110-117.

79. Lillo MA, Nichols C, Perry C, et al. Methylparaben stimulates tumor initiating cells in ER+ breast cancer models. *J Appl Toxicol.* 2017;37(4):417-425.

80. Nutrition C for FS and A. *Parabens in Cosmetics.* FDA https://www.fda.gov/cosmetics/cosmetic-ingredients/parabens-cosmetics#are_parabens_safe. Published online. Accessed March 8, 2022.

81. Rubin CB, Brod B. Natural does not mean safe - the dirt on clean beauty products. *JAMA Dermatol.* 2019;155(12):1344-1345.

82. *Teaching Your Child Healthy Hair Care Habits.* https://www.aad.org/public/everyday-care/hair-scalp-care/hair/hair-care-habits. Accessed February 16, 2022.

6

Wigs and Hair Prosthetics

Molly Stout and Omer Ibrahim

KEY POINTS

- Patients with androgenetic alopecia and other types of alopecia may turn to hair prosthetics when other medical and procedural interventions have been aesthetically unsatisfying and hair loss negatively affects their quality of life.
- When recommending a wig style to a patient, it is important to consider the patient's face shape, lifestyle, goals, and environment.
- Wigs and hair prosthetics should be considered important therapeutic treatment options for many diagnoses and severities of scarring and nonscarring alopecia.
- Synthetic wigs are usually less expensive, less prone to environmental wear, and easier to maintain than natural wigs. However, natural wigs may look more natural and are less susceptible to damage from heat-styling.
- Wigs are often categorized by the type of foundation to which the hair is attached. Wig foundations include wefted (less expensive, less natural looking) and netted or lace (more expensive, more natural looking).
- For patients with patchy hair loss, beneficial hair prosthetics include demi wigs, toupees, lace fronts, and integration wigs.
- Adverse events with respect to wigs and hair prostheses typically occur as a result of improper fixation to the scalp or existing hair. Hair extensions and partial prostheses may cause traction alopecia if the braids to which they are affixed are too tight, or the extensions themselves are too heavy.

BACKGROUND, DEFINITIONS, AND HISTORY

Wigs and hair prosthetics have been used for centuries to conceal hair disorders and to enhance existing hair. The earliest wigs date back to Ancient Egypt, where they were worn by nobility to dually signify elite social status and confer sun protection.[1] Since then, they have been worn as status symbols throughout history by Roman emperors and European royalty.[1] The word "wig" derives from the word "periwig," which first came into use in the English language in the 1670s. King Louis XIII of France, who reportedly wore a wig to cover his premature balding, is credited with popularizing the wearing of powdered wigs, which were dusted with white starch to combat odor and parasites. During the late 18th century, wealthy women in Western Europe fashioned their hair in elaborate arrangements with decorations that sometimes even included birdcages.[2]

Wigs may also have religious significance, as is the case with sheitels for married women in Orthodox Jewish communities. Today, the wigs and hair prosthetics market forms a multimillion-dollar industry. Hair prosthetics include, but are not limited to, wefted wigs, netted wigs, integration wigs, partial hair pieces, and hair extensions or weaves.

Patients with androgenetic alopecia (AGA) and inflammatory alopecia may turn to hair prosthetics when other medical and procedural interventions have been aesthetically unsatisfying and hair loss negatively affects their quality of life. Therefore, it is critical that dermatologists are aware of characteristics and variations of wigs and hair prosthetics.[3]

INDICATIONS AND PATIENT SELECTION

Rather than a mere cosmetic accessory, wigs and hair prosthetics should be considered important therapeutic treatment options for many diagnoses and severities of scarring and nonscarring alopecia. The recommendation of a hair prosthetic is not mutually exclusive of continuing medical or procedural therapy for hair loss. Some patients may want to save wispy strands even as they realize that hope for regrowth to the effect of a socially acceptable natural hairstyle is unattainable.

Many patients may initially present with personal experience of using hair prosthetics prior to any prescribed medical or procedural intervention for hair loss. Providers should feel comfortable asking about a history of prior wig or hair prosthetic use when considering adding a hair prosthetic to the treatment plan for hair loss.

Some patients may use hair prosthetics as a bridge until medical or procedural therapies for their alopecia take effect. In the case of chemotherapy-induced hair loss, wigs typically serve as a temporary solution to alopecia during treatment.

When recommending a wig style to a patient, it is important to consider the patient's face shape, lifestyle, goals, and even environment. For example, patients living in a warmer climate may be best suited with lower-density and shorter wigs to avoid overheating and perspiration of the scalp under the wig. Patients with drug-induced hair loss and progressive hair loss disorders may often want to recapitulate the texture, color, and length of their natural hair style. Human hair wigs can be dyed, cut, and styled, while synthetic hair wigs may have more limited flexibility of daily styling.

Wig cap sizing is also important, and the authors recommend patients have measurements of head circumference, frontal hairline to occiput, and coronally from ear to ear to ensure a proper fit. The typical wig cap size is about 22 inches for an adult.

Patients with chronic and progressive forms of hair loss, such as AGA, may view wigs and hair prosthetics as a sign of giving up on treating their hair loss, and the contrary should be emphasized. Initiating a discussion on wigs and hair prosthetics early on in the course of disease is important, as end-stage scarring alopecia or severe AGA may progress to a state where there is little hope for aesthetically acceptable regrowth, despite maximizing medical and procedural therapy.

Just like any other medical or dermatologic treatment, dermatologists recommending wigs and hair prosthetics must take into account a patient's natural anatomy, lifestyle, goals, and profession, and ensure that the patient is happy with the treatment, that the treatment is effective, and, most of all, that the treatment fits seamlessly into their life.

EXPECTED OUTCOMES

Hair loss has the capacity to significantly affect all aspects of a patient's quality of life, regardless of the cause or severity of alopecia. Numerous studies have demonstrated the negative effect of hair loss on quality of life, including emotional well-being and financial potential. Studies have demonstrated increased prevalence of psychological disorders in patients with alopecia. Patients may experience depression, anxiety, and neuroticism scales, regardless of the duration of the disease, age at disease onset, number of relapses, and intensity of disease.

Considering economic stability of patients with hair loss, the Canadian Hair Research Foundation found that, among 1502 men and women responders, 1 in 8 believed hair loss to be a barrier to getting hired.[4] In addition, studies have shown it is important to patients that the wig or hair prosthetic look as close as possible to natural hair with minimal noticeability for strangers and acquaitenances.[5] The ideal outcomes with use of a wig or hair prosthetic are improved quality of life in all aspects of a patient's well-being and reduction of stigma.

Wigs have demonstrated positive effects on social anxiety in patients with alopecia areata and may be an important coping strategy to dealing with hair loss disorders. Wearing wigs has been associated with increased social confidence in patients with alopecia, and patient concerns about not being able to wear a wig when needed have been associated with higher levels of depression and anxiety.[6]

TREATMENT TECHNIQUES AND BEST PRACTICES

Wig Hair Composition

Wig hair may be synthetic or natural (Pearl 6.1). Among synthetic wigs, the hair material is typically composed of uniform fibers of nylon acetate or Dynel, which is a copolymer of acrylonitrile and vinyl chloride.[6] Benefits of synthetic hair wigs include that they are typically less expensive than natural hair, less prone to environmental wear, and easier to maintain.[7] The pitfalls of synthetic hair wigs are their unnatural look as a result of uniform fiber diameter and their lower melting point, which makes them vulnerable to damage with heat styling.[8] The benefits of wigs containing human hair fibers are their natural look and ability to be heat styled (Fig. 6.1, Pearl 6.2). They are typically more expensive and must be replaced more frequently because of their susceptibility to environmental damage, such as UV-induced fading.[3] Human hair fibers are most frequently sourced from China, Thailand, Indonesia, and India, and more expensive hair fibers are sourced from Europe.[9]

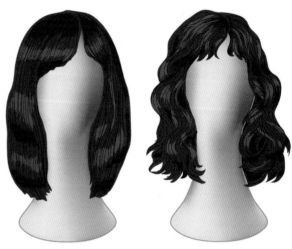

Fig. 6.1 Examples of human hair wigs demonstrating flexibility of styling. (Courtesy of Sheila Macomber.)

PEARL 6.2: Wigs from human hair may be styled with heat and look more natural, but they are more expensive and must be replaced more often than synthetic wigs.

PEARL 6.1: Wigs may be categorized by hair fiber: synthetic or natural.

PEARL 6.3: Wig foundations include wefted (less expensive, less natural looking) and netted or lace (more expensive, more natural looking).

Wig Foundations

Wigs are most frequently categorized by the type of foundation to which the hair is attached (Pearl 6.3). Wefted foundations are composed of a base of synthetic rows to which the hairs are attached by a machine. In contrast, net foundations are composed of a mesh base to which the hair fibers are attached by hand-tied knots (Fig. 6.2). Net wigs may also contain a lace cap component, where hairs are hand-tied to small fenestrations. This component may be present at the frontal hairline to mimic a naturally irregular contour (Fig. 6.3). Foundations containing a mix of polyurethane, lace, wefted, and net may achieve a natural look balanced with improved durability.

Wigs may be fashioned as full caps or partial systems depending on the pattern of hair loss requiring concealment. Partial systems include demiwigs, lace fronts, and hair extensions (Figs. 6.4 and 6.5, Pearl 6.4). In patients with female-pattern hair loss and a preserved frontal hairline, a demiwig prothesis that covers the entire scalp excluding the frontal hairline may be a viable option.[6] Demiwigs also include toupees, which are typically used by men with AGA. Lace fronts are partial hair prostheses used to cover the frontal hairline and have particular use for patients with frontal fibrosing alopecia (FFA). Hair extensions may be made from natural or synthetic hair fibers and are used to add volume and/or length to existing hair. Integrated foundations use a patient's own remaining hairs pulled through a fenestrated wig cap (Fig. 6.6). This type of foundation is only practical for patients with thinning hair and without total alopecia.

PEARL 6.4: Hair prosthetics, including demi wigs, toupees, lace fronts, and integration wigs, may be appropriate for patients with patchy hair loss.

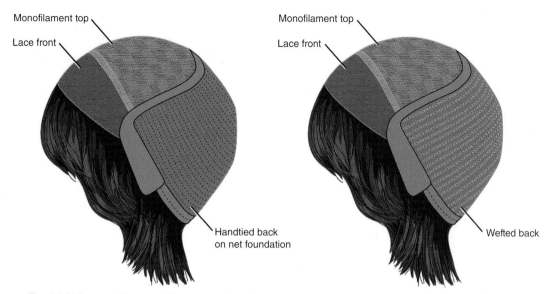

Fig. 6.2 Wig cap with a monofilament top, lace front, and hand-tied back with silicone around the perimeter to allow for better grip of scalp for individuals with total hair loss. (Courtesy of Sheila Macomber.)

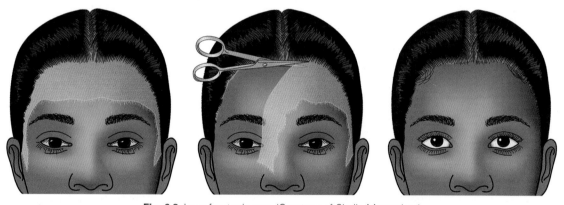

Fig. 6.3 Lace-front wig cap. (Courtesy of Sheila Macomber.)

Wig and Prosthetic Attachments

Wigs may be further characterized into the method of attachment of the wig cap to the scalp. All forms of wig attachment may lead to traction alopecia in the remaining hairs. Wigs containing clips are easily removable but require some of the patient's own hair to fasten. The main advantage of clip wigs is the ability to easily remove the wig or hair prosthesis to continue any topical treatment to the scalp. Hair extensions may contain clips or glues or may be sewn into braided tracks in the scalp (weaves).

Fixed wigs use bonding glues or tapes to adhere to the scalp. A fixed foundation allows a wig to be worn continuously for up to 30 days through bathing, exercise, and sleeping. Though rare, components of these adhesives, including cyanoacrylate, hydroquinone, polymethyl methacrylate, and sulfonic acid, may cause contact dermatitis.[10]

Vacuum-attached wigs are the most expensive option, as they are made from custom molds of a patient's scalp fit to a silicone or polyurethane base. Vacuum wigs do not require any adhesives or clips to remain in place. Creation of vacuum wigs may take up to 6 months.[9]

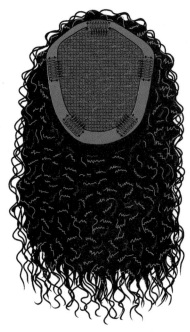

Fig. 6.4 Example of a partial wig. (Courtesy of Sheila Macomber.)

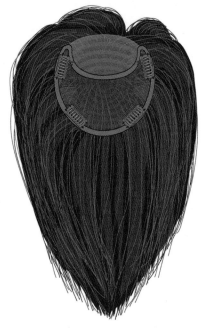

Fig. 6.5 Example of a partial wig. (Courtesy of Sheila Macomber.)

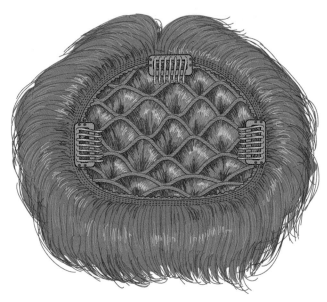

Fig. 6.6 Integration wig. (Courtesy of Sheila Macomber.)

PREVENTION AND MANAGEMENT OF ADVERSE EVENTS

Adverse events with respect to wigs and hair prostheses typically occur as a result of improper fixation to the scalp or existing hair. Hair extensions and partial prostheses may cause traction alopecia if the braids to which they are affixed are too tight, or if the extensions themselves are too heavy.[11] As mentioned, contact dermatitis to synthetic wig materials and adhesives may rarely occur in susceptible patients (Pearl 6.5).

PEARL 6.5: The main adverse outcomes associated with wigs and prosthetics are contact dermatitis from adhesives and traction alopecia from attachments that are too tight.

FUTURE DIRECTIONS

Transparency and improved social consciousness regarding the sourcing of human hair for wigs would be a positive direction. Sourcing of human hair has long been considered an exploitive and unbalanced market. Temples in India dedicated to the Hindu deity

Venkateshwara are sites of pilgrimage for thousands of men and women each day for the purpose of hair tonsuring. The hair offerings amass tons, which must be cleaned, dried, processed, and sold at auction. Although the auctions garner millions of dollars for the temples and a small number of distributors, the original owners of the hair see zero share of the compensation and are often unaware of the profit from their own hair.[12] The hair is then sewn into wigs in factories in India and China before they are sold around the world for thousands of dollars. In the worst cases motivated by the high return on hair, criminal hair theft by attacking women has been a disturbing trend in South Africa, Myanmar, and Venezuela.[13-15] Synthetic wigs and hair prosthetics with improved quality and aesthetics to behave more like human hair wigs may help to mitigate this problem.

Although wigs can be an important treatment and coping strategy for patients with alopecia, often the cost of the wig presents a financial burden to the patient not covered like other medical expenses. Patients may solicit donations from charitable wig suppliers or use crowdfunding (the use of social media to solicit funding) to finance hair loss treatments.[16] Recognition of alopecia as a medical condition and not merely a cosmetic issue by insurance providers and society at large is an ongoing advocacy initiative for the field of dermatology and patients with hair loss.

EVIDENCE SUMMARY

- Wigs and hair prosthetics can be recommended as a treatment option to patients with all etiologies of hair loss (strength of recommendation: D).
- Human hair wigs are more natural appearing than synthetic fiber wigs and have the advantage of heat styling. However, they are more expensive (strength of recommendation: D).
- When considering a wig and hair prosthetic attachment style, traction alopecia should be considered to avoid unnecessary progressive hair loss (strength of recommendation: D).

REFERENCES

1. Hafouda Y, Yesudian PD. Unraveling the locks of wigs: a historical analysis. *Int J Trichology.* 2019;11(4):177-178.
2. Weitz R. *Rapunzel's Daughters: What Women's Hair Tells Us About Women's Lives.* New York: Farrar, Strauss and Giroux; 2004.
3. Donovan JC, Shapiro RL, Shapiro P, Zupan M, Pierre-Louis M, Hordinsky M. A review of scalp camouflaging agents and prostheses for individuals with hair loss. *Dermatol Online J.* 2012;18(8):1.
4. Tischer B. *Influence of Hair Loss on Employment Decisions.* Abstract presented at: American Academy of Dermatology Meeting. March 2000; San Francisco, CA; 2000.
5. Wiggins S, Moore-Millar K, Thomson A. Can you pull it off? Appearance modifying behaviours adopted by wig users with alopecia in social interactions. *Body Image.* 2014;11(2):156-166.
6. Montgomery K, White C, Thompson AA. Mixed methods survey of social anxiety, anxiety, depression and wig use in alopecia. *BMJ Open.* 2017;7:e015468.
7. Love T. *The World of Wigs, Weaves & Extensions.* Albany NY: Milady; 2002:49-69.
8. Weffort F, Martins SS, Plata GT, et al. Do you know how to recommend a wig to a patient? *J Cosmet Dermatol.* 2021;20:724-728.
9. Saed S, Ibrahim O, Bergfeld WF. Hair camouflage: a comprehensive review. *Int J Womens Dermatol.* 2017;3(suppl 1):S75-S80.
10. Sornakumar L, Shanmugasekar C, Rai R, Priya S. Allergic contact dermatitis to superglue. *Int J Trichology.* 2013;5(1):43-44.
11. Yang A, Iorizzo M, Vincenzi C, Tosti A. Hair extensions: a concerning cause of hair disorders. *Br J Dermatol.* 2009;160(1):207-209.
12. Rai S. A religious tangle over the hair of pious Hindus. *The New York Times.* 14 July, 2004, Section A, Page 3.
13. Long-haired women face threat of hair thieves. IOL. https://www.iol.co.za/news/world/long-haired-women-face-threat-of-hair-thieves-352744. Accessed April 8, 2021.
14. Fihlani P. *South Africa's Dreadlock Thieves.* Johannesburg: BBC News; February 27, 2013.
15. Lopéz V. Venezuelan women get short, sharp shock as hair thieves cut and run. *The Guardian.* August 15, 2013.
16. Desai S, Manjaly P, Lee KJ, et al. Utilization of crowdfunding for expenses related to medical hair loss. *J Am Acad Dermatol.* 2020;86(5):1109–1110. doi:10.1016/j.jaad.2020.09.008.

7

Micropigmentation and Microblading

Katherine Almengo, Sara Salas, and Valerie D. Callender

KEY POINTS

- Androgenetic alopecia is a frequent cause of hair loss and hair thinning for both men and women, and it has the potential to negatively affect self-esteem, psychosocial functioning, and quality of life.
- Micropigmentation, also known as medical tattooing or dermatography, conveys the aesthetic use of tattooing for medical purposes.[1,2]
- Scalp micropigmentation is a cosmetic procedure used as a concealer to address hair loss involving the scalp, and it can be used to lessen the contrast
between the hair and skin colors to create the illusion of hair density (level of evidence: 4).[3]
- The scalp micropigmentation procedure uses a device with needles to implant metabolically inert pigment granules into the upper and mid-papillary dermis, and it is this level of placement that is the determining factor for the pigment to be retained uniformly.
- Scalp micropigmentation can be used as an adjunct to hair transplantation and medical therapies and to cover unwanted scars on the scalp.

BACKGROUND, DEFINITIONS, AND HISTORY

Androgenetic alopecia (AGA) affects millions of men and women around the world. The hair loss or hair thinning that results from AGA may inflict psychological comorbidities and thus diminish quality of life (QoL) (level of evidence: 5).[4] Curative options for AGA are not currently available; however, dermatologists and hair transplant surgeons should discuss all potential treatment modalities to mitigate the effects of AGA. Cosmetic approaches to scalp and hair deformities offer additional therapeutic options to medical and surgical treatments generally used by clinicians. This chapter will focus on scalp micropigmentation (SMP) and microblading as cosmetic camouflaging options for AGA and thinning eyebrows, and the necessary variables to ensure positive outcomes for patients with hair loss.

SMP was first introduced as a safe and effective technique to conceal hair and scalp deformities by Traquina in 2001 (level of evidence: 4).[5,6] SMP is a noninvasive procedure that may be used in any type of alopecia regardless of etiology, gender, or extent of hair loss (Video 7.1). The technique requires inserting a specialized ink into the upper dermis in a stippling pattern (level of evidence: 4).[1,7] The stippling pattern resembles painted dots that mimic hair follicles and aims to visually camouflage any areas of alopecia. The illusion of increased hair density created by SMP reduces the skin-to-hair color contrast.[1] SMP differs from body tattooing in that the anatomy of the scalp differs from that of the skin on the body.[1]

One of the oldest uses of the word "tattoo" is in the Polynesian language.[6] The Polynesians defined tattoos as black pigment placed under the skin.[6] Medical tattooing involves implantation of exogenous, metabolically inert, colorfast pigments into the scalp (SMP) or skin, and it is used to address a loss of pigment on other areas of the body.[1] Medical tattooing may be used as a cosmetic treatment to conceal scars from varying etiologies such as alopecic scars, vermillion scars, hypopigmented scars, and nipple-areolar reconstructive surgery after mastectomy (level of evidence: 4).[8] A case report in 2009 detailed how a decorative tattoo was designed to conceal a scar on the abdomen from a transverse rectus abdominis (TRAM) flap procedure after breast reconstruction in a patient who had breast cancer (level of evidence: 5).[6,9] Medical tattooing may also be considered as a treatment modality for dermatologic conditions such as vitiligo (level of evidence: 4)[10] and piebaldism (level of evidence: 4).[11]

Eyebrow restoration via the technique of microblading was first reported by Van der Velden et al for the treatment of alopecia areata (AA) of the eyebrow in 1998 (level of evidence: 3b).[6,12] Microblading is a cosmetic procedure that is becoming increasingly popular and involves superficial micropigmentation. In microblading, the pigment is deposited into the papillary dermis using a manual device with a single needle or a blade with a varying number of stacked needles (Pearl 7.1) (level of evidence: 5).[12,13]

INDICATIONS AND PATIENT SELECTION

SMP may be used as a noninvasive method to camouflage a variety of scalp and hair loss conditions. It is well documented that QoL in patients who experience hair loss is negatively affected (Pearl 7.2).[4] Providing a procedural intervention to conceal hair and scalp deformities through the appearance of a fuller head of hair breaks the cycle of psychological stressors that patients experience in their daily lives. After the diagnosis of a scalp or

---

PEARL 7.1: Scalp micropigmentation utilizes a device with one or more needles to implant metabolically inert pigment granules into the upper and midpapillary dermis, and it is this level of placement that is the determining factor for the pigment to be retained uniformly.

PEARL 7.2: Hair loss negatively affects patient quality of life.

---

hair deformity, patients are educated on the therapeutic options that are available. In a combination treatment regimen, SMP is part of the initial treatment as the medical treatment regrows the hair, or as a permanent solution if the area to be treated is stable.[5] SMP is not a recommended treatment modality for patients with progressive hair loss or those who change their hair color frequently.[5,12] Patients with the indications listed in Table 7.1 are the best candidates for SMP (Pearl 7.3).[3,7]

In microblading, the design of the eyebrow is dependent on the natural growth of the hair follicle (Fig. 7.1). Anatomically, the eyebrow is divided into four sections: head, body, arch, and tail.[13] These sections should be taken into careful consideration when shaping the eyebrow, as certain facial structures align best with different eyebrow variations.[13]

At the initial consultation, it should be determined whether the patient is a good candidate for the procedure. Indications for microblading include AGA, traumatic scars, madarosis in hypothyroidism, trichotillomania, scarring alopecias (e.g., frontal fibrosing alopecia), alopecia totalis, and chemotherapy-induced hypotrichosis (level of evidence: 4).[6,12-16] Notable contraindications for microblading are keratosis pilaris, psoriasis, and chronic acne or oily skin, especially near the eyebrows (Pearl 7.4). Providers should advise patients of the potential adverse effects associated with microblading, such as infection and contact dermatitis, as they may lead to negative outcomes in terms of patient self-esteem.[13,14] Patients should also be made aware that the pigment is semipermanent and is likely to fade over time.[12,14] Touch-ups to maintain pigment intensity are common and may be started two to three weeks after the initial procedure.[12]

EXPECTED OUTCOMES

A critical step for a successful SMP outcome is the selection of the proper patient for the procedure and the establishment of realistic expectations. During the initial consultation, a detailed medical history is obtained to verify whether SMP would be an appropriate procedure for the patient. At the first consult, it is important to note current medications such as blood thinners; allergies to medications; previous treatment for hair loss including medications (e.g., minoxidil, spironolactone, finasteride), scalp surgery (e.g., hair transplant, scalp reduction); and any history of relevant dermatoses (e.g.,

TABLE 7.1   Indications for Scalp Micropigmentation (SMP): A Patient With Any of the Following Indications May Be a Good Candidate for SMP

Androgenetic alopecia in men
Female pattern hair loss
Scarring alopecia
Alopecia areata[12]
Traction alopecia
Cosmetic (chemical) alopecia
Trichotillomania
Anagen effluvium
Telogen effluvium
Traumatic or surgical scars
Insufficient amount of donor hair to qualify for hair transplantation
Individuals who do not want to undergo hair transplantation
Individuals who are experiencing regional balding or thinning of hair and want the appearance of a fuller head of hair
Unsatisfactory coverage with medical therapy and/or hair transplantation

Rassman, WR, Pak JP, Kim J. Scalp Micropigmentation. *Facial Plast Surg Clin North Am.* 2013;21(3):497-503; Rassman WR, Pak JP, Kim J, Estrin NF. Scalp micropigmentation: a concealer for hair and scalp deformities. *J Clin Aesthet Dermatol.* 2015;8(3):35-42.

PEARL 7.3: Scalp micropigmentation is not a recommended treatment modality for patients with progressive hair loss or those who change their hair color frequently.

PEARL 7.4: Indications for microblading include androgenetic alopecia, traumatic scars, madarosis in hypothyroidism, trichotillomania, scarring alopecias, alopecia totalis, and chemotherapy-induced hypotrichosis. Contraindications include keratosis pilaris, psoriasis, and chronic acne or oily skin near the treatment site.

seborrheic dermatitis, psoriasis, or hypertrophic or keloid scars). The outcome the patient interprets and the work performed by the physician must be designed to align with the patient's initial objectives. The next step is to address the areas that require coverage with SMP and to determine the total treatment surface area. In addition, the patient must be informed on approximately how long the session will last and the number of sessions needed to achieve the desired camouflaging effect. Most patients will require two to three SMP sessions at 4 to 6 week intervals (Pearl 7.5). Each session is often lengthy, normally 4 to 8 hours, depending on how

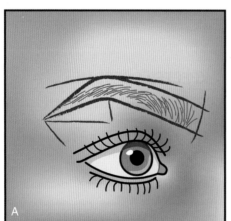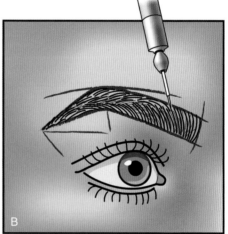

Fig. 7.1 Microblading. Before (A) and after (B) microblading. Before, eyebrows are marked at the desired length and thickness. After, eyebrows are filled in with a single tip. The tip of the instrument is maneuvered in a stippling pattern in the direction of the hair follicle to provide a natural appearance. (Courtesy of Sheila Macomber.)

PEARL 7.5: Depending on the total treatment area and desired level of camouflage, most patients require two or three scalp-micropigmentation sessions. Each session may take 4 to 8 hours.

PEARL 7.6: The goal of SMP is to attain results that look 100% natural.

PEARL 7.7: Scalp micropigmentation typically fades completely after 5 years. Frequent sun exposure may cause the intensity of pigment to fade more quickly.

TABLE 7.2 Factors That Determine the Outcome of SMP

Angle of needle	Needle insertion at different angles
Depth of needle	Insertion at varying depths ranging from 0.3–1.2 mm
Pattern of dot placement (of pigment)	Placement of pigment in regular versus random manner
Tattoo ink used	Jet black versus black-brown in a ratio of 2:1
Contact time of the needle	Different contact times in correlation with pigment deposition
Resistance of scalp	Effect of skin suppleness/elasticity/turgidity on pigment deposition
Speed of rotor	Effect of varying rotor speed on pigment deposition
Viscosity of dye	Fluidity of dye affecting outcome
Needle number	• Single-pronged needle used for hairline designing • Triple-pronged needle for the rest of the scalp
Level of expertise of the operator - technical and artistic skill, proper training	Length of exposure (amount of time the needle is in contact with the scalp)

Dhurat RS, Shanshanwal SJS, Dandale AL. Standardization of SMP procedure and its impact on outcome. *J Cutan Aesthet Surg* 2017;10(3):145-149; Rassman WR, Pak, JP, Kim J. Scalp Micropigmentation. *Facial Plast Surg Clin North Am.* 2013;21(3):497-503; Rassman WR, Pak JP, Kin J, Estrin NF. Scalp micropigmentation: a concealer for hair and scalp deformities. *J Clin Aesthet Dermatol.* 2015;8(3):35-42.

extensive the area of alopecia is, the presenting diagnosis, and if the treated area is normal scalp or in an area of scar tissue (level of evidence: 5).[16,17]

After the consultation, the scalp is evaluated to select the optimal pigment for SMP. The size of the dots or lines are assessed, and necessary adjustments are made. It is important to keep in mind that the goal is to attain results that look completely natural (Pearl 7.6). The color typically stays intact for 1 to 2 years, then slowly fades with time. It is estimated that the pigment will disappear by the fifth year. If the patient consistently takes part in outdoor activities, the intensity of pigment may decrease before the estimated timeframe. To mitigate a decrease in pigment, additional sessions may be required to reinforce pigment intensity (Pearl 7.7).

There are several variables that determine the outcome of SMP (Table 7.2). Authors of a study involving 30 patients with AGA, cicatricial alopecia, and AA examined these variables and ideal parameters to standardize the SMP procedure and correlate it with reproducible results.[1] Patients were assessed by clinical photography and trichoscopy at 1 month, and by clinical photography at 6 months after the SMP procedure. The treated area was evaluated by the physician using a seven-point scale and by the patient using a three-point satisfaction scale, both at 6 months. In addition, a histopathologic examination was performed to determine the ideal depth of pigment deposition. Results suggested that patients with AGA had better outcomes than those with AA or cicatricial alopecia, and that patient satisfaction was high. Adverse events included transient edema and redness.[1]

TREATMENT TECHNIQUE/BEST PRACTICES

Preoperative Care

Preoperative instructions and the surgical instruments used for SMP are presented in Tables 7.3 and 7.4, respectively. Preoperative photographs are recommended to document the treatment area and to monitor success

TABLE 7.3 Preoperative Care Instructions for Patients Undergoing Treatment With Scalp Micropigmentation

Patient should avoid blood thinners, including aspirin, nonsteroidal anti-inflammatory drugs, vitamin E, ginkgo biloba, and ginseng[1]
Patient should be advised to not change hairstyle
Instruct patient to shampoo hair day of procedure
Patient should avoid using hair products before the procedure
After the procedure, patients should not wash their hair for 48 hours
Patients may wear a hat after the procedure, if desired

TABLE 7.4 Surgical Instruments and Supplies Used for Scalp Micropigmentation

Markers
Antiseptic and alcohol solution (e.g., Microdacyn, to cleanse the scalp)
Vibrating devices
Loupe with magnification
Dermatoscope
Topical anesthetic (e.g., Emla cream)
Xylocaine 1% with epinephrine (1:100,000); 0.25% bupivacaine can also be used and can last up to 8 hours[3]
Bicarbonate (dilutes epinephrine)
Syringe with 30G and 33G needles
25G cannula (nerve block)
Elastic tape
Sterile gauze
Sterile drapes
Dermograph instrument that supports one to six needles
Pigments (colors vary)

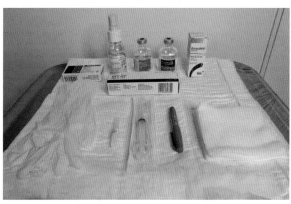

Fig. 7.2 Preoperative Anesthesia. Preoperative anesthetics used for scalp micropigmentation. Top row from left to right: sublingual ketorolac (systemic medication for pain relief), microdacyn, bicarbonate, lidocaine with epinephrine 2%, bupivacaine, and Emla cream (topical anesthetic). Bottom row from left to right: gloves, 33g needle, 5cc syringe, and marker.

of the procedure. Video 7.2 provides a visual of the preoperative process. The area of hair loss that will be treated should be cleansed with antiseptic and alcohol solutions (Fig. 7.2), then marked with a surgical pen based on the preoperative consultation. A vibrating device is given to the patient to hold onto their chest, and two more vibrators are placed around the patient's forehead.

One of the authors (SS) uses these maneuvers to minimize the patient's discomfort with the procedure.

Local anesthesia is achieved by injecting 1% xylocaine with epinephrine using a 33-gauge needle into three different injection sites on the scalp. These three areas will be the entry points for the 25-gauge cannula used to perform a nerve block.

Pigment Selection

A nonvisible area of the scalp is selected for a pigment color test. Whether or not the same color should be continued or changed to a lighter or more intense pigment is decided at this point. Different pigments can be mixed to match the color of the patient's hair. A test is recommended prior to performing the entire procedure to ensure that the right color is used to produce a natural result. Most pigments (Fig. 7.3) are composed of iron oxide, glycerin, and isopropyl alcohol.[5]

Procedural Technique

Fig. 7.4 illustrates a dermographic instrument with a single-needle tip. This device is used to insert microdroplets of pigment through the skin and into the upper dermis (Fig. 7.5), approximately 1.5-2 mm from the surface of the skin.[2] This machine can also support one to six needles and cycles between 100 to 150 cycles per second in normal skin. The cycle velocity correlates with the quality of the dots: a slow velocity results in larger

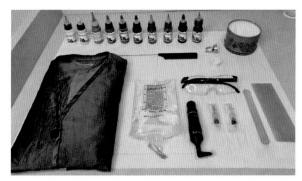

Fig. 7.3 Surgical Tray. Top row from left to right: pigments (range of tones), hair comb, pigment containers, and Vaseline (to moisturize the scalp). Bottom row from left to right: dressing gown, sterile solution (to dilute pigment), dermograph instrument, magnifying glasses, two needles (single-needle tip and three-needle tip), sterile spatula for Vaseline, sterile protection for scalp micropigmentation machine.

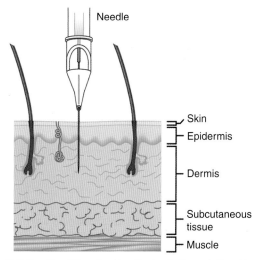

Fig. 7.5 Depth of Needle. Needle depth through the skin and epidermis into the upper dermis.

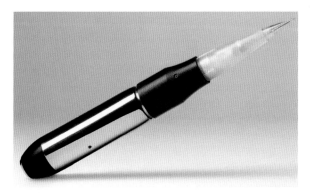

Fig. 7.4 Dermograph Sevice. Instrument used to conduct scalp micropigmentation with a single-needle tip. (Courtesy Goldeneye Micropigmentation.)

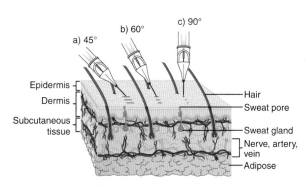

Fig. 7.6 Angle of Single Needle Tip Relative to Scalp. (A) 45-degree angle, (B) 60-degree angle, (C) 90-degree angle. Smaller angles result in more superficial pigment. (Courtesy of Sheila Macomber.)

dots, and a fast velocity results in a dot that appears dull with little uniformity. Video 7.3 further illustrates the technique in which pigment is deposited into the scalp.

The technique used to cover the area of hair loss depends on several factors. If the patient has short hair, small dots (points) of pigment are used, in contrast to patients with long hair that will require small dots and small lines. In addition, when placing the dots of pigment into the scalp, avoid superimposing the dots or placing them too close together. This will result in patchy areas of pigment on the scalp that can produce an unnatural appearance.[6] The dots should be placed in an irregular pattern and not in a continuous line.[1,6] The

angle of the needle relative to the scalp can vary between 45, 60, and 90 degrees[1] (Fig. 7.6). Larger angles result in deeper penetration, darker tone, and longer duration of the pigment, while smaller angles result in a more superficial implantation with a lighter tone, opaque hue, and less durability of the pigment (Pearl 7.8). In addition, the needle should be positioned at a more perpendicular angle (90 degrees) when a dot is needed, and at a 60-degree angle for a line. Moderate pressure throughout the entire procedure should be used to obtain uniformity in color, and special attention should be made to any changes in angulation and/or depth of the needle.

PEARL 7.8: Larger angles result in deeper penetration, darker tone, and longer duration of the pigment. Smaller angles result in more superficial implantation with a lighter tone, opaque hue, and less durability of the pigment.

PEARL 7.9: When the needle is inserted deeper than necessary, even by a minimal amount, the pigment may spread to neighboring tissue.

Postoperative Care

Postoperative photography is recommended to monitor clinical success of SMP treatment. Immediately after the SMP procedure, the treated area of the scalp will appear red and inflamed for approximately 3 to 4 days. Petrolatum (e.g., Aquaphor or Vaseline) may be applied immediately after the procedure, then daily.[1] Hair washing with a mild shampoo is allowed after 2 to 3 days.[7]

A superficial crust will develop over the tattooed (pigmented) areas. This will resolve slowly over the next week, resulting in a lightened tone after the scabs and excess pigment have been expelled from the skin surface (stratum corneum and stratum granulosum).[7] The patient must be cautioned not to remove the scabs and to allow the scabs to fall off naturally. The remaining pigment is in the stratum spinosum within the track created by the needles, and in the papillary dermis.[7]

After 3 to 4 weeks, and when the scabs have completely healed, a second procedure to darken any areas of alopecia is recommended. In general, it is common for the pigment to fade over time. Patients should be advised that additional SMP procedures may be necessary in the future to enhance pigment intensity and if hair loss worsens.[6] As natural hair may become gray with time, patients should also be informed that it may be in their best interest to dye their hair a dark color if they develop many gray hairs that do not blend with the SMP pigment.[6]

Scar Correction Procedure

Correcting scars on the scalp with SMP is less invasive than surgery and thus is beneficial in patients who may develop a phobia of surgery.[6] SMP can be used to camouflage scars on the scalp with different causes. Examples include scars from a hair transplant procedure, rhytidectomy, surgical excision/biopsy, or trauma.[5,6]

In a study conducted by Park et al., 43 Korean patients underwent SMP for AGA and scalp scars.[6,16] There were six patients treated for scalp scars, five of whom had scars from previous hair transplants, and one of whom had a scar from an accidental fall.[6] Favorable outcomes were achieved among all six patients undergoing micropigmentation to cover their scars.[6] The evaluation of outcome was determined by satisfaction of cosmetic appearance according to the patient and surgeon.[6]

The procedure to camouflage scar tissue is complicated. The operator performing this technique should have ample experience performing SMP on patients with AGA and gauging needle depth.[6] The needle needs to penetrate at an adequate level of the scar tissue or else the outcome will not be favorable.[6] When the needle is deeper than necessary, even by a minimal amount, the pigment may spread to neighboring tissue (Pearl 7.9).[6] Conversely, if the needle is placed superficially, the pigment may not hold within the tissue.[6]

The scar correction procedure is depicted in Video 7.4. The first step in this procedure is to select the pigment that matches the skin surrounding the scar. Position the dermograph device with linear or circular three or five-pointed needles at an angle of 45 degrees (Fig. 7.7). Set the dermograph to a medium velocity, and use a scanning method to place

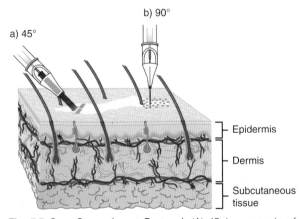

Fig. 7.7 Scar Concealment Protocol. (A) 45-degree angle of three- to five-tip needle to cover hypopigmented scar in a scanning motion. (B) 90-degree angle of a single-tip needle to add dots or lines to cover scar tissue. (Courtesy of Sheila Macomber.)

the pigment superficially over the scar. Once the hue of the scar is blended with the scalp, position the dermograph at an angle of 90 degrees with a single needle tip to create pigmented dots on the scalp. The dots should follow an irregular stippling pattern that matches the direction of hair growth (see Fig. 7.7). Once the scar is completely covered, randomly add dots around the scar into the normal tissue to blend the scarred tissue with the normal tissue, creating a "feathering" effect.[5] This is achieved by gradually decreasing pigment and the number of dots placed at the ends of the scar tissue.[5]

Clinical Correlates

Videos 7.5 and 7.6 and Figs. 7.8-7.15 depict clinical cases provided by one of the authors (SS). Each case

provides pre- and postoperative photography for SMP, microblading, or scar concealment.

PREVENTION AND MANAGEMENT OF ADVERSE EVENTS

Table 7.5 lists the complications that may occur after SMP. Many of the complications can be avoided through use of carefully selected pigment and a good understanding of the variables in the skin that can change from patient to patient. Complications after SMP usually result from improper technique. Improper needle insertion can result in pigment bleeding.[3,5] This results in leaking of the color from the original site of implantation. Other adverse events include postoperative edema and redness, which are usually transient and can

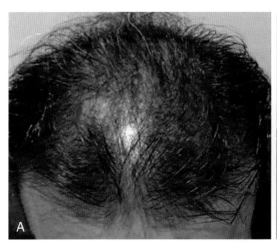
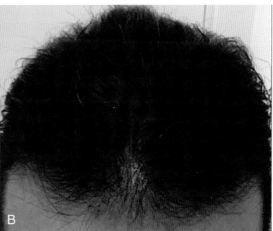

Fig. 7.8 Clinical Correlate: Androgenetic alopecia. (A) Male patient with androgenetic alopecia. (B) Results after three scalp micropigmentation sessions.

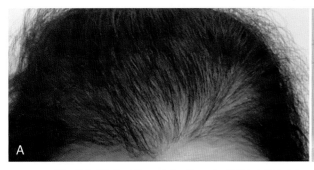
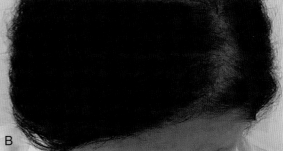

Fig. 7.9 Clinical Correlate: Female Pattern Hair Loss. (A) Patient with female pattern hair loss. (B) Added density after one scalp micropigmentation session.

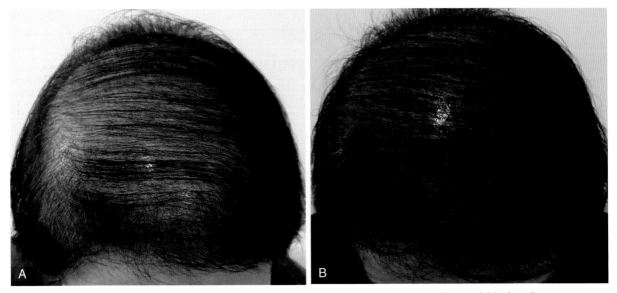

Fig. 7.10 Clinical Correlate: Hypothyroidism. (A) Female patient with hypothyroidism and thinning all over the head. (B) Results after three scalp micropigmentation sessions.

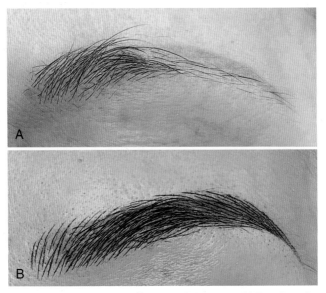

Fig. 7.11 Clinical Correlate: Microblading for Thinning Eyebrows. (A) Female patient with thinning eyebrows. (B) After two scalp micropigmentation sessions. (Image courtesy Dr. Mary Matsuda, Brazil)

be treated with systemic corticosteroids (level of evidence: 5)[1,18]. If a skin infection occurs postoperatively, systemic or topical antibiotic therapy is initiated. Color changes may occur with repeated sun exposure. Iron oxide-based inks usually turn a reddish tinge. In this case, strict sun protection is recommended to maintain pigment color in the skin. This unwanted pigment can be lightened by laser surgery with a Q-switched Nd:YAG laser on a low fluence setting using a spot size of 3 to 4 mm (level of evidence: 4)[19-21]. Skin pigment can be lightened with a Q-switch laser.[3,7,19,21] Rare complications include allergic reaction to the ink, koebnerization,

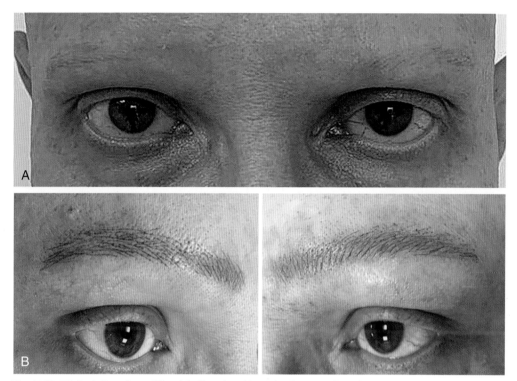

Fig. 7.12 Clinical Correlate: Microblading for Alopecia Areata. (A) Male patient with alopecia areata. (B) After one scalp micropigmentation session. (Image courtesy Dr. Mary Matsuda, Brazil)

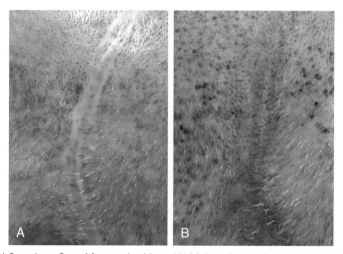

Fig. 7.13 Clinical Correlate: Scar After an Accident. (A) Male patient with linear scars on both sides of the head from an accident. (B) The scars have been concealed after one scalp micropigmentation session.

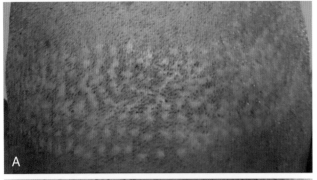

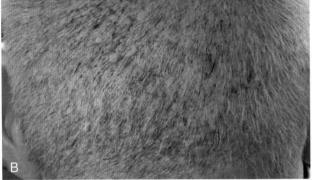

Fig. 7.14 Clinical Correlate: Scar from Previous Hair Transplant. (A) Male patient with numerous 4-mm scars after an old hair transplant technique. (B) Results after one scalp micropigmentation session; all scars have been covered.

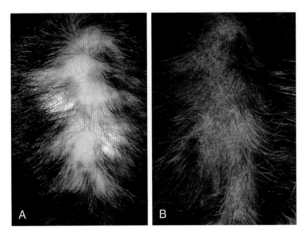

Fig. 7.15 Clinical Correlate: Systemic Lupus. (A) Female patient with systemic lupus and scar tissue on the crown of the scalp. (B) Results after three scalp micropigmentation sessions.

TABLE 7.5 Complications That May Occur After Scalp Micropigmentation
Pigment bleeding or blurring (leaking of color from site of insertion)
Postoperative edema
Redness
Blurring of pigment
Color changes with repeated sun exposure
Allergic reaction to the ink[a]
Koebnerization[a]
Granulomatous reactions[a]
Sarcoidal Granuloma[a]
Scarring[a]

[a]Rare complications of scalp micropigmentation
Dhurat RS, Shanshanwal SJS, Dandale AL. Standardization of SMP procedure and its impact on outcome. *J Cutan Aesthet Surg.* 2017;10(3):145-149; LeBlanc PM, Hollinger KA, Klontz KC. Tattoo ink–related infections — awareness, diagnosis, reporting, and prevention. *N Engl J Med.* 2012;367(11):985-987.

granulomatous reaction, sarcoidal granuloma (level of evidence: 4),[22] and scarring[15] (level of evidence: 5).[1,18]

FUTURE DIRECTIONS

SMP is a relatively new cosmetic procedure used to address hair loss involving the scalp. It can be used in patients with AGA to conceal or camouflage an area of alopecia, alongside medical or surgical treatment. This procedure is also an excellent alternative to improve the appearance of scars on the scalp, especially in patients who are not surgical candidates for scar revision. Dermatologists interested in increasing their scope of services to patients with alopecia or other scalp-related deformities may be motivated to acquire SMP skills.

Future directions include the expansion of various pigment shades to match all skin tones, the development of specific lasers that can target and easily remove unwanted pigment from the skin, the use of SMP for other indications (AA, scarring alopecias, off-scalp locations), and combining SMP with other aesthetic procedures such as platelet-rich plasma injections and follicular unit excision transplantation (level of evidence: 4).[23]

EVIDENCE SUMMARY

- Scalp micropigmentation should only be performed by a trained operator who has an artistic eye for detail (strength of recommendation: D).
- Avoid superimposing the dots of pigment into the scalp, as it may lead to an unnatural appearance (strength of recommendation: D).
- It is recommended to use small dots (points) for patients with short hair. In contrast, patients with long hair require small dots and small lines (strength of recommendation: C).
- The needle should be positioned at a perpendicular angle (90 degrees) when a dot is needed, and at a 60-degree angle for a line (strength of recommendation: D).
- Moderate pressure should be used throughout the entire procedure to obtain uniformity in color (strength of recommendation: D).
- The area that underwent scalp micropigmentation will produce a superficial scab. Patients should be instructed to not remove this superficial layer, as it will resolve on its own (strength of recommendation: D).
- Over time, the pigment will fade. Touch-ups are recommended to maintain the intensity of the pigment (strength of recommendation: D).
- Once a scar is completely covered, randomly add dots around the scar into the normal tissue to blend the scarred tissue with the normal tissue, creating a "feathering" effect (strength of recommendation: D).

REFERENCES

1. Dhurat R, Shanshanwal SJS, Dandale AL. Standardization of SMP procedure and its impact on outcome. *J Cutan Aesthet Surg.* 2017;10(3):145. Available at: https://doi.org/10.4103/jcas.jcas_116_16.
2. Garg G, Thami GP. Micropigmentation. *Dermatol Surg.* 2005;31(8):928-931. Available at: https://doi.org/10.1097/00042728-200508000-00007.
3. Rassman WR, Pak JP, Kim J. Scalp micropigmentation: a useful treatment for hair loss. *Facial Plast Surg Clin North Am.* 2013;21(3):497-503. Available at: https://doi.org/10.1016/j.fsc.2013.05.010.
4. Davis DS, Callender VD. Review of quality of life studies in women with alopecia. *Int J Womens Dermatol.* 2018;4(1):18-22. Available at: https://doi.org/10.1016/j.ijwd.2017.11.007.
5. Traquina AC. Micropigmentation as an adjuvant in cosmetic surgery of the scalp. *Dermatol Surg.* 2001;27(2):123-128. Available at: https://doi.org/10.1097/00042728-200102000-00005.
6. Park JH, Moh JS, Lee SY, You SH. Micropigmentation: camouflaging scalp alopecia and scars in Korean patients. *Aesthetic Plast Surg.* 2013;38(1):199-204. Available at: https://doi.org/10.1007/s00266-013-0259-1.
7. Rassman WR, Pak JP, Kim J, Estrin NF. Scalp micropigmentation: a concealer for hair and scalp deformities. *J Clin Aesthet Dermatol.* 2015;8(3):35-42.
8. Kim EK, Chang TJ, Hong JP, Koh KS. Use of tattooing to camouflage various scars. *Aesthetic Plast Surg.* 2011;35(3):392-395. Available at: https://doi.org/10.1007/s00266-011-9698-8.
9. Spyropoulou GA, Fatah F. Decorative tattooing for scar camouflage: patient innovation. *J Plast Reconstr Aesthet Surg.* 2009;62(10). Available at: https://doi.org/10.1016/j.bjps.2008.01.043.
10. Halder RM, Pham HN, Breadon JY, Johnson BA. Micropigmentation for the treatment of Vitiligo. *J Dermatol Surg Oncol.* 1989;15(10):1092-1098. Available at: https://doi.org/10.1111/j.1524-4725.1989.tb03129.x.
11. Offidani A, Cellini A, Peramezza C, Di Giuseppe A, Di Benedetto G. Tattooing: an alternative treatment for piebaldism. *Eur J Dermatol.* 1993;3:508.
12. Van der Velden EM, Drost BH, Ijsselmuiden OE, Baruchin AM, Hulsebosch HJ. Dermatography as a new treatment for alopecia areata of the eyebrows. *Int J Dermatol.* 1998;37(8):617-621. Available at: https://doi.org/10.1046/j.1365-4362.1998.00540.x.
13. Marwah MK, Kerure AS, Marwah GS. Microblading and the science behind it. *Indian Dermatol Online J.* 2021;12(1):6. Available at: https://doi.org/10.4103/idoj.idoj_230_20.
14. Donovan JC, Shapiro RL, Shapiro P, Zupan M, Pierre-Louis M, Hordinsky MK. A review of scalp camouflaging agents and prostheses for individuals with hair loss. *Dermatol Online J.* 2012;18(8). Available at: https://doi.org/10.5070/d38h70t82k.
15. Motoki THC, Isoldi FC, Ferreira LM. Pathologic scarring after eyebrow micropigmentation: a case report and systematic review. *Adv Skin Wound Care.* 2020;33(10):1-4. Available at: https://doi.org/10.1097/01.asw.0000672496.83825.75.
16. Okereke UR, Simmons A, Callender VD. Current and emerging treatment strategies for hair loss in women of color. *Int J Womens Dermatol.* 2019;5(1):37-45. Available at: https://doi.org/10.1016/j.ijwd.2018.10.021.
17. Saed S, Ibrahim O, Bergfeld WF. Hair camouflage: a comprehensive review. *Int J Womens Dermatol.* 2016;2(4):122-127. Available at: https://doi.org/10.1016/j.ijwd.2016.09.002.

18. LeBlanc PM, Hollinger KA, Klontz KC. Tattoo ink–related infections — awareness, diagnosis, reporting, and prevention. *N Engl J Med.* 2012;367(11):985-987. Available at: https://doi.org/10.1056/nejmp1206063.

19. Goldman A, Wollina U. Severe unexpected adverse effects after permanent eye makeup and their management by Q-Switched Nd:YAG Laser. *Clin Interv Aging.* 2014;2014:1305. Available at: https://doi.org/10.2147/cia.s67167.

20. Mao JC, DeJoseph LM. Latest innovations for tattoo and permanent makeup removal. *Facial Plast Surg Clin North Am.* 2012;20(2):125-134. doi:10.1016/j.fsc.2012.02.009.

21. Wu DC. Successful treatment of scalp micropigmentation with 1064 nm picosecond nd:YAG laser. *Lasers Surg Med.* 2020;53(7):935-938. Available at: https://doi.org/10.1002/lsm.23364.

22. Valbuena MC, Franco VE, Sánchez L, Jiménez HD. Sarcoidal granulomatous reaction due to tattoos: report of two cases. *An Bras Dermatol.* 2017;92(5 suppl 1):138-141. Available at: https://doi.org/10.1590/abd1806-4841.20175860.

23. Rassman W, Pak J, Kim J. Combining follicular unit extraction and scalp micropigmentation for the cosmetic treatment of alopecias. *Plast Reconstr Surg Glob Open.* 2017;5(11):e1420. Available at: https://doi.org/10.1097/gox.0000000000001420.

Medical Treatments for Hair Loss

8

Minoxidil, Finasteride, and Dutasteride

Wilma F. Bergfeld and Claudia M. Ricotti

KEY POINTS

- Androgenetic alopecia is the most common cause of alopecia in both men and women; however, approved therapeutic treatment options are limited.
- Patients should be counseled that treatment of androgenetic alopecia is directed toward prevention of further hair thinning and loss, as complete hair regrowth may not be achieved.
- Topical minoxidil is an Food and Drug Administration–approved, first line treatment for androgenetic alopecia in both men and women. Oral low-dose minoxidil is not Food and Drug Administration approved for the treatment of androgenetic alopecia but may be considered in patients who are unwilling or unable to use the topical formulation.

- The enzyme 5α-reductase converts testosterone to dihydrotestosterone, thereby inducing hair follicle miniaturization in androgenetic alopecia. Inhibition of this pathway is the target of the 5α-reductase inhibitors finasteride and dutasteride.
- Oral finasteride is a type II 5α-reductase inhibitor that is Food and Drug Administration–approved and a first line treatment for androgenetic alopecia in men. Oral dutasteride is a type I and type II 5α-reductase inhibitor that is not Food and Drug Administration approved; however, it can be considered a second-line treatment for androgenetic alopecia in men.
- Topical 5α-reductase inhibitors are a promising area of investigation for the treatment of androgenetic alopecia.

BACKGROUND, DEFINITIONS, AND HISTORY

Androgenetic alopecia (AGA) is the most common cause of alopecia in both men and women.[1] Despite its high prevalence, approved therapeutic options for AGA are limited.[2] Treatment of AGA is directed toward prevention of further hair thinning and loss, which can affect both quality of life and self-esteem (level of evidence: 1).[1,3] This chapter discusses the U.S. Food and Drug Administration (FDA)-approved treatment options for AGA, including topical minoxidil and oral finasteride.[3] Non-FDA approved treatment options including oral dutasteride, oral minoxidil, and topical finasteride are also discussed.

Minoxidil (Rogaine [topical]), the first FDA-approved treatment for AGA in men and women, was originally developed as an oral hypertension medication.[4] Its possible use in AGA was incidentally discovered as a result of its side effect of increased hair growth.[4] The exact mechanism by which minoxidil promotes hair growth remains unclear, but it is thought to be partly caused by potassium channel opening.[4] Minoxidil is an inactive metabolite transformed into its active metabolite, minoxidil sulfate, by the enzyme sulphotranspherase.[4] Minoxidil sulfate then opens adenosine triphosphate (ATP)-sensitive potassium channels in cell membranes, leading to vasodilation.[4] Other mechanisms by which minoxidil is thought to promote hair growth include stimulation of vascular endothelial growth factor and increased prostaglandin synthesis.[5]

The 5α-reductase inhibitors finasteride (Propecia [oral]) and dutasteride (Avodart [oral]) were initially developed and approved for the treatment of benign prostatic hyperplasia.[4] The enzyme 5α-reductase converts testosterone to the more potent dihydrotestosterone (DHT), which induces characteristic miniaturization of the hair follicles in AGA (Fig. 8.1).[3] There are type I and type II isoenzymes of 5α-reductase, and their expression varies depending on body location.[6] Hair follicles express higher concentrations of the type I isoenzyme, suggesting a key role in androgen-regulated hair growth.[6,7] Finasteride is a type II 5α-reductase inhibitor that decreases serum DHT levels by about 65% (see Fig. 8.1).[4] In contrast, dutasteride inhibits both type I and type II isoenzymes, further reducing serum DHT levels by 90% (see Fig. 8.1).[1,8]

INDICATIONS AND PATIENT SELECTION

Topical minoxidil is the first line treatment for AGA in both men and women (level of evidence: 1) (Pearl 8.1).[3,4,9-12] For men, the 2% solution was approved in 1988, the 5% solution in 1991, and the 5%

> **PEARL 8.1:** Topical minoxidil is first line for the treatment of androgenetic alopecia in both men and women.

foam in 2016.[1] For women, the 2% solution was approved in 1991, and the 5% foam was approved in 2014.[1] Topical minoxidil 2-5% solution or 5% foam twice daily is recommended for treatment of mild-to-moderate AGA in men ages 18 and older (Table 8.1).[4] Topical minoxidil 2% solution twice daily or 5% topical foam once daily is recommended for treatment of mild-to-moderate AGA in women ages 18 and older (see Table 8.1).[4] Topical minoxidil is not advised for use in women who are pregnant or breastfeeding.[4,12]

Oral finasteride is FDA approved for treatment of AGA in men and is also considered a first-line therapy (level of evidence: 1) (Pearl 8.2).[3,9] The recommended dose of finasteride is 1 mg once daily for men older than 18 years of age to prevent progression or to improve mild-to-moderate AGA (Table 8.2) (level of evidence: 1).[4] Oral dutasteride is not currently FDA approved for treatment of AGA but can be considered a second-line treatment in men older than 18 years of age who have failed previous treatment over 12 months

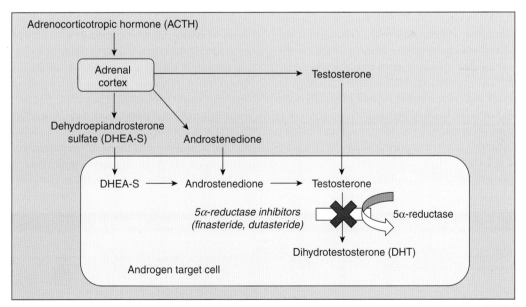

Fig. 8.1 The enzyme 5α-reductase converts testosterone to the more potent dihydrotestosterone (DHT), inducing characteristic miniaturization of the hair follicles in androgenetic alopecia (AGA). Inhibition of this pathway is the target of the 5α-reductase inhibitors finasteride and dutasteride.

TABLE 8.1 Summary of Topical Treatments for Androgenetic Alopecia

Medication	Dosage	Side Effects
Topical minoxidil	2% solution twice daily, 5% solution twice daily (men), 5% foam twice daily (men), or once daily (women)	Transitory increase in hair shedding, scalp irritation and erythema, facial hypertrichosis
Topical finasteride	0.25% solution once daily	Scalp irritation and erythema, testicular pain, headaches, presyncope

PEARL 8.2: The 5α-reductase inhibitors include finasteride and dutasteride. Finasteride is FDA-approved and a first-line treatment for androgenetic alopecia in men, whereas dutasteride is not FDA-approved and considered a second-line treatment.

with finasteride (level of evidence: 1).[4] The recommended dose of dutasteride is 0.5 mg once daily (see Table 8.2).[4] Finasteride and dutasteride are contraindicated in pregnancy and women of childbearing age.[13]

EXPECTED OUTCOMES

The efficacy of topical minoxidil in treating male and female AGA has been established by numerous double-blind, randomized, placebo-controlled trials and meta-analyses.[1] Kanti et al. assessed the efficacy of topical minoxidil in 48 studies of AGA in men and 19 studies AGA in women.[4] The majority of trials reported findings on the efficacy of topical minoxidil 2% solution, 5% solution, or 5% foam.[4] In male AGA, randomized controlled trials confirmed minoxidil 5% solution and 5% foam are more effective for hair regrowth than the 2% solution (Figs. 8.2 and 8.3) (level of evidence: 1b).[1,14,15] In female AGA, once-daily 5% foam was similar in efficacy

compared with the 2% solution twice daily (level of evidence: 1b) (Fig. 8.4).[1,16,17] In all studies, topical minoxidil led to significant increases in total hair count when compared with placebo. The mean changes from baseline total hair count were 5.4 hairs/cm^2 and 29.9 hairs/cm^2 at 4 and 6 months, followed by counts between 15.5 hairs/cm^2 and 83.3 hairs/cm^2 at 12 months (level of evidence: 1b).[1,18-35] Visible hair growth was most apparent at four to six months with continuous application of topical minoxidil.[5] To maintain any beneficial effect, applications must continue indefinitely to prevent hair loss.[4,10,36] If topical minoxidil treatment is stopped, clinical regression occurs within six months.[10,36]

Systematic reviews of long-term use of finasteride 1 mg daily for treatment of male AGA report noticeable improvement in 30% of patients at 3 months of use (level of evidence: 1a).[1,37] Kanti et al. reviewed 25 studies assessing the efficacy of finasteride as a monotherapy for treatment of AGA in males.[4] In all included trials, finasteride 1 mg daily led to a significant increase in total hair count compared to placebo.[4] The mean change from baseline total hair count was 7.0 hairs/cm^2 in the frontal and centroparietal regions and 13.5 hairs/cm^2 in the vertex at 6 months (level of evidence: 1b).[4,38,39] The mean increase from baseline total hair counts at 12 months was between 9.3 hairs/cm^2 and 9.6 hairs/cm^2

TABLE 8.2 Summary of Systemic Treatments for Androgenetic Alopecia

Medication	Dosage	Side Effects
Oral finasteride	1 mg once daily	Decreased libido, erectile dysfunction, decreased ejaculation volume, depression, hypersensitivity reactions, breast tenderness, gynecomastia
Oral dutasteride	0.5 mg once daily	
Oral minoxidil	0.25–2.5 mg once daily	Hypertrichosis, hypotension, bradycardia, pedal edema, electrocardiogram changes

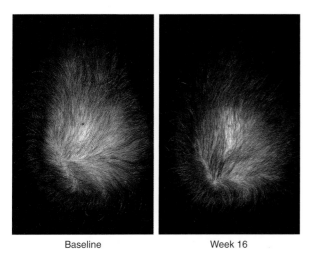

Baseline Week 16

Fig. 8.2 A 41-year-old male with androgenetic alopecia (AGA) treated with daily application of topical minoxidil 5% foam, at baseline (A) and with moderate hair growth at week 16, rated by an expert panel (B). (Reprinted with permission from Olsen E, Whiting D, Bergfeld W, et al. A multicenter, randomized, placebo-controlled, double-blind clinical trial of a novel formulation of 5 % minoxidil topical foam versus placebo in the treatment of androgenetic alopecia in men. *J Am Acad Dermatol.* 2007;57:767-774. Copyright Elsevier 2007.)

in the frontal and centroparietal region and 7.2 hairs/cm^2 and 36.1 hairs/cm^2 in the vertex (level of evidence: 1b).[4,40-46] In general, daily use for 3 months or more is necessary before benefit is observed (Figs. 8.5 and 8.6).[4] Continued use is recommended to sustain the benefit, as withdrawal of treatment leads to gradual hair loss and return to the pretreatment status within 1 year.[1,47] For greater efficacy, oral finasteride 1 mg may be combined with topical minoxidil.[4]

In comparison with minoxidil and finasteride, fewer randomized controlled studies have analyzed the efficacy of dutasteride to treat AGA in males.[1] In 2006, the first randomized controlled trial compared the effect of dutasteride 0.05, 0.1, 0.5, and 2.5 mg, finasteride 5 mg, and placebo in 416 men with AGA over 24 weeks (level of evidence: 1b).[1,48] Dutasteride 2.5 mg was shown to be superior over finasteride 5 mg in increasing hair count (level of evidence: 1b).[1,48] In 2014, a randomized controlled trial comparing dutasteride 0.02, 0.1, and 0.5 mg daily with finasteride 1 mg daily and placebo in 917 men over 24 weeks revealed that dutasteride 0.5 mg was statistically superior than finasteride 1 mg and placebo at increasing hair count after 24 weeks (level of evidence: 1b)

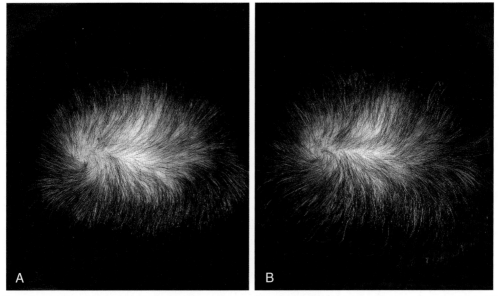

Fig. 8.3 A 33-year-old male with androgenetic alopecia (AGA) treated with daily application of topical minoxidil 5% foam, at baseline (A) and with moderate hair growth at week 16, rated by an expert panel (B). (Reprinted with permission from Olsen E, Whiting D, Bergfeld W, et al. A multicenter, randomized, placebo-controlled, double-blind clinical trial of a novel formulation of 5 % minoxidil topical foam versus placebo in the treatment of androgenetic alopecia in men. *J Am Acad Dermatol.* 2007;57:767-774. Copyright Elsevier 2007.)

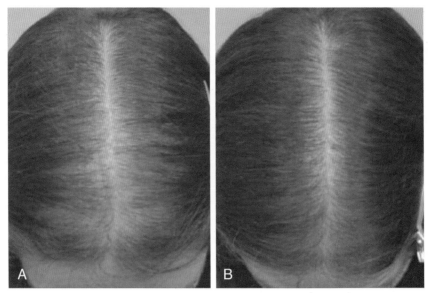

Fig. 8.4 Before (A) and after (B) use of topical 5% minoxidil for 6 months. (Reprinted with permission from Rogers NE. Medical Therapy for Female Pattern Hair Loss. *Hair Transplant Forum International.* 2014;24(3): 81–88. Copyright The International Society of Hair Restoration Surgery 2014.)

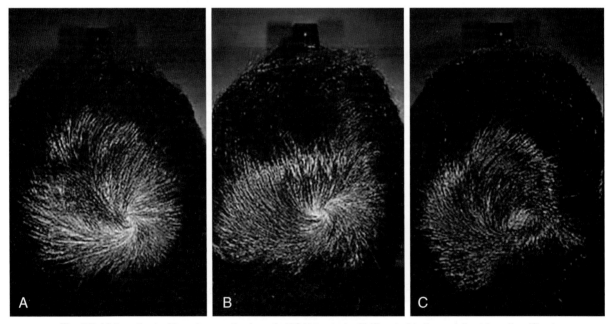

Fig. 8.5 Male patient with androgenetic alopecia (AGA) treated with finasteride 1 mg daily at baseline (A), at 12 months with moderately increased hair growth (B), and at 24 months with greatly increased hair growth (C). (Reprinted with permission from Kaufman KD, Olsen EA, Whiting D, et al. Finasteride in the treatment of men with androgenetic alopecia. *J Am Acad Dermatol.* 1998;39(4):578-589. Copyright Elsevier 1998.)

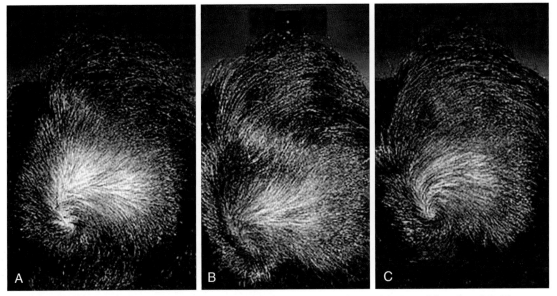

Fig. 8.6 Male patient with androgenetic alopecia (AGA) treated with finasteride 1 mg daily at baseline (A), at 12 months with slightly increased hair growth (B), and at 24 months with moderately increased hair growth (C). (Reprinted with permission from Kaufman KD, Olsen EA, Whiting D, et al. Finasteride in the treatment of men with androgenetic alopecia. *J Am Acad Dermatol.* 1998;39(4):578-589. Copyright Elsevier 1998.)

(Fig. 8.7).[1,49] Based on systematic reviews and meta-analyses, dutasteride may provide better efficacy compared to finasteride for treatment of male AGA (level of evidence: 1a).[50] Further case series have shown efficacy of dutasteride in males with AGA who have failed prior treatment with oral finasteride over 12 months (level of evidence: 4).[1,52,52]

TREATMENT TECHNIQUE AND BEST PRACTICES

For men, twice-daily application of topical minoxidil 2% solution, 5% solution, or 5% foam in the morning and evening is recommended.[4,53] For women, twice-daily application of topical minoxidil 2% solution or once daily 5% foam is recommended.[4] The 5% solution or 5% foam are generally recommended for greater efficacy.[4] To prepare for application, hair should be parted in the area of thinning or loss.[53] Minoxidil should be applied as 1 mL of solution with a pipette or half a cap of foam to dry hair and scalp.[4] After application, the hands should be washed with warm water.[4] Shampooing the hair is not recommended for

4 hours after applying treatment.[53] Generally, normal hair-care practices can be continued during treatment.[53] If one or two daily doses of minoxidil are missed, treatment should continue with the next dose, and the patient should not make up for missed doses.[53] It is not recommended to use minoxidil more than twice daily.[53]

The recommended dose of finasteride for treatment of AGA in males is one tablet (1 mg) daily.[4,47] Finasteride can be taken with or without food, and no pertinent drug interactions have been identified.[47] However, caution should be exercised in patients with liver dysfunction, as finasteride is metabolized by the liver.[47] The recommended dose of dutasteride for treatment of AGA in males is one capsule (0.5 mg) daily.[13] The capsule should be swallowed whole and not chewed or opened, as contact with capsule contents can result in irritation of the oropharyngeal mucosa.[13] Dutasteride may be administered with or without food.[13] Dutasteride is extensively metabolized by the CYP3A4 and CYP3A5 isoenzymes, and caution should be used in patients taking CYP3A4 enzyme inhibitors (e.g., ritonavir).[13]

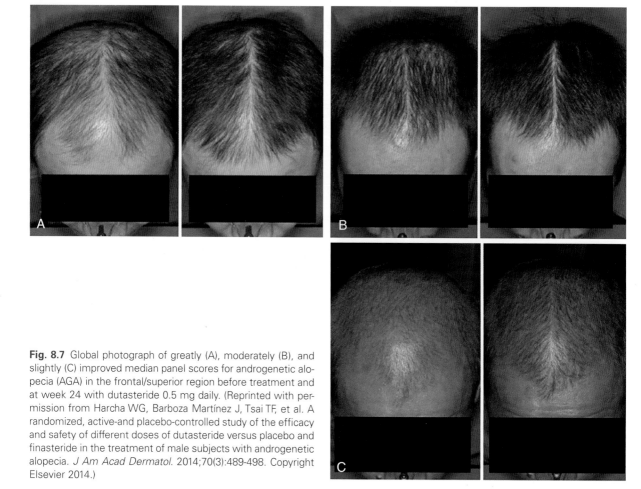

Fig. 8.7 Global photograph of greatly (A), moderately (B), and slightly (C) improved median panel scores for androgenetic alopecia (AGA) in the frontal/superior region before treatment and at week 24 with dutasteride 0.5 mg daily. (Reprinted with permission from Harcha WG, Barboza Martínez J, Tsai TF, et al. A randomized, active-and placebo-controlled study of the efficacy and safety of different doses of dutasteride versus placebo and finasteride in the treatment of male subjects with androgenetic alopecia. *J Am Acad Dermatol.* 2014;70(3):489-498. Copyright Elsevier 2014.)

Baseline prostate specific antigen (PSA) levels are recommended in men older than 50 years of age prior to initiating treatment with 5α-reductase inhibitors.[1] Total serum PSA levels may be reduced by up to 50% when taking finasteride or dutasteride.[4,13] For accurate interpretation of test results, the PSA level should be doubled.[4,13] Any increase from the lowest PSA value may signal the presence of prostate cancer, even if levels are within normal range for men not taking 5α-reductase inhibitors.[47] High-grade prostate cancers (e.g., Gleason score 8–10) are also reported with increased incidence in men taking 5α-reductase inhibitors.[4,47] However, this is not thought to affect survival outcomes in comparison with patients who have low-grade prostate cancers.[4,47]

PREVENTION AND MANAGEMENT OF ADVERSE EVENTS

Topical minoxidil has exceptional safety and tolerability. Minor adverse effects of topical minoxidil include a transitory increase in hair shedding, contact dermatitis, and facial hypertrichosis (Pearl 8.3). Patients should be counseled on transitory hair shedding, which can be seen within the first few weeks of treatment.[1,4] Therapy should be maintained through shedding, as telogen

> **PEARL 8.3:** Minor adverse effects of topical minoxidil include transitory increase in hair shedding, contact dermatitis, and facial hypertrichosis.

follicles are reentering the anagen phase, indicating efficacy.[1] The most common side effect of topical minoxidil is hypertrichosis, usually seen in women using the 5% preparations.[4] Hypertrichosis related to minoxidil therapy is most often caused by incorrect application or inadvertent contact with the face.[4] To avoid contamination of the pillow and subsequent contact with the face, patients should apply minoxidil at least 2 hours before going to bed.[4] Hypertrichosis usually resolves 1 to 3 months after discontinuation of therapy.[1] Irritant and allergic contact dermatitis may also occur with topical minoxidil and are often caused by ingredients of the vehicle, particularly propylene glycol.[1,4] The foam formulation is an option in the case of suspected contact dermatitis, as it does not contain propylene glycol.[1] If contact dermatitis is suspected, confirmation with patch testing is recommended (Fig. 8.8).[4]

The most common adverse reactions associated with 5α-reductase inhibitors include decreased libido, erectile dysfunction, and decreased ejaculation volume (Pearl 8.4).[47] In three controlled clinical trials of finasteride, 1.4% of patients taking finasteride discontinued use as a result of medication-related adverse reactions.[47] Resolution of sexual dysfunction most often occurred in men who discontinued therapy (level of evidence: 1b).[47] Several published case series have reported sexual dysfunction and loss

> **PEARL 8.4:** The most common adverse reactions associated with 5α-reductase inhibitors include decreased libido, erectile dysfunction, and decreased ejaculation volume.

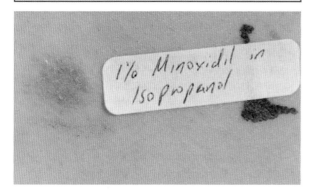

Fig. 8.8 Positive allergic contact reaction to 1% minoxidil in isopropanol, demonstrated by patch testing. (Reprinted with permission from Friedman ES, Friedman PM, Cohen DE, Washenik K. Allergic contact dermatitis to topical minoxidil solution: etiology and treatment. *J Am Acad Dermatol.* 2002;46(2):309-312. Copyright Elsevier 2002.)

of libido persisting for months or years after discontinuation of finasteride (level of evidence: 4).[4,54-59] This has been referred to as "postfinasteride syndrome" (PFS), although a clear causal relationship with finasteride use has not yet been established.[4] Sexual dysfunction associated with dutasteride is reported more frequently within the first 6 months of therapy.[1] However, at the end of 24 months, the onset of new adverse effects was reported as similar to those not taking dutasteride (level of evidence: 1a).[1,60] Less common adverse reactions of 5α-reductase inhibitors reported in postmarketing data include hypersensitivity reactions (e.g., rash, pruritus, urticaria, swelling of the lips or face), breast tenderness or gynecomastia, and depression.[47]

Finasteride and dutasteride are contraindicated in women who are pregnant or may become pregnant as a result of their teratogenicity.[13,47] Due to a lack of data in nursing mothers, these medications are also not indicated for use in breastfeeding women. By inhibiting the conversion of testosterone to DHT, 5α-reductase inhibitors may cause abnormalities of the external genitalia of a male fetus if taken by a pregnant woman.[13,47] Men taking 5α-reductase inhibitors should not donate blood, in order to prevent transmission to a pregnant woman during blood transfusion.[1,61] Men taking finasteride should wait 1 month after the last dose to donate blood, whereas those taking dutasteride should wait 6 months after the last dose.[62] Finasteride and dutasteride are also contraindicated in patients who have had clinically significant hypersensitivity reactions (e.g., angioedema) to 5α-reductase inhibitors.[13,47]

FUTURE DIRECTIONS

Although oral minoxidil (Loniten) is not FDA approved for the treatment of AGA, clinical trials have displayed effectiveness and safety using oral minoxidil at various low doses of 0.25 to 2.5 mg daily.[63] In an open-label, prospective, single-arm study, 5 mg oral minoxidil was evaluated for the treatment of AGA in men (level of evidence: 1b).[4,64] After 24 weeks of treatment, total hair count showed a statistically significant increase of 35.1 hairs/cm^2, only slightly higher compared with topical administration (level of evidence: 1b).[4,64] A 24-week, randomized controlled trial additionally concluded that 1 mg oral minoxidil for the treatment of female AGA was comparable in efficacy to the topical 5% solution (level of evidence: 1b).[65] Adverse effects include hypertrichosis (most common), decreased blood pressure, decreased heart rate, pedal edema, and electrocardiogram

> **PEARL 8.5:** Low-dose oral minoxidil and topical finasteride are promising therapeutic options in the treatment of androgenetic alopecia that have shown considerable safety and efficacy.

changes (level of evidence: 1b).[4,64] Significant adverse effects were not reported with low-dose oral minoxidil, indicating its potential use as a reasonable alternative in those intolerant of or unwilling to use the topical preparation.[64,65]

Current data suggest that there is promising therapeutic potential for topical finasteride in the treatment of AGA (Pearl 8.5).[66] A 2018 randomized, double-blind controlled study reviewed the efficacy and safety of topical finasteride 0.25% solution in 40 men with AGA (level of evidence: 1b).[67] Participants were randomized to 24 weeks of treatment with finasteride 0.25% solution with minoxidil 3% solution or minoxidil 3% solution twice daily.[67] At week 24, the combined solution of finasteride and minoxidil was significantly superior to minoxidil alone in improvements of hair density, hair diameter, and global photographic assessment (level of evidence: 1b).[67] Studies comparing topical finasteride 0.25% solution to oral finasteride 1 mg have shown that both significantly suppress plasma DHT levels (level of evidence: 1a).[66,68] However, topical finasteride was shown to have decreased systemic absorption, indicating a lower risk of adverse effects when compared to oral finasteride.[66] Serious or life-threatening adverse effects have not been reported with topical finasteride.[65] Minor adverse effects include scalp irritation and erythema, increased liver enzymes, testicular pain, headaches, and presyncope.[66,68-70] Currently, topical finasteride 0.25% solution applied once daily appears to be the most efficacious concentration and frequency (level of evidence: 1a) (see Table 8.1).[66] Further studies are warranted to determine the efficacy, therapeutic safety, cost-effectiveness, and patient tolerability and satisfaction.[66]

Finally, the janus kinase (JAK) inhibitors have emerged as highly effective treatment options for alopecia areata (AA) through inhibition of inflammatory signaling pathways in hair follicles.[71-73] JAK inhibitors have also been considered for treatment of other types of hair loss disorders, including AGA.[72,73] At the time of this publication, an open-label study to assess the safety, tolerability, and efficacy of the investigational JAK 1/3 inhibitor, topical ATI-50002 0.46% solution, in male and female subjects with AGA is undergoing clinical trial.[74]

EVIDENCE SUMMARY

For men with androgenetic alopecia, treatment with twice-daily application of topical minoxidil 5% solution or 5% foam is recommended (strength of recommendation: A). For women, twice-daily application of topical minoxidil 2% solution or once daily 5% foam is recommended (strength of recommendation: A). The 5% solution or 5% foam is generally recommended for greater efficacy (strength of recommendation: B). Low-dose oral minoxidil may be considered for use in the treatment of androgenetic alopecia for males and females (strength of recommendation: B). Oral finasteride 1 mg once daily is recommended for treatment of male androgenetic alopecia (strength of recommendation: A). Oral dutasteride 0.5 mg once daily may be used as a second-line treatment for male androgenetic alopecia and may be superior in efficacy when compared to finasteride (strength of recommendation: B). Novel therapies, including low-dose oral minoxidil and topical finasteride, are not currently Food and Drug Administration approved for treatment of androgenetic alopecia but show considerable safety, tolerability, and efficacy (strength of recommendation: C).

REFERENCES

1. Kelly Y, Blanco A, Tosti A. Androgenetic alopecia: an update of treatment options. *Drugs.* 2016;76(14):1349-1364.
2. Varothai S, Bergfeld WF. Androgenetic alopecia: an evidence-based treatment update. *Am J Clin Dermatol.* 2014;15(3):217-230.
3. Adil A, Godwin M. The effectiveness of treatments for androgenetic alopecia: a systematic review and meta-analysis. *J Am Acad Dermatol.* 2017;77(1):136-141.
4. Kanti V, Messenger A, Dobos G, et al. Evidence based (s3) guidelines for the treatment of androgenetic alopecia in women and in men. *J Eur Acad Dermatol Venereol.* 2017. Available at: https://turkderm.org.tr/turkdermData/Uploads/files/S3_guideline_androgenetic_alopecia_update_final-version.pdf. Accessed April 20, 2021.
5. Messenger AG, Rundegren J. Minoxidil: mechanisms of action on hair growth. *Br J Dermatol.* 2004;150(2):186-194.
6. Martinez-Jacobo L, Villarreal-Villarreal CD, Ortiz-López R, Ocampo-Candiani J, Rojas-Martínez A. Genetic and

molecular aspects of androgenetic alopecia. *Indian J Dermatol Venereol Leprol*. 2018;84(3):263.

7. Liu S, Yamauchi H. Different patterns of 5alpha-reductase expression, cellular distribution, and testosterone metabolism in human follicular dermal papilla cells. *Biochem Biophys Res Commun*. 2008;368:858-864.

8. Clark RV, Hermann DJ, Cunningham GR, Wilson TH, Morrill BB, Hobbs S. Marked suppression of dihydrotestosterone in men with benign prostatic hyperplasia by dutasteride, a dual 5-alpha-reductase inhibitor. *J Clin Endocrinol Metab*. 2004;89:2179-2184.

9. Goren A, Naccarato T. Minoxidil in the treatment of androgenetic alopecia. *Dermatol Ther*. 2018;31(5):e12686.

10. Sinclair RD. Female pattern hair loss: a pilot study investigating combination therapy with low-dose oral minoxidil and spironolactone. *Int J Dermatol*. 2018;57(1):104-109.

11. DeVillez RL, Jacobs JP, Szpunar CA, Warner ML. Androgenetic alopecia in the female: treatment with 2% topical minoxidil solution. *Arch Dermatol*. 1994;130(3):303-307.

12. Murase JE, Heller MM, Butler DC. Safety of dermatologic medications in pregnancy and lactation: part I. Pregnancy. *J Am Acad Dermatol*. 2014;70(3):401.e1-414.

13. Dutasteride. *Highlights of Prescribing Information*. Available at: https://www.accessdata.fda.gov/drugsatfda_docs/label/2011/021319s023s025lbl.pdf. Accessed April 20, 2021.

14. Olsen EA, Dunlap FE, Funicella T, et al. A randomized clinical trial of 5% topical minoxidil versus 2% topical minoxidil and placebo in the treatment of androgenetic alopecia in men. *J Am Acad Dermatol*. 2002;47(3):377-385.

15. Olsen E, Whiting D, Bergfeld W, et al. A multicenter, randomized, placebo-controlled, double-blind clinical trial of a novel formulation of 5 % minoxidil topical foam versus placebo in the treatment of androgenetic alopecia in men. *J Am Acad Dermatol*. 2007;57:767-774.

16. Blume-Peytavi U, Hillmann K, Dietz E, Canfield D, Bartels NG. A randomized, single-blind trial of 5 % minoxidil foam once daily versus 2 % minoxidil solution twice daily in the treatment of androgenetic alopecia in women. *J Am Acad Dermatol*. 2011;65:1126-1134.

17. Rogers NE. Medical Therapy for Female Pattern Hair Loss (FHPL). *Hair Transplant Forum International*. 2014;24(3):81-88.

18. Tsuboi R, Arano O, Nishikawa T, Yamada H, Katsuoka K. Randomized clinical trial comparing 5% and 1% topical minoxidil for the treatment of androgenetic alopecia in Japanese men. *J Dermatol*. 2009;36(8):437-446.

19. Karam P. Topical minoxidil therapy for androgenic alopecia in the Middle East. The Middle-Eastern Topical Minoxidil Study Group. *Int J Dermatol*. 1993;32(10):763-766.

20. Califano A, Virgili A, Caputo R, et al. 2% Minoxidil topical solution in the treatment of alopecia androgenetica.

A controlled clinical study. *G Ital Dermatol Venereol*. 1991;126(3):V-X.

21. Anderson CD, Hansted B, Abdallah MA, et al. Topical minoxidil in androgenetic alopecia. Scandinavian and Middle East experience. *Int J Dermatol*. 1988;27(6):447-451.

22. Dutree M, Nieboer C, Koedijk FHJ, Stolz E. Treatment of male pattern alopecia using topical minoxidil in The Netherlands. *Int J Dermatol*. 1988;27(6):435-440.

23. Petzoldt D, Borelli S, Braun-Falco O, et al. The German double-blind placebo-controlled evaluation of topical minoxidil solution in the treatment of early male pattern baldness. *Int J Dermatol*. 1988;27(6):430-434.

24. Olsen EA, DeLong ER, Weiner MS. Dose-response study of topical minoxidil in male pattern baldness. *J Am Acad Dermatol*. 1986;15(1):30-37.

25. Lopez-Bran E, Robledo A, Aspiolea F, et al. Multicenter comparative study of the efficacy of topical 2% minoxidil (Rogaine) versus placebo in the treatment of male baldness. *Adv Ther*. 1990;7(3):159-168.

26. Civatte J, Degreef H, Dockx P, et al. Topical 2% minoxidil solution in male pattern alopecia: the initial European experience. *Int J Dermatol*. 1988;27(6):424-429.

27. Alanis A, Barbara F, Meurehg C, Montes D, Ramirez L. Double-blind comparison of 2% topical minoxidil and placebo in early male pattern baldness. *Curr Ther Res Clin Exp*. 1991;49(5):723-730.

28. Olsen EA, Weiner MS, Delong ER, Pinnell SR. Topical minoxidil in early male pattern baldness. *J Am Acad Dermatol*. 1985;13(2):185-192.

29. Savin RC. Use of topical minoxidil in the treatment of male pattern baldness. *J Am Acad Dermatol*. 1987;16(3):696-704.

30. Kreindler TG. Topical minoxidil in early androgenetic alopecia. *J Am Acad Dermatol*. 1987;16(3):718-724.

31. Hillmann K, Garcia Bartels N, Stroux A, Canfield D, Blume-Peytavi U. Investigator-initiated double-blind, two-armed, placebo-controlled, randomized clinical trial with an open-label extension phase, to investigate the efficacy of 5% Minoxidil topical foam twice daily in men with androgenetic alopecia in the fronto-temporal and vertex regions regarding hair volume over 24/52 weeks. *J Invest Dermatol*. 2013;133(5):1400.

32. Rietschel RL, Duncan SH. Safety and efficacy of topical minoxidil in the management of androgenetic alopecia. *J Am Acad Dermatol*. 1987;16(3):677-685.

33. Roberts JL. Androgenetic alopecia: treatment results with topical minoxidil. *J Am Acad Dermatol*. 1987;16(3):705-710.

34. Saraswat A, Kumar B. Minoxidil vs finasteride in the treatment of men with androgenetic alopecia. *Arch Dermatol*. 2003;139(9):1219-1221.

35. Reygagne P, Assouly P, Catoni I, et al. Male androgenic alopecia. Randomized trial versus 2% minoxidil. *Les nouvelles dermatologiques*. 1997;16(2):59-63.

36. Olsen EA, DeLong ER, Weiner MS. Long-term follow-up of men with male pattern baldness treated with topical minoxidil. *J Am Acad Dermatol*. 1987;16:688-695.

37. Mella JM, Perret MC, Manzotti M, Catalano HN, Guyatt G. Efficacy and safety of finasteride therapy for androgenetic alopecia: a systematic review. *Arch Dermatol*. 2010;146:1141-1150.

38. Leyden J, Dunlap F, Miller B, et al. Finasteride in the treatment of men with frontal male pattern hair loss. *J Am Acad Dermatol*. 1999;40(6):930-937.

39. Roberts JL, Fiedler V, Imperato-McGinley J, et al. Clinical dose ranging studies with finasteride, a type 2 5alpha-reductase inhibitor, in men with male pattern hair loss. *J Am Acad Dermatol*. 1999;41(4):555-563.

40. Kaufman KD, Olsen EA, Whiting D, et al. Finasteride in the treatment of men with androgenetic alopecia. *J Am Acad Dermatol*. 1998;39(4):578-589.

41. Stough DB, Rao NA, Kaufman KD, Mitchell C. Finasteride improves male pattern hair loss in a randomized study in identical twins. *Eur J Dermatol*. 2002;12(1):32-37.

42. Van-Neste D, Fuh V, Sanchez-Pedreno P, et al. Finasteride increases anagen hair in men with androgenetic alopecia. *Br J Dermatol*. 2000;143(4):804-810.

43. Leyden J, Dunlap F, Miller B, et al. Finasteride in the treatment of men with frontal male pattern hair loss. *J Am Acad Dermatol*. 1999;40(6):930-937.

44. Whiting DA, Waldstreicher J, Sanchez M, Kaufman KD. Measuring reversal of hair miniaturization in androgenetic alopecia by follicular counts in horizontal sections of serial scalp biopsies: results of finasteride 1 mg treatment of men and postmenopausal women. *J Invest Dermatol*. 1999;4(3):282-284.

45. Brenner S, Matz H. Improvement in androgenetic alopecia in 53-76-year-old men using oral finasteride. *Int J Dermatol*. 1999;38(12):928-930.

46. Price VH, Menefee E, Sanchez M, Ruane P, Kaufman KD. Changes in hair weight and hair count in men with androgenetic alopecia after treatment with finasteride, 1 mg, daily. *J Am Acad Dermatol*. 2002;46(4):517-523.

47. Finasteride. *Highlights of Prescribing Information*. Available at: https://www.accessdata.fda.gov/drugsatfda_docs/label/2012/020788s020s021s023lbl.pdf. Accessed April 20, 2021.

48. Olsen EA, Hordinsky M, Whiting D, et al. The importance of dual 5alpha-reductase inhibition in the treatment of male pattern hair loss: results of a randomized placebo-controlled study of dutasteride versus finasteride. *J Am Acad Dermatol*. 2006;55:1014-1023.

49. Harcha WG, Barboza Martínez J, Tsai TF, et al. A randomized, active-and placebo-controlled study of the efficacy and safety of different doses of dutasteride versus placebo and finasteride in the treatment of male subjects with androgenetic alopecia. *J Am Acad Dermatol*. 2014;70(3):489-498.

50. Zhou Z, Song S, Gao Z, Wu J, Ma J, Cui Y. The efficacy and safety of dutasteride compared with finasteride in treating men with androgenetic alopecia: a systematic review and meta-analysis. *Clin Interv Aging*. 2019;14:399.

51. Boyapati A, Sinclair R. Combination therapy with finasteride and low-dose dutasteride in the treatment of androgenetic alopecia. *Australas J Dermatol*. 2013;54(1):49-51.

52. Jung JY, Yeon JH, Choi JW, et al. Effect of dutasteride 0.5 mg/d in men with androgenetic alopecia recalcitrant to finasteride. *Int J Dermatol*. 2014;53(11):1351-1357.

53. *Minoxidil* [package insert]. Skillman, NJ: Johnson & Johnson Healthcare Products; 2014.

54. Irwig MS, Kolukula S. Persistent sexual side effects of finasteride for male pattern hair loss. *J Sex Med*. 2011;8(6):1747-1753.

55. Irwig MS. Depressive symptoms and suicidal thoughts among former users of finasteride with persistent sexual side effects. *J Clin Psychiatry*. 2012;73(9):1220-1223.

56. Irwig MS. Persistent sexual side effects of finasteride: could they be permanent? *J Sex Med*. 2012;9(11):2927-2932.

57. Ganzer CA, Jacobs AR, Iqbal F. Persistent sexual, emotional, and cognitive impairment post-finasteride: a survey of men reporting symptoms. *Am J Mens Health*. 2015;9(3):222-228.

58. Chiriacò G, Cauci S, Mazzon G, Trombetta C. An observational retrospective evaluation of 79 young men with long-term adverse effects after use of finasteride against androgenetic alopecia. *Andrology*. 2016;4(2):245-250.

59. Traish AM, Hassani J, Guay AT, Zitzmann M, Hansen ML. Adverse side effects of 5α-reductase inhibitors therapy: persistent diminished libido and erectile dysfunction and depression in a subset of patients. *J Sex Med*. 2011;8(3):872-884.

60. Andriole GL, Kirby R. Safety and tolerability of the dual 5alpha-reductase inhibitor dutasteride in the treatment of benign prostatic hyperplasia. *Eur Urol*. 2003;44(1):82-88.

61. Becker CD, Stichtenoth DO, Wichmann MG, Schaefer C, Szinicz L. Blood donors on medication—an approach to minimize drug burden for recipients of blood products and to limit deferral of donors. *Transfus Med Hemother*. 2009;36(2):107-113.

62. *Medication Deferral List*. Available at: https://www.redcrossblood.org/donate-blood/manage-my-donations/rapidpass/medication-deferral-list.html. Accessed April 20, 2021.

63. Badri T, Nessel TA, Kumar D. *Minoxidil*. Treasure Island, FL: StatPearls Publishing; 2020.

64. Panchaprateep R, Lueangarun S. Efficacy and safety of oral minoxidil 5 mg once daily in the treatment of male patients with androgenetic alopecia: an open-label and global photographic assessment. *Dermatol Ther.* 2020;10(6):1345-1357.

65. Sinclair RD. Female pattern hair loss: a pilot study investigating combination therapy with low-dose oral minoxidil and spironolactone. *Int J Dermatol.* 2018;57(1):104-109.

66. Lee SW, Juhasz M, Mobasher P, Ekelem C, Mesinkovska NA. A systematic review of topical finasteride in the treatment of androgenetic alopecia in men and women. *J Drugs Dermatol.* 2018;17(4):457.

67. Suchonwanit P, Srisuwanwattana P, Chalermroj N, Khunkhet S. A randomized, double-blind controlled study of the efficacy and safety of topical solution of 0.25% finasteride admixed with 3% minoxidil vs. 3% minoxidil solution in the treatment of male androgenetic alopecia. *J Eur Acad Dermatol Venereol.* 2018;32(12): 2257-2263.

68. Caserini M, Radicioni M, Leuratti C, Annoni O, Palmieri R. A novel finasteride 0.25% topical solution for androgenetic alopecia: pharmacokinetics and effects on plasma androgen levels in healthy male volunteers. *Int J Clin Pharmacol Ther.* 2014;52(10):842-849.

69. Hajheydari Z, Akbari J, Saeedi M, Shokoohi L. Comparing the therapeutic effects of finasteride gel and tablet in treatment of the androgenetic alopecia. *Exp Gerontol.* 2002;37:981-990.

70. Tanglertsampan C. Efficacy and safety of 3% minoxidil versus combined 3% minoxidil/0.1% finasteride in male pattern hair loss: a randomized, double-blind, comparative study. *J Med Assoc Thai.* 2012;95(10):1312-1316.

71. Phan K, Sebaratnam DF. JAK inhibitors for alopecia areata: a systematic review and meta-analysis. *J Eur Acad Dermatol Venereol.* 2019;33(5):850-856.

72. Yale K, Pourang A, Plikus MV, Mesinkovska NA. At the crossroads of 2 alopecias: androgenetic alopecia pattern of hair regrowth in patients with alopecia areata treated with oral Janus kinase inhibitors. *JAAD Case Rep.* 2020;6(5):444.

73. Ocampo-Garza J, Griggs J, Tosti A. New drugs under investigation for the treatment of alopecias. *Expert Opin Investig Drugs.* 2019;28(3):275-284.

74. *A Study in Male and Female Subjects with Androgenetic Alopecia Treated with Ati-50002 Topical Solution.* Updated December 9, 2020. Available at: https://clinicaltrials.gov/ct2/show/study/NCT03495817. Accessed April 20, 2021.

9

Topical Immunotherapies

Cynthia Truong, Katharina Shaw, Kristen Lo Sicco, and Jerry Shapiro

KEY POINTS

- Androgenetic alopecia is the most common cause of hair loss and arises from androgen-dependent hair follicle miniaturization on the scalp.
- Several studies have suggested that follicular microinflammation is implicated in the pathogenesis of androgenetic alopecia, but to date, no immune modulatory therapies have been investigated for use in androgenetic alopecia alone.
- Androgenetic alopecia can arise in the setting of other forms of alopecia such as alopecia areata and cicatricial alopecias. As such, therapy for patients with

- androgenetic alopecia superimposed on other alopecias should be guided by the best-practice standards for all etiologies of hair loss.
- Topical immunotherapies and topical or intralesional corticosteroids are appropriate treatments for alopecia areata, while intralesional steroids are appropriate for frontal fibrosing alopecia.
- In this chapter, we discuss the use of topical and intralesional immunomodulatory agents for the treatment of alopecia areata or frontal fibrosing alopecia that may present in concert with androgenetic alopecia.

BACKGROUND, DEFINITIONS, AND HISTORY

Androgenetic alopecia (AGA), otherwise known as male or female pattern hair loss, is the most common cause of hair loss, affecting 50% of men and 40% women by the age of 50 (level of evidence; 1a).[1,2] Despite its prevalence, only one medical treatment for women and two for men are currently approved by the U.S. Food and Drug Administration (FDA) for the treatment of AGA: topical minoxidil for both and oral finasteride for men. Additionally, several low-level laser therapy (LLLT) devices have received 510(k) premarket medical device approval from the FDA for use in both men and women with AGA (level of evidence: 3b).[3] Response to these treatments can vary and may achieve partial response in some, highlighting the need for therapies that target alternative mechanisms in the pathophysiology of alopecia and those that may work synergistically with the standard-of-care therapies already available.

AGA specifically arises in the setting of androgen-dependent hair follicle miniaturization on the scalp. Notably, histopathologic examination of the scalp skin of males and females with AGA demonstrates activated T cells, macrophages, and mast cells infiltrating the hair follicle region, suggesting that microinflammation could be implicated in the cause or occur as a consequence of miniaturization (level of evidence: 5).[4-7] In one study, AGA patients with follicular microinflammation experienced hair regrowth after combination therapy with topical steroids, minocycline, and red light.[7] Another study found that the histologic patterns of early AGA lesions were indistinguishable from those seen in lichen planopilaris (LPP), suggesting the lichenoid reaction leading to follicular destruction in these patients may be related to the underlying mechanisms driving AGA (level of evidence: 4).[8] Although therapies targeting the immune system are widely used for alopecia areata (AA) or cicatricial alopecias such as LPP or central centrifugal cicatricial alopecia (CCCA), their utility in AGA requires further exploration. Given the potential immune mechanisms involved in AGA pathogenesis, immune modulation may represent a novel therapeutic avenue for some patients with AGA.

AGA often presents in combination with other forms of alopecia. For instance, AGA has been observed in both men and pre- and postmenopausal women diagnosed with frontal fibrosing alopecia (FFA) (level of evidence: 4).[9-11] Oral 5α-reductase inhibitors are commonly used as part of a multitherapy approach to halt hair loss in FFA, suggesting that concurrent treatment of underlying AGA may be responsible for a portion of the response (level of evidence: 3a).[12,13] AA can also present concurrently with AGA or can present with hair loss in the androgen-dependent areas, effectively mimicking AGA (level of evidence: 4).[14-16] As such, recognition and treatment of all underlying pathomechanisms of hair loss is paramount to achieving optimal hair regrowth and maximizing patient satisfaction. Herein we discuss the evidence behind and best practices for immunomodulatory therapies, with a specific focus on therapies that may be of use in patients with AGA and comorbid AA or cicatricial alopecia.

TOPICAL IRRITANTS AND SENSITIZERS

Topical immunotherapy has proven to be an effective first-line treatment for autoimmune, noncicatricial alopecias such as AA. Current methods include application of an irritant (anthralin) or an allergic sensitizer (squaric acid dibutylester [SADBE] or diphenylcyclopropenone [DPCP]). The notable difference between irritant and allergic contact dermatitis is that once the topical agent is applied to the skin, the latter requires both a sensitization phase *and* an elicitation phase. Although the mechanisms of action of these therapies are not fully understood, they are believed to modulate proinflammatory cytokines (level of evidence: 5).[17] Allergic sensitization is believed to also induce antigenic competition, reduce the CD4+/CD8+ T cell ratio, and lead to apoptosis of autoreactive T cells (level of evidence: 5).[18]

Indications and Patient Selection

Use of topical immunotherapy should be limited to patients who have AA. Although distinction between AGA and AA is typically possible via history and clinical examination, diagnosis may be difficult if there is diffuse AA, or if AGA presents in the androgen-dependent areas

> **PEARL 9.1:** Distinguishing between alopecia areata (AA) and androgenetic alopecia (AGA) may be challenging if a patient presents with diffuse AA or with AGA in androgen-dependent areas. For presentations that are clinically equivocal, biopsy showing highly positive CD3 infiltration or CD8 T-cell infiltration, especially in the intrafollicular region, is suggestive of AA.[15,16]

(level of evidence: 5).[19] For presentations that are clinically equivocal, biopsy may be necessary. The presence of highly positive CD3 infiltration or CD8 T-cell infiltration, especially in the intrafollicular region, is suggestive of AA (Pearl 9.1).[15,16] For patients with AA, topical sensitizers (SADBE and DPCP) are first-line for moderate-to-severe hair loss (>10% of the scalp) or for those with chronic-relapsing AA (level of evidence: 5).[20] Topical irritants (anthralin) remain a second-line option for moderate disease (level of evidence: 5).[21] Generally, patients experiencing acute or rapidly progressive hair loss are not good candidates for topical irritants or sensitizers. Though the majority of higher-level evidence supports the use of topical immunotherapy for AA patients, at least one study showed that patients with patchy AA did not experience significant benefit (level of evidence: 3b).[22] For these patients, intralesional steroids may be beneficial, as discussed later in this chapter.[20] Notably, patients with serious concurrent medical illnesses and women who are pregnant or breastfeeding should not be treated with topical sensitizers (level of evidence: 4).[23]

Expected Outcomes

Although no randomized controlled trials evaluating the efficacy of topical sensitizers exist to date, the largest review of the use of topical sensitizers in AA estimated that 50% to 60% of patients with moderate-to-severe AA could be treated effectively with DPCP or SADBE (level of evidence: 4).[24] However, the range of responses reported in the individual studies varied widely (9% to 87%).[24] An observational study revealed that 77.9% of participants treated with DPCP experienced clinically significant hair growth at 32 months, defined as patient-reported cosmetically acceptable regrowth or regrowth resulting in more than 75% of scalp terminal hair coverage.[23] These patients began to see hair growth at an average of 3 months after treatment initiation and achieved clinically significant regrowth at a median of 12.2 months (Fig. 9.1). In general, patients who demonstrated

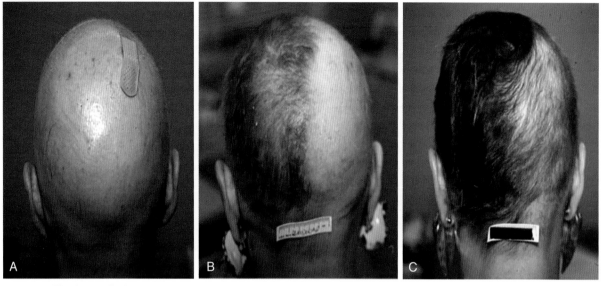

Fig. 9.1 (A) Patient with alopecia areata prior to treatment with topical immunotherapy. (B) Four months after treatment of alopecia areata with topical immunotherapy. (C) Seven months after treatment of alopecia areata with topical immunotherapy.

terminal hair regrowth earlier in treatment or with fewer treatments had more favorable outcomes.[23] Patients with earlier onset of hair loss or larger areas of hair loss at baseline were less likely to respond. Additionally, patients requiring higher peak concentration of therapy (>2.0% solution) had a decreased chance of significant regrowth. Unfortunately, response to treatment is often transient. One study found that after achieving clinically significant regrowth, 62.5% of patients experienced relapse, with a median time to relapse of 2.5 years.[23] For patients with recalcitrant alopecic patches, concomitant intralesional steroids may be of use, as discussed later in this chapter.[23]

Of note, one randomized controlled trial exists for topical anthralin, in which 0.5% anthralin was used as the "positive control" to study the efficacy of 20% azelaic acid in AA. This study found that cosmetically acceptable regrowth after anthralin treatment was achieved in 56.2% of patients who presented with patch-type alopecia with no evidence of relapse 8 weeks after completion of the treatment. This study was not placebo-controlled, however, making these results difficult to interpret (level of evidence: 1b).[25] Similarly, there is observational evidence that 0.5% to 1.0% anthralin elicits a cosmetic response in 75% of patients with patch-type AA and 25% of patients with AA totalis

(level of evidence: 4).[21,26] In one patient with long standing AA who failed several years of treatment with intralesional steroids and a trial of whole scalp anthralin 1% cream, treatment with anthralin 1% cream combined with calcipotriene 0.005% cream achieved visible hair regrowth that was maintained through follow-up at 8 months posttreatment (level of evidence: 5).[27]

Treatment Techniques and Best Practices

DPCP is the most commonly used topical sensitizer, though efficacy studies have shown that DPCP and SADBE are equally effective in treating AA (level of evidence: 4).[24,28] The patient can be sensitized with a patch containing a 2% solution of DPCP or SADBE diluted in acetone. The patch is applied to a small, 4-cm-diameter circular area on the scalp.[23] The patient is instructed to avoid washing their head or removing the patch for 48 hours. After this time, the patch is removed. Approximately 2 weeks later, an allergic contact dermatitis should appear on the scalp (Fig. 9.2). Three weeks after the sensitization, the patient should return to the office, either to have the clinician apply the topical immunotherapy or accompanied by someone who will apply the topical immunotherapy for them. Patients can also be instructed to apply the therapy themselves; however, they should be made

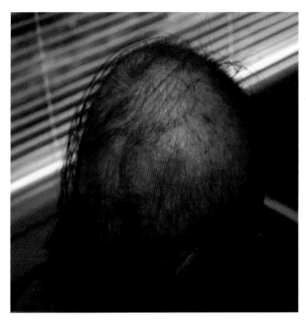

Fig. 9.2 Approximately 2 weeks after sensitization of the scalp with a 2% solution of diphenylcyclopropenone (DPCP) or squaric acid dibutylester (SADBE), an allergic contact dermatitis should appear.

aware of the severe allergic reactions that can occur in the case of a spill. The scalp is first treated with a weak solution of DPCP or SADBE using a cotton swab, starting as low as a 0.001% solution. Many clinicians initially choose to treat half of the scalp to distinguish treatment response versus spontaneous regrowth. A reinforced cotton applicator is saturated with the treatment chemical and applied to the scalp, first antero-posteriorly, then laterally (Fig. 9.3).[23] At weekly intervals, the concentration is increased until a mild dermatitis reaction is observed (Pearl 9.2). The concentration that produces this dermatitis reaction is used as the maintenance concentration for subsequent treatments (level of evidence: 4).[29] As such, the final concentration of solution varies by patient. In cases of excess inflammation, the concentration can be reduced. Similarly, in the case of insufficient response, the concentration can be increased. Communication with the patient about the degree of dermatitis experienced is extremely important. Once the correct concentration has been chosen, the application area can be gradually expanded until all alopecic areas are covered.

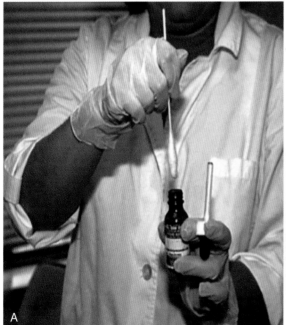
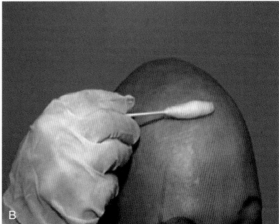

Fig. 9.3 (A-D) A cotton-reinforced applicator is used to apply topical immunotherapy to alopecic areas. For treatment of the scalp, the solution is applied antero posteriorly and then laterally. Proper personal protective equipment, including gloves, should be worn by the provider, family member, or patient who is applying the immunotherapy. Care should be taken to avoid spills, which can cause severe allergic reactions.

(Continued)

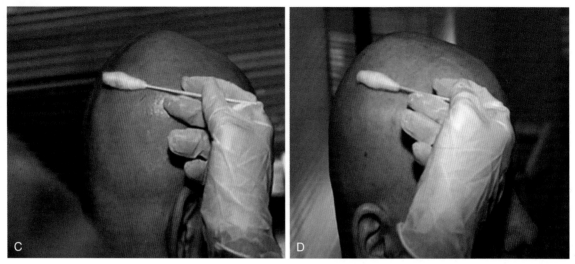

Fig. 9.3, cont'd

PEARL 9.2: After the sensitization period, treatment is initiated with a weak solution of diphenylcycloprope-none (DPCP) or squaric acid dibutylester (SADBE), starting as low as a 0.001% solution and increasing in concentration at weekly intervals until contact dermatitis is elicited.

Once all alopecic areas are treated with adequate response, visits can be scheduled at 3-month intervals. Treatment efficacy should be evaluated at 18 months. Afterward, maintenance therapy every 1 to 4 weeks may be beneficial for patients who exhibit clinically significant hair regrowth[23] (Fig. 9.4).

Treatment with anthralin similarly involves inducing a dermatitis reaction on the scalp. Anthralin cream 0.5% to 1.0% is commonly used, although these concentrations are not currently commercially available and may need to be prepared by a compounding pharmacy, which may not be cost effective for the patient. The compound can be applied daily to affected areas for 15 to 20 minutes, then washed off. On a weekly basis, the amount of time the cream is applied is increased by 5 minutes up to a maximum of 1 hour, or until a low-grade dermatitis develops. Once the optimal contact time is determined, the patient should continue to apply anthralin daily to the affected area for that fixed contact time. Clinical response should be evaluated at 3 months.[21] For patients with recalcitrant AA who have

failed anthralin alone, anthralin plus calcipotriene may be tried. For these patients, anthralin 1% cream and calcipotriene 0.005% cream should initially be applied for 5 minutes, increasing in duration to 90 minutes as tolerated for 5 days a week.[27]

Prevention and Management of Adverse Events

For both topical sensitizers and irritants, avoidance of sun exposure to the area is highly recommended for the entire treatment period. Though topical sensitizers are generally well tolerated, clinically significant adverse events have occurred in 56.8% of patients undergoing DPCP for AA, with the most common adverse effects including blistering (45.3%), hyperpigmentation (12.2%), autoeczematization (10.1%), hypopigmentation (2.0%), and symptomatic lymphadenopathy (2.0%).[23] Anecdotally, the authors have rarely observed facial edema. Blistering and autoeczematous reactions are often caused by incorrect selection of concentration, and management includes washing off the treatment and applying topical corticosteroids (Fig. 9.5). In severe cases, oral corticosteroids may be used. Cervical and occipital lymphadenopathy are common and resolve with decreasing concentration; however, they should be reviewed with the patient to avoid any potentially unnecessary anxiety (Fig. 9.6). Hyper- or hypopigmentation may occur, especially in darker skin, and, rarely, vitiligo affecting the treatment

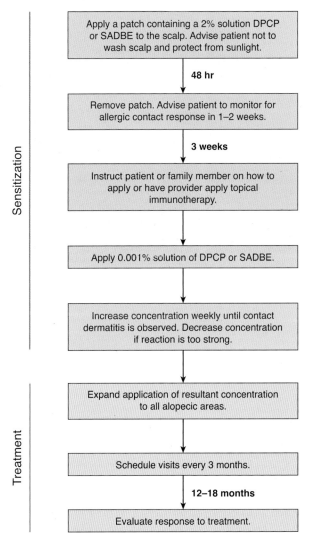

Sensitization

Apply a patch containing a 2% solution DPCP or SADBE to the scalp. Advise patient not to wash scalp and protect from sunlight.

↓ **48 hr**

Remove patch. Advise patient to monitor for allergic contact response in 1–2 weeks.

↓ **3 weeks**

Instruct patient or family member on how to apply or have provider apply topical immunotherapy.

↓

Apply 0.001% solution of DPCP or SADBE.

↓

Increase concentration weekly until contact dermatitis is observed. Decrease concentration if reaction is too strong.

Treatment

↓

Expand application of resultant concentration to all alopecic areas.

↓

Schedule visits every 3 months.

↓ **12–18 months**

Evaluate response to treatment.

Fig. 9.4 Treatment algorithm for topical immunotherapy for alopecia areata.

area can occur (level of evidence: 4)[20,30] (Fig. 9.7). In the case of therapy-induced vitiligo, treatment should be immediately discontinued and topical steroids applied. Phototherapy (PUVA or nb-UVB) may be used with variable response. Complete repigmentation in these cases is rare.[30]

Adverse outcomes associated with anthralin treatment include severe irritation, folliculitis, regional lymphadenopathy, and brown staining of skin, clothes, and hair.[20,26] Contact with eyes should be avoided.[21]

TOPICAL AND INTRALESIONAL STEROIDS

Corticosteroids are immunosuppressive agents with great clinical utility in facilitating scalp hair regrowth in AA and halting progression in cicatricial alopecias such as FFA. For AA, while the application of *topical* corticosteroids has demonstrated relatively modest efficacy, *intralesional* corticosteroids, by contrast, have emerged as a first-line treatment. For FFA, both topical and intralesional corticosteroids are first-line treatments.[20] For many of these patients, topical or intralesional steroids are combined with a 5α-reductase inhibitor.

Indications and Patient Selection

As with topical immunotherapy, corticosteroids can be used for patients with either comorbid AA or FFA/LPP. Topical steroids may be a good option for AA patients who have failed topical immunotherapy. Studies have found that both clobetasol propionate 0.05% ointment applied under occlusion and betamethasone butyrate propionate 0.05% ointment were effective in subsets of patients resistant to topical immunotherapy (level of evidence: 4).[31,32] Intralesional steroids are considered a first-line treatment for AA when less than 50% of the scalp is involved. However, they may also be used as an adjunctive agent in those on systemic therapy such as oral tofacitinib (Pearl 9.3) (level of evidence: 5).[33] As an isolated therapy, intralesional steroids are most effective in patients with limited AA, patchy AA, or those with a shorter duration of disease. For patients with FFA, topical or intralesional steroids and systemic therapy are often initiated on the first visit to prevent any further hair loss. Regimens including a combination of these therapies can be modified and simplified as the patient improves.

Expected Outcomes

Outcomes with use of topical corticosteroids in AA are variable. One randomized controlled trial found that treatment of patients with moderate-to-severe AA with clobetasol 0.05% foam resulted in 47% of patients demonstrating more than 25% hair regrowth, and 25% of patients with more than 50% hair regrowth (level of evidence: 1b).[34] Clobetasol propionate 0.05% ointment applied under occlusion achieved almost complete regrowth in 28.5% of patients in one study, though only 17.8% had long-term benefits.[31] Another randomized controlled trial found more than 50% regrowth in 61%

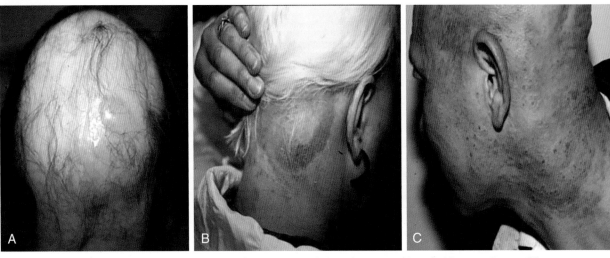

Fig. 9.5 (A) Severe blistering reaction after treatment of alopecia areata with topical immunotherapy. Blistering and autoeczematous reactions are often caused by incorrect selection of treatment concentration. Management involves washing off the treatment, application of topical corticosteroids, and, in severe cases, oral corticosteroids. (B-C) Autoeczematous reactions after treatment with topical immunotherapy.

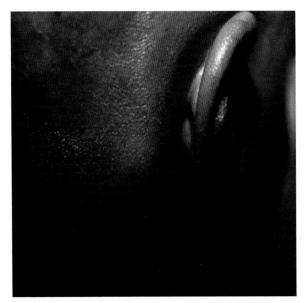

Fig. 9.6 Cervical lymphadenopathy resulting from topical immunotherapy treatment in a patient with alopecia areata. Lymphadenopathy may be alarming to the patient but most often resolves with decreasing the concentration of immunotherapy.

PEARL 9.3: Intralesional steroids are considered a first-line treatment for alopecia areata when less than 50% of the scalp is involved; however, it may also be used as an adjunctive agent in those on systemic therapy such as oral tofacitinib.[33]

of patients with mild-to-moderate AA after treatment with betamethasone valerate 0.1% foam compared with more than 50% regrowth in 27% of patients treated with betamethasone dipropionate 0.05% lotion, although a therapeutic effect of the vehicle could not be excluded (level of evidence: 1b).[35] For patients who failed topical immunotherapy, response to topical betamethasone butyrate propionate 0.05% lotion was seen after 3 to 5 months of treatment and lasted between 10 to 51 months.[32] Unfortunately, relapse rates vary from 37% to 63% after topical corticosteroids are stopped, or even with continuation of therapy.[21]

Intralesional steroids for patients with limited AA may result in better outcomes. Prospective studies of intralesional steroids, primarily triamcinolone acetonide (5 to 10 mg/mL) injected intradermally every 2 to 6 weeks, showed local regrowth of 60% to 67% at injection sites (level of evidence: 4).[36,37] A systematic review of intralesional triamcinolone acetonide revealed

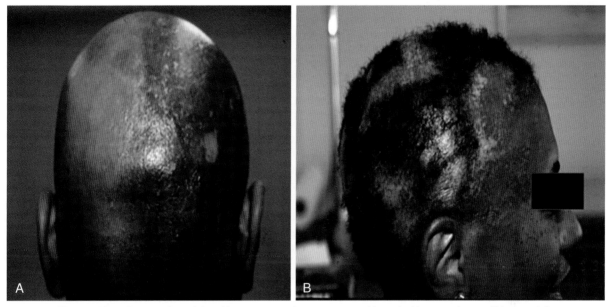

Fig. 9.7 Hypopigmentation of the skin can occur after treatment with topical immunotherapy (A), especially in patients with darker skin subtypes (B).

pooled rates of regrowth to be 62.3% with less than 5 mg/mL concentration, 80.9% with 5 mg/mL, and 76.4% with 10 mg/mL (level of evidence: 4).[38] Although few studies followed patients for long enough to ascertain maintenance of regrowth, one study found that at 18 months, 54% of patients had continued hair growth at the sites of injection (level of evidence: 3a).[39] Those with more extensive AA or longer duration of disease (greater than 1 year) tend to be more treatment refractory.[39]

For patients with FFA, intralesional corticosteroids are more effective at halting the progression of hair loss than topical corticosteroids. A systematic review found that intralesional steroids alone were the second-most effective treatment for FFA, after oral finasteride or dutasteride +/- topical minoxidil or intralesional steroids, resulting in partial clinical response in approximately 60% of patients (Pearl 9.4).[12] Of note, 93% of patients treated with moderate- or high-potency topical steroids alone had no response.[12]

PEARL 9.4: Intralesional steroids alone are the second most effective treatment for frontal fibrosing alopecia, after oral 5α-reductase inhibitors +/- topical minoxidil or intralesional steroids.[12]

Treatment Techniques and Best Practices

For treatment of AA with topical corticosteroids, 2.5 g of clobetasol propionate 0.05% ointment can be applied to the scalp every night under occlusion with a plastic film such as a shower cap. Patients with more scalp hair may find ointment solutions messy and may prefer solution or foam formulations, in which case clobetasol 0.05% solution or foam can be used. Providers may consider applying the steroid on one side of the scalp to assess treatment efficacy versus spontaneous regrowth; however, this is not cosmetically ideal for those without spontaneous regrowth on the untreated side of the scalp. In the morning, the scalp should be washed with mild shampoo.[34] Treatment is performed 6 days a week and assessed at 6 months.[34]

If treatment of AA with intralesional steroids is desired, triamcinolone acetonide is generally preferred to triamcinolone hexacetonide because of the lower risk of atrophy (level of evidence: 5).[40] In a single visit, a concentration of 10 mg/mL with a maximum total of 2 mL or 5 mg/mL with a maximum total of 4 mL can be used on the scalp to optimize response while minimizing adverse effects.[40] Similarly, a concentration of 2.5 mg/mL is recommended for the face or along the frontal hairline.[21,38] Topical anesthetic can be used prior to injection to minimize patient discomfort. Triamcinolone acetonide is injected in the deep dermal/upper subcutaneous plane using a jet injector or a 0.5-inch 30-gauge needle. Injections of 0.1 mL per site can be performed at 0.5-1 cm intervals. Treatments are repeated every 4 to 6 weeks for 6 months. If no response is noted after 6 consecutive months, treatment should be discontinued.

For patients with FFA of the scalp, a concentration of 10 mg/mL of triamcinolone acetonide can be used on top of the scalp and 2.5 mg/mL along the hairline, with a maximum total of 0.5 ml to 3 mL per session. Injections can be scheduled every 6 to 12 weeks (level of evidence: 3b).[41] If there is involvement of the eyebrow, a concentration of 10 mg/mL with a total of 0.125 mL per eyebrow can be injected at the same interval (level of evidence: 4).[42] Systemic treatment with an oral agent can be considered for all patients but should be initiated in symptomatic patients or those with perifollicular scaling. Treatment should be continued until hairline recession halts and evidence of active inflammation, such as perifollicular scaling or erythema, resolves. The mean number of treatments in one retrospective study was eight per patient.[10] To monitor the efficacy, it is recommended to systematically measure frontotemporal hairline recession and degree of perifollicular inflammation by trichoscopy at 3- to 6-month intervals.[20] After a response is seen, patients should be placed on oral treatment until there is stabilization of hair loss and cessation of inflammation. The length of treatment will vary by patient, with some patients reaching remission within 1 year and others requiring several years of treatment (level of evidence: 5).

Prevention and Management of Adverse Events

In rare cases, topical steroids may cause skin atrophy and telangiectasias.[21] If atrophy occurs, treatment should be discontinued at those sites. Skin atrophy was the most commonly observed adverse effect in a systematic review of intralesional steroids for AA, occurring in 3.33% of patients treated with a concentration of 5 mg/mL and 20% of those treated with 10 mg/mL.[38] This atrophy tends to be transient and can be prevented by the use of smaller volumes and concentrations, minimizing the number of injections per site, and ensuring that injections are not made too superficially (i.e., intraepidermally).[21] Transient telangiectasias may also occur after treatment with intralesional steroids.[21]

TOPICAL PROSTAGLANDIN ANALOGS

Prostaglandins play an important role in the regulation of the hair cycle. Prostaglandin D2 (PGD2) inhibits hair growth, while prostaglandin F2 (PGF2) and prostaglandin E2 (PGE2) work synergistically to stimulate hair growth. Increased levels of PGD2 and decreased levels of PGF2 and PGE2 have been demonstrated on the scalps of patients with AGA (level of evidence: 5).[43] Although PGF2 analogs such as topical bimatoprost and topical latanoprost are typically used in the treatment of eyelash hypotrichosis and have been used in the treatment of eyelash AA, their role in the treatment of AGA is under investigation (level of evidence: 1a).[44,45] To date, results are mixed regarding the efficacy of topical PGF2 analogs and PGD2 antagonists for AGA.[20]

Indications and Patient Selection

Studies showing efficacy for topical prostaglandin analogs have included men aged 18 to 50 years with Hamilton-Norwood II-, IIIv-, IV-, V-, and Va-grade hair loss. To date, no studies have demonstrated efficacy in women. Importantly, patients with a history of glaucoma or elevated intraocular pressure should not be treated with prostaglandin analogs (level of evidence: 1b).[46] Additionally, bimatoprost is classified as a category C drug according to use-in-pregnancy FDA ratings and should be avoided in pregnant women if possible.[44]

Expected Outcomes

Preliminary results from a multicenter, randomized, controlled trial of patients with AGA found that treatment with different formulations of bimatoprost solution resulted in a greater change from baseline in Target Area Hair Count (TAHC) compared with vehicle after 6 months of application, with the most effective formulation increasing TAHC by 13.1 terminal hairs/cm^2. Notably, topical minoxidil 5% solution still outperformed bimatoprost (TAHC 21.9) (level of evidence: 1b).[47] Another randomized controlled trial compared two formulations of bimatoprost to vehicle, and the authors found that after 6 months of application, the two formulations increased TAHC by 12.7 and 9.3 hairs/cm^2, respectively, while the vehicle increased TAHC by 5.8 hairs/cm^2 (level of evidence: 1b).[48] Commercially available PGF2 analogs such as topical bimatoprost 0.03% (trade names Lumigan or Latisse) have been shown to increase TAHC from baseline compared with vehicle after 16 weeks (TAHC 27.4 vs. -2.6) (level of evidence: 1b).[49] One study used TrichoScan imaging, which combines epiluminescence microscopy and digital image analysis to measure hair growth rate, density, diameter, and anagen/telogen ratio to assess response to topical latanoprost 0.1% solution (trade name Xalatan) (level of evidence: 1b).[50] By this measure, Xalatan, another PGF2 analog, increased hair growth from baseline by 22% at 24 weeks of treatment when compared with placebo, which increased hair growth by 10% (level of evidence: 1b).[50] Cetirizine is a second-generation histamine H1 receptor antagonist that has been shown to reduce inflammatory cell infiltrate and PGD2 production. Topical cetirizine 1% applied daily for 6 months in patients with AGA showed an increase in total and terminal hair density (level of evidence: 2b).[51] Use of PGE2 analogs such as transdermal viprostol 0.4% have shown limited results for men with AGA (level of evidence: 1b).[49] Only one clinical trial to date has included women with AGA, and it revealed no significant hair regrowth after application of bimatoprost formulation for 6 months.[47]

Treatment Techniques and Best Practices

Several formulations of bimatoprost used in the aforementioned trials are not commercially available, and compound preparations can be cost-prohibitive. The bimatoprost 0.03% solution (Lumigan or Latisse) or latanoprost 0.1% solution (Xalatan) are commercially available options; however, they are often not covered by insurance and pose an out-of-pocket cost to the patient. Clinical trials evaluating bimatoprost have patients apply bimatoprost solution to the affected areas twice daily for 6 months. However, because trials have not shown improved efficacy of prostaglandin analogs over topical minoxidil, many clinicians prefer to use it alongside topical minoxidil or, in the case of contact dermatitis, secondary to topical minoxidil (Pearl 9.5).[20] This contact dermatitis is often caused by the propylene glycol-based vehicles of topical minoxidil solutions, which can cause irritation,

itching, and decreased patient compliance (level of evidence: 5).[52] It is unclear whether topical prostaglandin analogs represent an effective alternative for patients that experience these side effects. Alternatively, 1 mL of topical cetirizine 1% can be applied daily to the affected areas, and treatment response can be assessed at 6 months. Currently there are no known side effects of this treatment.[51]

Prevention and Management of Adverse Events

In a pooled safety analysis of bimatoprost 0.03% solution for eyelash hypotrichosis, most of the reported adverse events were mild, localized to the site of application, and reversible with cessation of treatment. Observed reactions include conjunctival hyperemia, eyelid pruritus, eyelid pigmentation, nasopharyngitis, erythema of the eyelid, punctate keratitis, and excessive growth and thickness of the eyelashes.[52] In some glaucoma patients treated with intraocular PGF2α, poliosis together with hypertrichosis were observed, without evidence of resolution 2 months after the cessation of therapy (level of evidence: 4).[53] Eyelid and periorbital lipodystrophy has been documented with use of topical prostaglandin analogs for both glaucoma and eyelash hypotrichosis, with its incidence likely underestimated in the latter group (level of evidence: 1a).[54,55] Side effects reported after bimatoprost use for AGA include dryness (6.56%), irritation (7.69%), contact dermatitis (7.69%), and pruritus (11.48%).[44,52] Erythema at the site of application may also be observed.[20]

FUTURE DIRECTIONS

Although both topical immunotherapies and corticosteroids have demonstrated clinical benefit for many patients with autoimmune or inflammatory alopecias, we recommend use of these agents in patients with AGA *only* if comorbid AA or cicatricial alopecia is observed. Well-designed randomized clinical trials are needed to validate use of these therapies in patients with AGA alone. Further evaluation of these therapies for female patients with AGA and those with nonwhite, ethnic skin (corresponding to a wider range of Fitzpatrick skin types and hair qualities, such as curly versus straight) is also needed to better stratify treatment response and predict and prevent adverse outcomes.

> **PEARL 9.5:** As trials have not shown improved efficacy of prostaglandin analogs over topical minoxidil for androgenetic alopecia, many clinicians prefer to use it alongside topical minoxidil or, in the case of contact dermatitis, secondary to topical minoxidil.[20]

EVIDENCE SUMMARY

- Of the topical immune modulatory therapies discussed in this chapter, only topical prostaglandin analogs are indicated for use in androgenetic alopecia alone. Although the prostaglandin analog formulations studied in the randomized controlled trials are not commercially available, agents commonly used for glaucoma and eyelash hypotrichosis (trade names Lumigan, Latisse, or Xalatan) have been shown to be effective for androgenetic alopecia when applied on the scalp (strength of recommendation: B).
- For alopecia areata patients with more than 10% scalp involvement, topical immunotherapy with allergic contact sensitizers (diphenylcyclopropenone or squaric acid dibutylester) is considered the first-line treatment. Contact irritants (anthralin +/- calcipotriene) can be considered for patients with more limited scalp involvement. Response to topical immunotherapies is usually robust, except in cases where larger areas of hair loss were present at baseline or in cases requiring higher concentrations of immunotherapy. Unfortunately, hair regrowth in most cases is temporary, requiring use of alternate second-line options (strength of recommendation: B).
- Intralesional corticosteroids are a first-line agent for alopecia areata patients with less than 50% scalp involvement, or those with recalcitrant alopecic patches after treatment with topical immunotherapy (strength of recommendation: B).
- For patients with frontal fibrosing alopecia, intralesional corticosteroids are the second most effective treatment, after oral 5α-reductase inhibitors. Intralesional corticosteroids can halt the progression of hair loss; however, regrowth of hair in cicatricial areas is not possible in some of these patients (strength of recommendation: A).

REFERENCES

1. Afifi L, Maranda EL, Zarei M, et al. Low-level laser therapy as a treatment for androgenetic alopecia. *Lasers Surg Med*. 2017;49(1):27-39. doi:10.1002/lsm.22512.
2. Severi G, Sinclair R, Hopper JL, English DR, Mccredie MRE. Epidemiology and Health Services Research Androgenetic alopecia in men aged 40 – 69 years : prevalence and risk factors. *Br J Dermatol*. 2003:1207-1213.
3. Wang S, Seth D, Ezaldein H, et al. Shedding light on the FDA's 510(k) approvals process: low-level laser therapy devices used in the treatment of androgenetic alopecia. *J Dermatolog Treat*. 2019;30(5):489-491. doi:10.1080/09546634.2018.1528327.
4. Jaworsky C, Kligman AM, Murphy GF. Characterization of inflammatory infiltrates in male pattern alopecia: implications for pathogenesis. *Br J Dermatol*. 1992;127(3):239-246. doi:10.1111/j.1365-2133.1992.tb00121.x.
5. Lattanand A, Johnson WC. Male pattern alopecia a histopathologic and histochemical study. *J Cutan Pathol*. 1975;2(2):58-70. doi:10.1111/j.1600-0560.1975.tb00209.x.
6. Young JW, Conte ET, Leavitt ML, Nafz MA, Schroeter AL. Cutaneous immunopathology of androgenetic alopecia. *J Am Osteopath Assoc*. 1991;91(8):765.
7. Magro CM, Rossi A, Poe J, Manhas-Bhutani S, Sadick N. The role of inflammation and immunity in the pathogenesis of androgenetic alopecia. *J Drugs Dermatol*. 2011;10(12):1404.
8. Zinkernagel M, Med C, Trueb RM. Fibrosing alopecia in a pattern distribution: patterned lichen planopilaris or androgenetic alopecia with a lichenoid tissue reaction pattern? *Arch Dermatol*. 2000;136(2):205-2111. doi:10.35541/cjd.20191142.
9. Moreno-Ramírez D, Martínez FC. Frontal fibrosing alopecia: a survey in 16 patients. *J Eur Acad Dermatol Venereol*. 2005;19(6):700-705. doi:10.1111/j.1468-3083.2005.01291.x.
10. Vañó-Galván S, Molina-Ruiz AM, Serrano-Falcón C, et al. Frontal fibrosing alopecia: a multicenter review of 355 patients. *J Am Acad Dermatol*. 2014;70(4):670-678. doi:10.1016/j.jaad.2013.12.003.
11. Kossard S, Lee MS, Wilkinson B. Postmenopausal frontal fibrosing alopecia: a frontal variant of lichen planopilaris. *J Am Acad Dermatol*. 1997;36(1):59-66. doi:10.1016/S0190-9622(97)70326-8.
12. Rácz E, Gho C, Moorman PW, Noordhoek Hegt V, Neumann HAM. Treatment of frontal fibrosing alopecia and lichen planopilaris: a systematic review. *J Eur Acad Dermatol Venereol*. 2013;27(12):1461-1470. doi:10.1111/jdv.12139.
13. Porriño-Bustamante ML, Fernández-Pugnaire MA, Arias-Santiago S. Frontal fibrosing alopecia: a review. *J Clin Med*. 2021;10(9):1805. doi:10.3390/jcm10091805.
14. Benigno M, Anastassopoulos KP, Mostaghimi A, et al. A large cross-sectional survey study of the prevalence of alopecia areata in the United States. *Clin Cosmet Investig Dermatol*. 2020;13:259-266. doi:10.2147/CCID.S245649.
15. Kamyab K, Rezvani M, Seirafi H, et al. Distinguishing immunohistochemical features of alopecia areata from androgenic alopecia. *J Cosmet Dermatol*. 2019;18(1):422-426. doi:10.1111/jocd.12677.

16. Kolivras A, Thompson C. Distinguishing diffuse alopecia areata (AA) from pattern hair loss (PHL) using CD3+ T cells. *J Am Acad Dermatol*. 2016;74(5):937-944. doi:10.1016/j.jaad.2015.12.011.

17. Tang L, Cao L, Pelech S, Lui H, Shapiro J. Cytokines and signal transduction pathways mediated by anthralin in alopecia areata-affected Dundee experimental balding rats. *J Investig Dermatol Symp Proc*. 2003;8(1):87-90. doi:10.1046/j.1523-1747.2003.12178.x.

18. Singh G, Lavanya M. Topical immunotherapy in alopecia areata. *Int J Trichology*. 2010;2(1):36-39. doi:10.4103/0974-7753.66911.

19. Werner B, Mulinari-Brenner F. Clinical and histological challenge in the differential diagnosis of diffuse alopecia: female androgenetic alopecia, telogen effluvium and alopecia areata - part I. *An Bras Dermatol*. 2012;87(5):742-747.

20. Tosti A, Asz-Sigall D, Pirmez R. *HAIR and Scalp Treatments:* Switzerland: Springer Nature; 2020.

21. Shapiro J. Current treatment of alopecia areata. *J Investig Dermatol Symp Proc*. 2013;16(1):S42-S44. doi:10.1038/jidsymp.2013.14.

22. Ro BI. Alopecia areata in Korea (1982–1994). *J Dermatol*. 1995;22(11):858-864. doi:10.1111/j.1346-8138.1995.tb03936.x.

23. Wiseman MC, Shapiro J, MacDonald N, Lui H. Predictive model for immunotherapy of alopecia areata with diphencyprone. *Arch Dermatol*. 2001;137(8):1063-1068.

24. Rokhsar CK, Shupack JL, Vafai JJ, Washenik K. Efficacy of topical sensitizers in the treatment of alopecia areata. *J Am Acad Dermatol*. 1998;39(5 Pt 1):751-761. doi:10.1016/S0190-9622(98)70048-9.

25. Sasmaz S, Arican O. Comparison of azelaic acid and anthralin for the therapy of patchy alopecia areata: a pilot study. *Am J Clin Dermatol*. 2005;6(6):403–406. doi:10.2165/00128071-200506060-00007.

26. Fiedler-Weiss VC, Buys CM. Evaluation of anthralin in the treatment of alopecia areata. *Arch Dermatol*. 1987;123(11):1491-1493. doi:10.1001/archderm.1987.01660350091020.

27. Krueger L, Peterson E, Shapiro J, Lo Sicco K. Case report of novel combination of anthralin and calcipotriene leading to trichologic response in alopecia areata. *JAAD Case Rep*. 2019;5(3):258-260. doi:10.1016/j.jdcr.2019.01.006.

28. Harries MJ, Sun J, Paus R, King LE. Management of alopecia areata. *BMJ*. 2010;341(7766):c3671. doi:10.1136/bmj.c3671.

29. Sutherland L, Laschinger M, Syed ZU, Gaspari A. Treatment of alopecia areata with topical sensitizers. *Contact Dermatitis*. 2015;26(1):26-31. doi:10.1097/DER.0000000000000094.

30. Kutlubay Z, Engin B, Songur A, Serdaroglu S, Tuzun Y. Topical immunotherapy with diphenylcyclopropenone-induced vitiligo. *J Cosmet Laser Ther*. 2016;18(4):245-246. doi:10.3109/14764172.2016.1157357.

31. Tosti A, Piraccini BM, Pazzaglia M, Vincenzi C. Clobetasol propionate 0.05% under occlusion in the treatment of alopecia totalis/universalis. *J Am Acad Dermatol*. 2003;49(1):96-98. doi:10.1067/mjd.2003.423.

32. Inui S, Itami S. Contact immunotherapy-resistant alopecia areata totalis/universalis reactive to topical corticosteroid. *J Dermatol*. 2015;42(9):937-939. doi:10.1111/1346-8138.12965.

33. Strazzulla LC, Avila L, Lo Sicco K, Shapiro J. Image gallery: treatment of refractory alopecia universalis with oral tofacitinib citrate and adjunct intralesional triamcinolone injections. *Br J Dermatol*. 2017;176(6):e125. doi:10.1111/bjd.15483.

34. Tosti A, Iorizzo M, Botta GL, Milani M. Efficacy and safety of a new clobetasol propionate 0.05% foam in alopecia areata: a randomized, double-blind placebo-controlled trial. *J Eur Acad Dermatol Venereol*. 2006;20(10):1243-1247. doi:10.1111/j.1468-3083.2006.01781.x.

35. Mancuso G, Balducci A, Casadio C, et al. Efficacy of betamethasone valerate foam formulation in comparison with betamethasone dipropionate lotion in the treatment of mild-to-moderate alopecia areata: a multicenter, prospective, randomized, controlled, investigator-blinded trial. *Int J Dermatol*. 2003;42(7):572-575. doi:10.1046/j.1365-4362.2003.01862.x.

36. Abell E, Munro DD. Intralesional treatment of alopecia areata with triamcinolone acetonide by jet injector. *Br J Dermatol*. 1973;88(1):55-60. doi:10.1111/j.1365-2133.1973.tb06672.x.

37. Kubeyinje EP, C'Mathur M. Topical tretinoin as an adjunctive therapy with intralesional triamcinolone acetonide for alopecia areata. Clinical experience in northern Saudi Arabia. *Int J Dermatol*. 1997;36(4):320. doi:10.1111/j.1365-4362.1997.tb03060.x.

38. Yee BE, Tong Y, Goldenberg A, Hata T. Efficacy of different concentrations of intralesional triamcinolone acetonide for alopecia areata: a systematic review and meta-analysis. *J Am Acad Dermatol*. 2020;82(4):1018-1021. doi:10.1016/j.jaad.2019.11.066.

39. Kassim JM, Shipman AR, Szczecinska W, et al. How effective is intralesional injection of triamcinolone acetonide compared with topical treatments in inducing and maintaining hair growth in patients with alopecia areata? A critically appraised topic. *Br J Dermatol*. 2014;170(4):766-771. doi:10.1111/bjd.12863.

40. Shapiro J, Price VH. Hair regrowth. *Dermatol Clin*. 1998;16(2):341-356. doi:10.1016/s0733-8635(05)70017-6.

41. Gamret AC, Potluri V, Krishnamurthy K, Fertig RM. Frontal fibrosing alopecia: efficacy of treatment

modalities. *Int J Womens Health.* 2019;11:273-285. doi:10.2147/IJWH.S177308.

42. Donovan JC, Samrao A, Ruben BS, Price VH. Eyebrow regrowth in patients with frontal fibrosing alopecia treated with intralesional triamcinolone acetonide. *Br J Dermatol.* 2010;163(5):1142-1144. doi:10.2147/IJWH.S177308. 10.1111/j.1365-2133.2010.09994.x

43. York K, Meah N, Bhoyrul B, Sinclair R. Treatment review for male pattern hair-loss. *Expert Opin Pharmacother.* 2020;21(5):603-612. doi:10.1080/14656566.2020.1721463.

44. Bratton EM, Davies BW, Hink EM, Durairaj VD. Bimatoprost in the treatment of hypotrichosis. *J Dermatol Nurses Assoc.* 2013;5(5):278-279. doi:10.1097/JDN.0b013e3182a52462.

45. Meah N, Wall D, York K, et al. The Alopecia Areata Consensus of Experts (ACE) study: results of an international expert opinion on treatments for alopecia areata. *J Am Acad Dermatol.* 2020;83(1):123-130. doi:10.1016/j.jaad.2020.03.004.

46. Olsen E. *Topical Bimatoprost Effect on Androgen Dependent Hair Follicles.* Duke University; 2014. Available at: https://clinicaltrials.gov/ct2/show/NCT02170662.

47. *Safety and Efficacy Study of Bimatoprost in the Treatment of Men with Androgenic Alopecia.* Allergan; 2012. Available at: https://clinicaltrials.gov/ct2/show/NCT01325337. Accessed August 5, 2021.

48. *A Safety and Efficacy Study of Bimatoprost in Men with Androgenic Alopecia.* Fridley, Minnesota: Allergan; 2016. Available at: https://clinicaltrials.gov/ct2/show/NCT01904721. Accessed August 5, 2021.

49. Olsen EA, DeLong E. Transdermal viprostol in the treatment of male pattern baldness. *J Am Acad Dermatol.* 1990;23(3):470-472. doi:10.1016/0190-9622(90)70242-A.

50. Blume-Peytavi U, Lönnfors S, Hillmann K, Garcia Bartels N. A randomized double-blind placebo-controlled pilot study to assess the efficacy of a 24-week topical treatment by latanoprost 0.1% on hair growth and pigmentation in healthy volunteers with androgenetic alopecia. *J Am Acad Dermatol.* 2012;66(5):794-800. doi:10.1016/j.jaad.2011.05.026.

51. Rossi A, Campo D, Fortuna MC, et al. A preliminary study on topical cetirizine in the therapeutic management of androgenetic alopecia. *J Dermatolog Treat.* 2018;29(2):149-151. doi:10.1080/09546634.2017.1341610.

52. Barrón-Hernández YL, Tosti A. Bimatoprost for the treatment of eyelash, eyebrow and scalp alopecia. *Expert Opin Investig Drugs.* 2017;26(4):515-522. doi:10.1080/13543784.2017.1303480.

53. Chen CS, Wells J, Craig JE. Topical prostaglandin f2α analog induced poliosis. *Am J Ophthalmol.* 2004;137(5):965-966. doi:10.1016/j.ajo.2003.11.020.

54. Sira M, Verity DH, Malhotra R. Topical bimatoprost 0.03% and iatrogenic eyelid and orbital lipodystrophy. *Aesthetic Surg J.* 2012;32(7):822-824. doi:10.1177/1090820X12455659.

55. Steinsapir KD, Steinsapir SMG. Revisiting the safety of prostaglandin analog eyelash growth products. *Dermatol Surg.* 2021;47:658-665. doi:10.1097/dss.0000000000002928.

10

Systemic Immunotherapies

Sarah Benton, Ronda Farah, and Maria Hordinsky

KEY POINTS

- The role of inflammation, including T cells, mast cells, prostaglandins, and cytokines, in the pathogenesis of androgenetic alopecia has been studied. Different approaches to address this inflammation have been recommended.
- Use of anti-inflammatory immunotherapy in androgenetic alopecia is primarily through topical treatment; systemic immunotherapy is rarely prescribed.

- When treated with systemic immunotherapy, patients who have both androgenetic alopecia and alopecia areata typically experience regrowth in a pattern that does not include regions affected by androgenetic alopecia.
- Future directions may include topical and systemic targeted anti-inflammatory therapies.

BACKGROUND, DEFINITIONS, AND HISTORY

Systemic immunotherapy is a class of medications characterized by their ability to affect the immune response. The specific mechanisms of drugs in this class can vary greatly depending on the immune cells that they target and the signaling molecules that they amplify or inhibit. It is notable that, historically, dermatopathologists have debated whether inflammation plays a role in androgenetic alopecia (AGA). The term "microinflammation" was penned to distinguish possible inflammatory pathways present in patients with AGA.[1,2] We now know that follicular microinflammation is driven by many factors, including perifollicular fibroblast activation, T-cell infiltration, prostaglandins, and mast cell degranulation (Pearl 10.1 and Fig. 10.1).[3-5] It is postulated that a combination of inflammatory, oxidative, and hormonal processes results in follicular miniaturization.[6,7] Scalp biopsies of male and female AGA frequently show chronic inflammation with the presence of lymphocytes and histiocytes, and a 2022 study located this perifollicular inflammation to be primarily at the isthmus and infundibulum of the hair follicle.[8] T-cell infiltration, mast

cell degranulation, and fibroblast activation have been postulated to lead to fibrosis of the perifollicular sheath and play a role in the abnormal hair cycle of AGA, which is characterized by a decreased anagen phase and normal or increased telogen phase.[9,10]

INDICATIONS AND PATIENT SELECTION

Systemic immunotherapy refers to a broad class of therapeutics, and thus selection of such treatment varies widely based on each patient's disease type, disease severity, and demographic factors. Of the nonscarring alopecias, treatment with systemic immunotherapy is more common in alopecia areata (AA) than in AGA or telogen effluvium (TE). In this chapter, we will discuss systemic immunotherapy as treatment for nonscarring alopecias and highlight the future directions of anti-inflammatory immunotherapy in AGA.

Androgenetic Alopecia

Though systemic immunotherapies have not been widely indicated for use in AGA, their anti-inflammatory activity has led to some clinical research in this area. For example, prostaglandins have been found to contribute

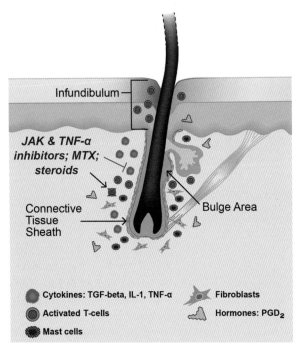

Fig. 10.1 The term "microinflammation" has been used to describe the possible inflammatory pathways present in androgenetic alopecia. Follicular microinflammation is multifactorial and involves perifollicular fibroblast activation, T-cell infiltration, prostaglandins, and mast cell degranulation. *JAK,* janus kinase; *MTX,* methotrexate; *TNF-α,* tumor necrosis factor alpha. (Courtesy of Sheila Macomber.)

to the inflammation of AGA, and the production of prostaglandin D(2) (PGD2) is upregulated in biopsies taken from a bald male-pattern scalp compared with a hair-bearing scalp (level of evidence: 4).[11] A clinical trial found that topical latanoprost, a prostaglandin F_2 analog, increases hair density in young men with mild AGA (level of evidence: 2b).[9,10] It has also been postulated that minoxidil may increase prostaglandin E_2. However, another clinical trial assessing setipiprant, a PGD2 antagonist, found no significant difference with treatment versus placebo in men with AGA (level of evidence: 2b).[12]

Inflammatory genes, such as *CASP7* and *TNF,* have also been shown to be overexpressed in male and female AGA tissue samples (level of evidence: 4).[13]

Many existing treatment methods for AGA also have anti-inflammatory mechanisms (Pearl 10.2). For example, treatment with the topical antihistamine cetirizine has been associated with clinical improvement in AGA, possibly related to the fact that mast cells produce PGD2, production of which is decreased with cetirizine (level of evidence: 2b).[14,15] Photobiomodulation is another expanding treatment modality for both male and female AGA and is postulated to work in part by reducing proinflammatory cytokines such as interleukin (IL)-6, tumor necrosis factor-alpha (TNF- α), and interferon-gamma.[16,17] Jimenez et al. found that treatment with a low-level laser device increased terminal hair density in male and female pattern hair loss.[18] As we understand more about the mechanism of platelet-rich plasma in the treatment of AGA, it appears that release of certain cytokines by platelets may also affect scalp inflammation.[19] In the 2020s, dexpanthenol, an anti-inflammatory molecule that is a precursor to coenzyme A, has been shown to improve outcomes in AGA when administered systemically (level of evidence: 4).[20,21] The use of both systemic and topical anti-inflammatory immunotherapies may play a more prominent role in the future treatment of AGA, likely as a component of combination therapy plans.[22]

Currently, the most commonly used systemic immunotherapies for the treatment of immune-mediated hair loss (e.g., AA) include oral steroids, janus kinase (JAK) inhibitors, and methotrexate (Pearl 10.3). Corticosteroids are steroid hormones that increase anti-inflammatory signaling and decrease proinflammatory signaling. JAK inhibitors act on the JAK-STAT pathway to inhibit proinflammatory cytokines, such as IL-15, and suppress T-cell activation. Methotrexate is an antifolate agent with multiple anti-inflammatory mechanisms, including the inhibition of T-cell activation. Less commonly used systemic immunotherapies include cyclosporine and biologics. Cyclosporine works as an immunosuppressive agent by decreasing T-cell activity, mostly through inhibition of IL-2 transcription, and by binding to ubiquitous cyclophilin.[23] Biologic drugs vary in their specific mechanisms.

There are also outcomes associated with topical immunotherapies that are encouraging for systemic therapy. When randomized controlled trials for finasteride featured the use of coal tar shampoo in both control and placebo groups, questions arose whether the anti-inflammatory nature of coal tar shampoo could have confounded the results. Patients have long turned to alternative anti-inflammatory botanical agents for treatment of male pattern baldness, even in the absence of robust clinical data on their efficacy in most cases.[24] Ginseng is a plant whose anti-inflammatory mechanisms have been studied in the setting of potential for hair growth (level of evidence: 5).[25] *Nigella sativa* is a plant containing the anti-inflammatory compound thymoquinone and has been hypothesized to be a potential treatment for AGA; however, it has only been studied in TE (level of evidence: 5).[14]

Other therapies discussed in this chapter, such as oral steroids, biologics, and cyclosporine, have not been demonstrated to have an effect on AGA.[26] Methotrexate was found in one case to partially reverse a patient's AGA after initiating the treatment for psoriasis.[27]

Androgenetic Alopecia and Alopecia Areata

Though systemic immunotherapy is commonly used in the treatment of cicatricial alopecias and certain nonscarring alopecias, such as AA, these therapies are not well studied in AGA. Treatment with systemic immunotherapy for AGA may be more relevant for patients with comorbid hair disease, such as in a patient with both AA and AGA. In these cases, treatment with systemic immunotherapy may need to be supplemented with targeted therapy for AGA.

Given the early positive response in AA patients to JAK inhibitor treatment, there was initial optimism that the treatment could be applied in other nonscarring alopecias. In a case series of four men with both AA and AGA, Yale et al. found that treatment with an oral JAK

1/2 inhibitor led to widespread scalp hair regrowth that spared the bitemporal regions (level of evidence: 4).[28] Thus, this immunotherapy did not counteract the miniaturization of hair follicles observed in AGA. Additionally, clinical trials for topical immunotherapy in the form of a JAK inhibitor for AGA were discontinued when no clear efficacy was observed.[29]

EXPECTED OUTCOMES

Androgenetic Alopecia

Current literature suggests that positive outcomes are not anticipated with the systemic immunotherapies that have been studied to date in AGA, including systemic corticosteroids, JAK inhibitors, and cyclosporine.[27] Outcomes have been better studied with topical immunotherapies for the management of AGA. Specifically, topical latanoprost and topical cetirizine have been associated with positive clinical outcomes.[9,15] Patients with concomitant AA and AGA may experience improvement of only their AA and not their AGA when treated with systemic immunotherapy (Pearl 10.4). In one case, a patient with AGA experienced partial regrowth with methotrexate use for psoriasis (level of evidence: 4).[26] However, we anticipate future clinical trials with systemic immunotherapy agents for use in AGA as our understanding of the inflammatory pathophysiology in AGA improves.

Alopecia Areata

In general, randomized clinical trials assessing the efficacy of treatment in AA are sparse, even for long-standing and gold-standard treatment methodologies such as intralesional steroid injections. Accordingly, there is no gold-standard metric against which to measure outcomes with new immunotherapy treatment methods.

Oral Corticosteroids

Oral corticosteroids for the treatment of AA are relatively well studied compared to many of the other systemic immunotherapies discussed in this chapter. Factors

---

PEARL 10.4: In patients with androgenetic alopecia, treatment with systemic immunotherapies may be indicated when there is comorbid immune-mediated hair loss (e.g., alopecia areata). However, in these patients, treatment with systemic immunotherapy may not lead to hair regrowth in areas affected by androgenetic alopecia.

> **PEARL 10.5:** In the treatment of alopecia areata, oral corticosteroids may lead to better outcomes in patients with decreased duration of disease and decreased disease surface area. Relapse is common after discontinuation of oral steroids.

associated with better outcomes from short-term or pulsed steroid treatment include decreased duration of disease and decreased disease surface area, and these patients may also experience disease relapse less frequently (Pearl 10.5). Ophiasis pattern hair loss and alopecia universalis are associated with poorer outcomes with oral steroid treatment (level of evidence: 4).[30] Studies on the effect of oral steroids for AA have a wide range of results, ranging from 0% to 100% efficacy, though these studies use varying metrics to assess for clinically significant regrowth (level of evidence: 5).[31-33] Time to clinically significant response is generally around three months (level of evidence: 4).[34] Response rates do not vary greatly for short-term treatment versus pulse treatment. Relapse rates are significant after discontinuation of oral steroid treatment, typically in at least half of patients discontinuing or tapering treatment (level of evidence: 4).[32,35]

Oral Janus Kinase Inhibitors

Results of the 2020 Alopecia Areata Consensus of Experts highlighted the increasing consensus regarding the efficacy of JAK inhibitors for AA (Pearl 10.6). Experts agreed that this method is the ideal second-line treatment and can be used as monotherapy for AA (level of evidence: 1a).[36] A 2019 meta-analysis of JAK inhibitors for AA found that 77.8% of patients responded to oral JAK inhibitors, which was greater than 22.2% of patients who responded to topical JAK inhibitor therapy (level of evidence: 1a).[37] The study found no significant difference in response between disease categories, such as alopecia universalis versus patchy AA. Time to clinically significant regrowth has been noted to be roughly 3 months. Notably, relapse can be observed in AA patients discontinuing or tapering use of oral JAK inhibitors (level of evidence: 1b).[38,39] Clinical trials for JAK inhibitors in AA are underway, and one can anticipate further outcome data to emerge.[40]

> **PEARL 10.6:** Janus kinase (JAK) inhibitors are efficacious second-line agents for the treatment of alopecia areata and may be used as monotherapy.

Methotrexate

A meta-analysis of the use of methotrexate for AA found the drug to be reasonably effective for treatment as monotherapy (level of evidence: 1b).[41] A greater than 50% regrowth response was observed in 63.2% of patients with AA treated with methotrexate in 16 studies. However, methotrexate was found to be significantly more effective when used as an adjunct with systemic corticosteroid therapy. The timeline to regrowth was similar to other immunotherapy treatments, with clinically evident regrowth at around 3 months into treatment. Adults were more likely to experience partial or complete regrowth than children with methotrexate treatment. Relapse poses a challenge to this treatment method, as nearly half of patients experienced hair loss when tapering or discontinuing treatment.

Cyclosporine

A meta-analysis of the use of cyclosporine for AA found the average response rate to cyclosporin monotherapy to be 57% across 14 studies (level of evidence: 1b).[42] Efficacy was best for patients with limited hair loss and worst for patients with alopecia universalis. In patients being treated with cyclosporine as an adjunct to systemic corticosteroids, the average response rate improved to 69%. Dual therapy also seems to decrease relapse rate, with fewer than half of patients experiencing relapse on dual therapy compared with the majority of patients who experience relapse on cyclosporin monotherapy. Time to treatment response ranged from 1 to 6 months. Though topical calcineurin inhibitors have been investigated for the pediatric AA population, their efficacy as systemic treatment in this population is not well known (level of evidence: 4).[43]

Biologics

Dupilumab is a monoclonal antibody against the IL-4 receptor. There are cases of patients with AA who experience hair regrowth after treatment with dupilumab for atopic dermatitis; however, there are also reports of patients experiencing new AA pattern hair loss after dupilumab treatment (level of evidence: 4).[44] Ustekinumab is another monoclonal antibody that targets IL-12 and IL-23, and it has been found to be effective in a case series of adults and children with AA.[44] Alefacept inhibits T-cell activation and is delivered intramuscularly; in a randomized controlled trial, no significant difference between alefacept and placebo was found in an adult population of patients with recalcitrant AA (level of evidence: 2b).[45] Of note, alefacept is no longer on the market in the United States. In general, TNF-α inhibitors may be more likely to cause nonscarring hair loss than treat it. A case series described eight patients treated with adalimumab and one patient with etanercept who developed AA at an average of 4 months into treatment with TNF-α inhibitors for various diseases (level of evidence: 4).[46] Two of the patients had previously been diagnosed with AA. It has been thought that this could be caused by self-reactive T cells activated by the anti-TNF-α mechanism. Histologically, the hair loss caused by TNF-α treatment appears to be distinct from true AA as a result of psoriasiform epidermal changes and the presence of dermal plasma cells (level of evidence: 4).[47] Nonetheless, TNF-α inhibitors have been trialed off-label for use in AA. One study investigated adalimumab in three patients with AA, one of whom experienced regrowth (level of evidence: 4).[48]

Other Immunomodulators

There are various other systemic immunotherapies of ranging mechanisms of action with reported use in AA. Azathioprine is a purine synthesis inhibitor. One small study found that 65% of patients with AA had a response to azathioprine, and another study reported four pediatric AA cases that improved with azathioprine (level of evidence: 4).[32,49] The following medications are no longer being studied for use in AA: Isoprinosine is a medication that stimulates cell-mediated immune response to viral infections. In a randomized control trial, 86.6% of AA patients aged 16 to 48 years experienced partial or complete response to isoprinosine (level of evidence: 2b).[50] Thymopentin is thymic polypeptide, which acts as an immunostimulant. It was studied as an intravenous therapy for AA, but no patients experienced regrowth (level of evidence: 5).[51]

TREATMENT TECHNIQUES AND BEST PRACTICES

Alopecia Areata
Oral Corticosteroids

Patients eligible for treatment with systemic steroids include adult and pediatric patients with acute or refractory AA, often with significant disease burden (level of evidence: 4) (Pearl 10.7).[33,52] However, patients with ophiasis or alopecia universalis hair loss may experience less robust responses. As a result of the poor metabolic, musculoskeletal, and dermatologic side-effect profile

> **PEARL 10.7:** Oral steroids are typically used to treat adults and children with significant disease burden, though treatment is limited to short-term or pulsed courses. Relapse after discontinuation of steroids is common.

> **PEARL 10.8:** Systemic janus kinase (JAK) inhibitors are typically used in adult patients, as additional research is needed to better understand the safety profile of these medications in the pediatric population.

with long-term use of oral corticosteroids, candidates must be carefully selected, and treatment is limited to short-term or pulsed courses. Typically, oral corticosteroids have been used for pediatric and adult patients with rapid hair loss and strong patient desire for medical treatment. Oral steroids should not be considered a first-line therapy, and one must consider the high rates of relapse with this treatment method.

Oral Janus Kinase Inhibitors

JAK inhibitors (e.g., tofacitinib and ruxolitinib) are emerging as safe and effective treatments for patients with AA (Pearl 10.8). Treatment with JAK inhibitors is typically reserved for adults rather than pediatric patients, as the safety profile in the pediatric population has not been fully elucidated. However, topical treatment has been studied in both children and adults. Treatment with oral JAK inhibitors is emerging as a second-line, off-label option for adults with AA.

Methotrexate

Methotrexate is available as a second-line treatment option for adult and pediatric patients with extensive AA. Methotrexate is sometimes used in combination with oral steroids and can be selected for steroid-sparing prevention of disease relapse.

Cyclosporine

Cyclosporine has been investigated in a few studies for second-line use in adult patients with AA, often in combination with systemic steroid treatment.

Biologics

Biologics that have been studied for use in nonscarring alopecias include dupilumab (a monoclonal antibody that blocks IL-4 and IL-13), ustekinumab (a monoclonal antibody that blocks IL-12 and IL-23), and alefacept (a fusion protein that inhibits T-cell activation) and TNF-α inhibitors including adalimumab, etanercept, and infliximab. Alefacept was withdrawn in 2011 and is no longer available for use. There is limited data regarding the efficacy of treatment with TNF-α inhibitors in adult patients with AA. In fact, many reports exist of patients treated with TNF-α inhibitors for nonhair loss diseases who secondarily developed AA.

Other Immunomodulators

Other systemic immunotherapies with limited data on the utility of treatment in adult AA include isoprinosine, thymopentin, and azathioprine. These should not be considered as first-line therapy, and more studies are required to understand the safety, efficacy, and target population of these treatment methods.

PREVENTION AND MANAGEMENT OF ADVERSE EVENTS (PEARL 10.9)

Oral Corticosteroids

Providers must take great care when providing oral corticosteroids to patients, as adverse effects are common and significant (Table 10.1). Reported side effects of treatment with oral steroids in AA include epigastric pain, weight gain, Cushing syndrome, striae, and irritability (level of evidence: 1b).[53,54] Higher rates of AA disease relapse have occurred in patients taking daily doses, thus pulsed or short-term doses are recommended (level of evidence: 2b).[55] Adverse events can also occur with topical use of corticosteroids, including atrophy, pigmentary changes, photosensitivity, and premature aging (level of evidence: 4).[56]

Oral Janus Kinase Inhibitors

In general, systemic therapy with JAK inhibitors has a safe treatment profile as an immunotherapy agent. Side effects in patients with AA include infections and laboratory abnormalities. Notably, increased incidence of herpes zoster infection has been observed in patients

TABLE 10.1 Adverse Events Associated With Systemic Immunotherapies Used for Hair Loss	
Systemic Immunotherapy	**Adverse events**
Oral corticosteroids	Acne Cushing syndrome Gastrointestinal discomfort Hypothalamic pituitary adrenal (HPA) axis suppression Hypertension Irritability Osteoporosis Striae Weight gain
Janus Kinase (JAK) inhibitors	Cardiovascular events (<1%) Infections, including herpes zoster (5%) Latent tuberculosis reactivation (<1%) Malignancy (<1%) Nasopharyngitis (3%–14%) Transaminitis Transient hyperlipidemia
Methotrexate	Alopecia (≤10%) Gastrointestinal discomfort (>10%) Hepatotoxicity Leukopenia (<5%) Pulmonary toxicity Stomatitis (≤10%) Transaminitis (<10%)
Cyclosporine	Gastrointestinal discomfort (<25%) Headache (>10%) Hirsutism (>10%) Hypertension, edema (>10%) Hypertrichosis (<20%) Infection (>10%) Tremor (>10%)
Biologics	Injection-site reactions Dupilumab – ophthalmologic events (≤10%) Ustekinumab – headache (<10%) and fatigue

Note that most systemic-steroid adverse events are dose and duration dependent.

PEARL 10.9: Each systemic immunotherapy drug has a unique side-effect profile. Prescribing physicians must be aware of common and severe adverse events and the risk factors for such events.

treated with JAK inhibitors. Laboratory abnormalities are mild and transient, such as mild elevations to liver function test values and lipid panel values.[37] It is important to consider that more serious adverse effects have been observed in patients treated with JAK inhibitors for rheumatoid arthritis, such as increased malignancy and cardiovascular events, resulting in updated warnings from the U.S. Food and Drug Administration. Before starting treatment with a JAK inhibitor, clinicians should obtain a baseline complete blood count, liver function tests, lipid panel, and screen for latent tuberculosis, hepatitis A, hepatitis B, and hepatitis C. The authors recommend obtaining safety labs every 3 months while patients are being treated with JAK inhibitors, including a comprehensive metabolic panel, complete blood count, lipid panel, and urinalysis.

Methotrexate

Adverse effects with the administration of methotrexate for hair loss include mild asymptomatic transaminitis and gastrointestinal discomfort (level of evidence: 4).[57] Patients may also experience asymptomatic leukopenia that can be treated with folic acid supplementation (level of evidence: 4).[58] Rarely, hepatotoxicity and pulmonary toxicity may be observed. The dose of methotrexate used for treatment of hair loss is lower than that used for malignancies. At higher doses, methotrexate can lead to morbid nephotoxicity.[59]

Cyclosporine

Adverse events reported by patients being treated with cyclosporine include gastrointestinal symptoms, hypertrichosis, and hypertension.[42] Cyclosporine has dose-dependent nephrotoxicity, which can be observed in transplant patients who are prescribed larger doses and undergo drug monitoring accordingly.[60]

Biologics

The most common adverse effects after dupilumab treatment include injection-site reaction and ophthalmologic events. Ustekinumab also causes injection-site reactions and may cause headache and fatigue.[44] In a case series of patients treated with adalimumab for AA, all experienced mild-to-moderate adverse effects, most common of which was injection-site reaction.[48] Patients treated with alefacept in a randomized controlled trial for AA only experienced mild adverse events and at a rate the same as in the placebo group.[45] In general, providers should monitor for

infection when treating patients with a TNF-α inhibitor. The adverse event profile of this class of medication seems to vary based on the disease for which it is being used; patients with rheumatoid arthritis experience more adverse events during treatment with TNF-α inhibitors than patients with psoriasis (level of evidence: 2a).[61]

Other Immunomodulators

When starting a patient on azathioprine, one typically starts at a low dose to minimize gastrointestinal symptoms.[32] Though adverse effects are not fully elucidated in the use of isoprinosine, no patients in a randomized controlled trial of its use for AA reported adverse symptoms.[50] Though not a systemic treatment, topical prostaglandin analogs including bimatoprost can be associated with erythema, pruritus, and hyperpigmentation (level of evidence: 4).[62]

FUTURE DIRECTIONS

Advancements in the field of systemic immunotherapy for AGA are likely in the coming years as we further understand the specific pathways in which cytokines, T-cells, mast cells, and fibroblasts lead to follicular microinflammation and follicle miniaturization in AGA. It is likely that anti-inflammatory immunotherapy will be used in combination with other targeted nonimmunotherapies (Pearl 10.10).

The study of systemic immunotherapies for other nonscarring alopecias, such as AA, is also actively growing. More robust data for current off-label treatment options, such as JAK inhibitors, are expected in the coming years given ongoing clinical trials for AA. Though currently the use of systemic immunotherapy is more efficacious in AA than AGA, there is hope that future studies may yield efficacious results for the use of systemic immunotherapy in AGA.

EVIDENCE SUMMARY

- Systemic immunotherapy is not a currently recommended treatment for androgenetic alopecia (strength of recommendation: D).

> **PEARL 10.10:** As the inflammatory pathways are better understood, there will likely be advancements in the utility of systemic immunotherapy medications for the treatment of androgenetic alopecia and other nonscarring alopecias.

- Topical immunotherapy may prove to be useful in the treatment of androgenetic alopecia, including in combination protocols (strength of recommendation: D).
- Systemic immunotherapy is useful in the treatment of alopecia areata (strength of recommendation: A).

REFERENCES

1. Sperling LC, Lupton GP. Histopathology of non-scarring alopecia. *J Cutan Pathol.* 1995;22(2):97-114.
2. Mahé YF, Michelet JF, Billoni N, et al. Androgenetic alopecia and microinflammation. *Int J Dermatol.* 2000;39(8):576-584.
3. Ramos PM, Brianezi G, Martins ACP, da Silva MG, Marques MEA, Miot HA. Apoptosis in follicles of individuals with female pattern hair loss is associated with perifollicular microinflammation. *Int J Cosmet Sci.* 2016;38(6):651-654.
4. El-Domyati M, Attia S, Saleh F, Abdel-Wahab H. Androgenetic alopecia in males: a histopathological and ultrastructural study. *J Cosmet Dermatol.* 2009;8(2):83-91.
5. Magro CM, Rossi A, Poe J, Manhas-Bhutani S, Sadick N. The role of inflammation and immunity in the pathogenesis of androgenetic alopecia. *J Drugs Dermatol.* 2011;10(12):1404-1411.
6. Kash N, Leavitt M, Leavitt A, Hawkins SD, Roopani RB. Clinical patterns of hair loss in men: is dihydrotestosterone the only culprit? *Dermatol Clin.* 2021;39(3):361-370.
7. Sadick N, Arruda S. Understanding causes of hair loss in women. *Dermatol Clin.* 2021;39(3):371-374.
8. Plante J, Valdebran M, Forcucci J, Lucas O, Elston D. Perifollicular inflammation and follicular spongiosis in androgenetic alopecia. *J Am Acad Dermatol.* 2022;86(2):437-438.
9. Blume-Peytavi U, Lönnfors S, Hillmann K, Garcia Bartels N. A randomized double-blind placebo-controlled pilot study to assess the efficacy of a 24-week topical treatment by latanoprost 0.1% on hair growth and pigmentation in healthy volunteers with androgenetic alopecia. *J Am Acad Dermatol.* 2012;66(5):794-800.
10. Nieves A, Garza LA. Does prostaglandin D2 hold the cure to male pattern baldness? *Exp Dermatol.* 2014;23(4):224-227.
11. Garza LA, Liu Y, Yang Z, et al. Prostaglandin D2 inhibits hair growth and is elevated in bald scalp of men with androgenetic alopecia. *Sci Transl Med.* 2012;4(126):126-134.
12. DuBois J, Bruce S, Stewart D, et al. Setipiprant for androgenetic alopecia in males: results from a randomized, double-blind, placebo-controlled phase 2a trial. *Clin Cosmet Investig Dermatol.* 2021;14:1507-1517.
13. Peyravian N, Deo S, Daunert S, Jimenez JJ. The inflammatory aspect of male and female pattern hair loss. *J Inflamm Res.* 2020;13:879-881.
14. Rossi A, Anzalone A, Fortuna MC, et al. Multi-therapies in androgenetic alopecia: review and clinical experiences. *Dermatol Ther.* 2016;29(6):424-432.
15. Rossi A, Campo D, Fortuna MC, et al. A preliminary study on topical cetirizine in the therapeutic management of androgenetic alopecia. *J Dermatolog Treat.* 2018;29(2):149-151.
16. Dodd EM, Winter MA, Hordinsky MK, Sadick NS, Farah RS. Photobiomodulation therapy for androgenetic alopecia: a clinician's guide to home-use devices cleared by the Federal Drug Administration. *J Cosmet Laser Ther.* 2018;20(3):159-167.
17. Fukuda TY, Tanji MM, Silva SR, Sato MN, Plapler H. Infrared low-level diode laser on inflammatory process modulation in mice: pro- and anti-inflammatory cytokines. *Lasers Med Sci.* 2013;28(5):1305-1313.
18. Jimenez JJ, Wikramanayake TC, Bergfeld W, et al. Efficacy and safety of a low-level laser device in the treatment of male and female pattern hair loss: a multicenter, randomized, sham device-controlled, double-blind study. *Am J Clin Dermatol.* 2014;15(2):115-127.
19. Gupta AK, Renaud HJ, Rapaport JA. Platelet-rich plasma and cell therapy: the new horizon in hair loss treatment. *Dermatol Clin.* 2021;39(3):429-445.
20. Kutlu Ö. Dexpanthenol may be a novel treatment for male androgenetic alopecia: analysis of nine cases. *Dermatol Ther.* 2020;33(3):e13381.
21. Kutlu Ö, Metin A. Systemic dexpanthenol as a novel treatment for female pattern hair loss. *J Cosmet Dermatol.* 2021;20(4):1325-1330.
22. Sadick NS, Callender VD, Kircik LH, Kogan S. New insight into the pathophysiology of hair loss trigger a paradigm shift in the treatment approach. *J Drugs Dermatol.* 2017;16(11):s135-s140.
23. Russell G, Graveley R, Seid J, al-Humidan AK, Skjodt H. Mechanisms of action of cyclosporine and effects on connective tissues. *Semin Arthritis Rheum.* 1992;21(6 suppl 3):16-22.
24. Hosking AM, Juhasz M, Atanaskova Mesinkovska N. Complementary and alternative treatments for alopecia: a comprehensive review. *Skin Appendage Disord.* 2019;5(2):72-89.
25. Choi BY. Hair-growth potential of ginseng and its major metabolites: a review on its molecular mechanisms. *Int J Mol Sci.* 2018;19(9):2703.
26. Green J, Sinclair RD. Oral cyclosporin does not arrest progression of androgenetic alopecia. *Br J Dermatol.* 2001;145(5):842-845.
27. Famenini S, Wu JJ. Partial reversal of androgenetic alopecia with methotrexate therapy for psoriasis. *Cutis.* 2013;92(3):127-128.

28. Yale K, Pourang A, Plikus MV, Mesinkovska NA. At the crossroads of 2 alopecias: androgenetic alopecia pattern of hair regrowth in patients with alopecia areata treated with oral Janus kinase inhibitors. *JAAD Case Rep.* 2020;6(5):444-446.

29. ClinicalTrials.gov. *A Study in Male and Female Subjects with Androgenetic Alopecia Treated with ATI-50002 Topical Solution.* U.S. National Library of Medicine. https://clinicaltrials.gov/ct2/show/results/NCT03495817?term=ATI-50002&draw=2&rank=1. Published 2020. Accessed April 1, 2022.

30. Friedli A, Labarthe MP, Engelhardt E, Feldmann R, Salomon D, Saurat JH. Pulse methylprednisolone therapy for severe alopecia areata: an open prospective study of 45 patients. *J Am Acad Dermatol.* 1998;39(4):597-602.

31. Kassira S, Korta DZ, Chapman LW, Dann F. Review of treatment for alopecia totalis and alopecia universalis. *Int J Dermatol.* 2017;56(8):801-810.

32. Cranwell WC, Lai VW, Photiou L, et al. Treatment of alopecia areata: An Australian expert consensus statement. *Australas J Dermatol.* 2019;60(2):163-170.

33. Trüeb RM, Dias MFRG. Alopecia areata: a comprehensive review of pathogenesis and management. *Clin Rev Allerg Immu.* 2018;54(1):68-87.

34. Sharma VK. Pulsed administration of corticosteroids in the treatment of alopecia areata. *Int J Dermatol.* 1996;35(2):133-136.

35. Alabdulkareem AS, Abahussein AA, Okoro A. Severe alopecia areata treated with systemic corticosteroids. *Int J Dermatol.* 1998;37(8):622-624.

36. Meah N, Wall D, York K, et al. The Alopecia Areata Consensus of Experts (ACE) study: results of an international expert opinion on treatments for alopecia areata. *J Am Acad Dermatol.* 2020;83(1):123-130.

37. Phan K, Sebaratnam DF. JAK inhibitors for alopecia areata: a systematic review and meta-analysis. *J Eur Acad Dermatol Venereol.* 2019;33(5):850-856.

38. Bokhari L, Sinclair R. Treatment of alopecia universalis with topical Janus kinase inhibitors - a double blind, placebo, and active controlled pilot study. *Int J Dermatol.* 2018;57(12):1464-1470.

39. Almutairi N, Nour TM, Hussain NH. Janus kinase inhibitors for the treatment of severe alopecia areata: an open-label comparative study. *Dermatol.* 2019;235(2):130-136.

40. Crowley EL, Fine SC, Katipunan KK, Gooderham MJ. The Use of Janus Kinase inhibitors in alopecia areata: a review of the literature. *J Cutan Med Surg.* 2019;23(3):289-297.

41. Phan K, Ramachandran V, Sebaratnam DF. Methotrexate for alopecia areata: a systematic review and meta-analysis. *J Am Acad Dermatol.* 2019;80(1):120-127.e2.

42. Nowaczyk J, Makowska K, Rakowska A, Sikora M, Rudnicka L. Cyclosporine with and without systemic corticosteroids in treatment of alopecia areata: a systematic review. *Dermatol Ther.* 2020;10(3):387-399.

43. Barton VR, Toussi A, Awasthi S, Kiuru M. Treatment of pediatric alopecia areata: a systematic review. *J Am Acad Dermatol.* 2022;86:1318-1334.

44. Pourang A, Mesinkovska NA. New and emerging therapies for alopecia areata. *Drugs.* 2020;80(7):635-646.

45. Strober BE, Menon K, McMichael A, et al. Alefacept for severe alopecia areata: a randomized, double-blind, placebo-controlled study. *Arch Dermatol.* 2009;145(11):1262-1266.

46. Le Bidre E, Chaby G, Martin L, et al. [Alopecia areata during anti-TNF alpha therapy: Nine cases]. *Ann Dermatol Venereol.* 2011;138(4):285-293.

47. Doyle LA, Sperling LC, Baksh S, et al. Psoriatic alopecia/alopecia areata-like reactions secondary to anti-tumor necrosis factor-α therapy: a novel cause of noncicatricial alopecia. *Am J Dermatopathol.* 2011;33(2):161-166.

48. Bolduc C, Bissonnette R. Safety and efficacy of adalimumab for the treatment of severe alopecia areata: case series of three patients. *J Cutan Med Surg.* 2012;16(4):257-260.

49. Saoji V, Kulkarni S, Madke B. Alopecia areata treated with oral azathioprine: a case series. *Int J Trichology.* 2019;11(5):219-222.

50. Georgala S, Katoulis AC, Befon A, Georgala K, Stavropoulos PG. Inosiplex for treatment of alopecia areata: a randomized placebo-controlled study. *Acta Derm Venereol.* 2006;86(5):422-424.

51. Tosti A, Manuzzi P, Gasponi A. Thymopentin in the treatment of severe alopecia areata. *Dermatologica.* 1988;177(3):170-174.

52. Friedland R, Tal R, Lapidoth M, Zvulunov A, Ben Amitai D. Pulse corticosteroid therapy for alopecia areata in children: a retrospective study. *Dermatol.* 2013;227(1):37-44.

53. Vañó-Galván S, Hermosa-Gelbard Á, Sánchez-Neila N, et al. Pulse corticosteroid therapy with oral dexamethasone for the treatment of adult alopecia totalis and universalis. *J Am Acad Dermatol.* 2016;74(5):1005-1007.

54. Shreberk-Hassidim R, Ramot Y, Gilula Z, Zlotogorski A. A systematic review of pulse steroid therapy for alopecia areata. *J Am Acad Dermatol.* 2016;74(2):372-374.e5.

55. Kurosawa M, Nakagawa S, Mizuashi M, et al. A comparison of the efficacy, relapse rate and side effects among three modalities of systemic corticosteroid therapy for alopecia areata. *Dermatol.* 2006;212(4):361-365.

56. Mehta AB, Nadkarni NJ, Patil SP, Godse KV, Gautam M, Agarwal S. Topical corticosteroids in dermatology. *Indian J Dermatol Venereol Leprol.* 2016;82(4):371-378.

57. Lim SK, Lim CA, Kwon IS, et al. Low-Dose systemic methotrexate therapy for recalcitrant alopecia areata. *Ann Dermatol.* 2017;29(3):263-267.

58. Hammerschmidt M, Mulinari Brenner F. Efficacy and safety of methotrexate in alopecia areata. *An Bras Dermatol*. 2014;89:729-734.
59. Howard SC, McCormick J, Pui CH, Buddington RK, Harvey RD. Preventing and managing toxicities of high-dose methotrexate. *Oncologist*. 2016;21(12):1471-1482.
60. Naesens M, Kuypers DR, Sarwal M. Calcineurin inhibitor nephrotoxicity. *Clin J Am Soc Nephrol*. 2009;4(2):481-508.
61. García-Doval I, Hernández MV, Vanaclocha F, Sellas A, de la Cueva P, Montero D. Should tumour necrosis factor antagonist safety information be applied from patients with rheumatoid arthritis to psoriasis? Rates of serious adverse events in the prospective rheumatoid arthritis BIOBADASER and psoriasis BIOBADADERM cohorts. *Br J Dermatol*. 2017;176(3):643-649.
62. Yoelin SG, Fagien S, Cox SE, et al. A retrospective review and observational study of outcomes and safety of bimatoprost ophthalmic solution 0.03% for treating eyelash hypotrichosis. *Dermatol Surg*. 2014;40(10):1118-1124.

11

Complementary and Alternative Medicine for Hair Loss

James T. Pathoulas and Maryanne M. Senna

KEY POINTS

- Patients with androgenetic alopecia may be interested in exploring complementary and alternative medicine, including supplements, specialty diets, and essential oils.
- There is insufficient evidence to support the use of any complementary and alternative medicine as monotherapy for androgenetic alopecia.
- Patients who wish to forgo traditional therapies in favor of complementary and alternative medicine should be counseled that the latter are not considered an appropriate monotherapy for alopecia. These patients can be directed toward efficacious treatments that may be similarly perceived as "natural," including platelet-rich plasma therapy, microneedling, and photobiomodulation.

- Although many complementary and alternative medicine therapies have roots in ancient culture and are generally considered safe, certain products and practices place patients at risk of serious harm.
- Patients with androgenetic alopecia and a serum ferritin less than 40 ng/mL should undergo repletion with an oral slow-release ferrous iron supplement for at least 3 to 6 months before laboratory reevaluation.
- Most individuals have adequate biotin intake, and biotin supplementation may invalidate laboratory tests such as cardiac troponin and thyroid panel assays.
- Alopecia patients experiencing psychosocial distress from hair loss may benefit from seeing a licensed mental-health professional, joining a patient support group, and scalp photography.

INTRODUCTION

Complementary and alternative medicine (CAM) includes treatments and practices that are distinct from traditional medical care. Patients with androgenetic alopecia (AGA) can feel distressed and may not respond to treatment, prompting them to explore CAM therapies. Many CAM therapies, including topical herbal preparations, massage, and specialty diets, have roots in ancient culture.[1] CAM treatments for AGA include natural herbal products, mind-body practices, and homeopathy.[1,2] Patients report turning to CAM to gain a sense of control over their condition and from concern with side effects of traditional medications (level of evidence: 5).[3,4]

Increasing patient interest in CAM mirrors trending consumer demand for "natural" products and is estimated to be an annual $30.2-billion industry.[1] However, less than half of patients using CAM therapies inform their physician (level of evidence: 2a).[5] Although CAM is generally considered safe, certain products and practices place patients at risk of serious harm (Pearl 11.1).[4,6,7] This chapter will provide an overview of the medical literature on CAM therapies for AGA.

DIET AND SUPPLEMENTS

Hair requires adequate intake of macronutrients and micronutrients for optimal growth. The association between nutrition and hair is so linked that anthropologists

> **PEARL 11.1:** Alopecia patients who wish to forgo tra-
> ditional therapies in favor of complementary and alter-
> native medicines (CAMs) should be counseled that
> CAMs are not considered an appropriate monotherapy
> for alopecia and can be directed toward efficacious
> treatments that may be similarly perceived as 'natural'
> including platelet-rich plasma treatment, micronee-
> dling, and photobiomodulation.

can measure the concentration of nitrogen isotopes specific to corn-fed animal-based proteins in a person's hair
and approximate their socioeconomic status (level of
evidence: 2c).[8] The well-known link between nutrition
and hair prompts many distressed alopecia patients to
start new diets and supplements, spurring the growth of
a massive hair-related diet and nutraceutical industry.[9]
However, the literature examining hair and nutrition is
conflicted. In this section, we review evidence regarding
diet and supplementation in AGA.

Protein

Hair primarily consists of protein. The importance of
dietary protein to hair growth is highlighted in conditions of inadequate protein intake. For example, children with kwashiorkor who have diets that are calori-
cally adequate but protein poor experience increased
hair shedding, decreased hair shaft diameter, hypopigmented fibers, and texture changes.[10] Although dietary
protein is readily available to people in developed countries, there is evidence to suggest that many patients
with AGA may not have adequate protein intake.

A small cross-sectional study of 20 patients with AGA
identified that 90% had inadequate protein intake and
that 55% were "severely deficient" (consumed <30 g/day)
despite self-reporting eating a regular diet (level of evidence: 4).[11] Histologic comparison revealed increased
perifollicular fibrosis in those with low dietary protein
compared with those with normal dietary protein. The
study found a positive association between consumption
of breakfast and overall protein intake. A similar case-
control study of 357 patients with AGA did not find a
significant association between protein intake and AGA
outcomes (level of evidence: 3b).[12] The small size of these
studies and conflicting results limit broad generalizations.
However, they demonstrate that patients who are food
secure may still have diets deficient in protein and could
benefit from nutrition counseling.

The dietary reference intake (DRI) for protein is
0.8 grams per kilogram of body weight for sedentary
adults.[13] However, this can be increased for adults who
are active.[14] Long-term dietary protein intake exceeding
2 grams per kilogram of body weight can cause renal,
cardiovascular, and gastrointestinal disease and should
be avoided.[14] The authors typically recommend 50 to
60 grams daily of dietary protein intake for patients
with AGA and normal renal function.

Cystine

Keratin is the primary hair protein. Although many oral
hair-growth supplements include keratin as an ingredient, it is poorly solubilized in water and not readily absorbed in the human digestive tract.[3] Supplementation
with keratin's constituent amino acids, namely cysteine,
to improve hair growth has been proposed in the treatment of AGA. Cystine is the oxidized form of cysteine
responsible for disulfide keratin cross-linking.[3] Various
studies have examined the use of cystine in AGA and
telogen effluvium (TE) and suggest a positive treatment
response (level of evidence: 1b).[15-17] However, cystine
was combined with other minerals, vitamins, and proprietary formulations in these studies, preventing true
determination of cystine's efficacy. There is not sufficient evidence to support routine cystine supplementation for the treatment of AGA.

Iron

Hair matrix cells undergo rapid division, facilitating
elongation of the anagen hair shaft.[18] Iron is a cofactor
of rate-limiting enzymes crucial to cell division and is
involved in the regulation of multiple genes along the
bulge region.[19,20] However, the mechanistic role of iron
in hair growth remains to be established.

Iron deficiency is common. In the United States 12%
to 16% of females ages 16 to 49 years and 2% of males
ages 16 to 69 years are iron deficient (level of evidence:
2c).[21] After age 50, fewer women are iron deficient (6%
to 9% total) as a result of decreased menstrual blood
loss, while more men (4% total) are iron deficient, pre-
sumably as a result of gastrointestinal blood loss.[21] Several laboratory tests can be used to estimate iron status.
However, serum ferritin is the most reflective of overall
iron status.[22]

It is important to distinguish iron depletion and iron
deficiency anemia (IDA). Iron depletion occurs when
total body iron reserves are decreased, indicated by a

low serum ferritin (typically <40 ng/mL but may be lab-specific) and normal hemoglobin.[22] There may not be overt clinical signs and symptoms in iron depletion. IDA is more severe and has the potential to cause functional limitations. In IDA, serum ferritin is less than 20 ng/mL, hemoglobin is low (9-12 g/dL), and total iron binding capacity (TIBC) is increased (350-400 mcg/dL).[19] IDA should always be treated, and prompt referral is needed to investigate the cause of anemia and to prevent end organ damage. However, there is no consensus regarding iron supplementation for the treatment of patients who are iron depleted and have AGA.

Studies examining the relationship between iron deficiency and hair loss have been conducted in women with AGA and TE. A case-control study of 52 women with AGA and 11 without found that those with AGA had significantly lower serum ferritin (level of evidence: 3b).[23] The association did not vary with respect to age, and there were no differences in hemoglobin between groups. A similar case-control study in 100 premenopausal women with AGA found that 72% had serum ferritin below the lowest serum ferritin of 40 ng/mL seen in the control group (n = 20) (level of evidence: 3b).[24] However, there are conflicting reports in the literature. A case-control study of 43 women with AGA and 43 controls found no difference in serum ferritin between groups (level of evidence: 3b).[25] A prospective cohort study identified 12 of 194 women with biopsy-proven AGA (level of evidence: 3b).[26] All patients underwent treatment with spironolactone 200 mg daily or cyproterone acetate 100 mg daily for 10 days each month. The 12 patients with AGA underwent treatment with iron supplementation for 6 months, and all achieved a target serum ferritin greater than 20 ng/mL. The study authors concluded that there was no significant benefit observed in those who underwent iron repletion. However, no statistical analysis was published.

Several case-control studies have demonstrated that patients with AGA have a higher incidence of iron depletion than those without AGA. However, conflicting reports remain. Although there is no consensus statement on universal screening for iron deficiency in those with AGA, it is frequently an expert recommendation (level of evidence: 5).[3,19] The treatment of IDA is necessary and requires referral for further workup. However, the treatment of iron depletion in those with AGA has not been extensively studied, and more research is needed. Despite this, iron repletion is not costly, and

> **PEARL 11.2:** Advise alopecia patients with iron depletion to purchase oral iron supplements with ferrous iron, as it is more readily absorbed than ferric iron.

the most common side effect is gastrointestinal intolerability.[19]

Given the potential for benefit with minimal serious side effects, we recommend patients at risk for iron depletion including premenopausal women, those with a restrictive diet or history of eating disorders, those with a family history of anemia, those with a history concerning for depletion (e.g., fatigue, headache, restless leg syndrome, pica, renal disease), and patients with malabsorptive disorders or a history of bariatric surgery be screened for iron deficiency. In those with iron depletion (ferritin <40 ng/mL with normal hemoglobin), we recommend treatment with an oral slow-release ferrous iron supplement for at least 3 to 6 months before laboratory reevaluation (Pearl 11.2).

Zinc

After iron, zinc is the most abundantly distributed trace element in the human body.[27] Zinc is critical to protein folding and nucleic acid synthesis, and it serves as a cofactor for many enzymes. True zinc deficiency, characterized by alopecia, glossitis, diarrhea, and nail dystrophy, is rare among people in developed countries.[3] However, there is some evidence to suggest that patients with AGA have decreased serum zinc compared with healthy controls.

A case-control study reported that serum zinc levels in 84 males and 77 females with AGA were significantly lower (range 10.2 to 17.3 μg/dL) than healthy controls (level of evidence: 3b).[28] However, the number of AGA patients with serum zinc levels below the established lower limit of normal (70 μg/dL) did not differ significantly between groups. A randomized controlled trial (RCT) comparing topical minoxidil 2% twice daily and oral zinc sulfate 50 mg once daily in 73 females with AGA found that oral zinc (n = 16) led to a significant improvement in hair density after 4 months of treatment (level of evidence: 2b).[29] However, density and diameter were greater for those using minoxidil.

Topical zinc preparations are commonly available as pyrithione zinc shampoos and indicated for antifungal treatment of seborrheic dermatitis. A single RCT evaluating daily use of pyrithione zinc 1% shampoo, placebo shampoo, twice daily use of topical minoxidil 5%, and combination treatment in 200 men with AGA found both interventions resulted in significantly increased hair density compared with placebo after 24 weeks (level of evidence: 2b).[30] However, only topical minoxidil resulted in significantly greater terminal hair diameter. The benefit seen with pyrithione zinc was only modest compared with minoxidil. Patients treated with both interventions did not have a greater benefit than those using only minoxidil.

The literature examining zinc in the treatment of AGA is limited. There is insufficient evidence to recommend oral zinc supplementation in those with AGA. Some evidence suggests pyrithione zinc shampoos may improve hair density in men with AGA. However, the literature is limited to a single controlled trial. Pyrithione zinc shampoo as monotherapy in AGA is not recommended. Instead, we recommend a low threshold for initiating treatment with pyrithione zinc shampoo at least twice weekly for AGA patients who have waxy scalp scale or other signs consistent with seborrheic dermatitis of the scalp. We recommend patients avoid shampoo formulations that contain formaldehyde releasers and other agents known to contribute to allergic contact dermatitis and potentially primary lymphocytic cicatricial alopecias (level of evidence: 2b).[31]

Biotin (Vitamin B$_7$)

Biotin is an essential cofactor for multiple metabolic reactions and is a transcriptional regulator. Most individuals in the developed world have adequate biotin intake through dietary sources. Additionally, the amount of biotin synthesized by symbiont intestinal bacteria exceeds daily intake requirements.[3] Inborn errors of biotin metabolism are rare and present with dermatitis, hair loss, and neurologic disease that require supplementation. Most dietary biotin is obtained from protein. Conversion of free biotin from dietary protein is decreased by isotretinoin and valproic acid.[32,33] Supplementation has been proposed in patients with alopecia on these medications. However, the evidence is limited to single cases (level of evidence: 4).[34,35]

A significant number of commercially available oral supplements and haircare products tout the benefit of biotin for improved hair density and texture. Patients and physicians alike are enthusiastic about biotin supplementation.[36-38] In a survey of 300 dermatologists,

66% reported recommending commercial supplements for hair, skin, and nails.[38] However, no RCTs have evaluated biotin for the treatment of hair loss, and there are concerns about its safety.

Biotin has the potential to invalidate biotinylated laboratory tests, such as cardiac troponin and thyroid panel assays.[9] The FDA has issued a warning regarding biotin supplementation and the risk of false laboratory findings, which have been implicated in at least one patient death.[39] Given the lack of evidence supporting the use of biotin for hair growth and potential risk, the authors do not recommend biotin therapy for the treatment of AGA.

Complex Nutraceuticals and Marine Peptides

A wide variety of commercial dietary supplements marketed to patients with hair loss contain multiple macronutrients, micronutrients, various phytochemicals, and proprietary ingredients. The evidence behind most constituent ingredients in complex nutraceuticals is limited. Proponents of these complex supplements argue that the benefit of numerous ingredients in proprietary formulations offer a beneficial synergistic effect. The best-studied complex nutraceuticals contain marine proteins. Complex nutraceuticals with 5α-reductase activity are explored in the following section.

Marine peptide complexes include extracellular matrix proteins derived from shark and mollusk sources.[40,41] However, ingredient specifications are limited by proprietary claims. The mechanism of marine peptide induced hair growth is unknown but may involve increased alkaline phosphatase activity at the dermal papillae (level of evidence: 5).[40] A double-blind study of 40 women with self-perceived hair thinning were randomized to treatment with twice daily marine protein supplementation or placebo for 6 months (level of evidence: 2b).[40] Those taking the proprietary supplement (n = 17) experienced a significantly greater increase in both hair density and diameter along the temporal hairline compared with those on placebo (n = 19). A larger double-blind RCT comparing the proprietary marine supplement against placebo in 96 women with self-perceived hair loss found supplementation three times daily resulted in increased vellus hair diameter only (level of evidence: 2b).[42] Supplement users experienced decreased shedding at 3 months. However, this difference was not significant between the interventions at

6 months, and early differences may be attributable to resolution of active TE. A similar RCT of marine protein in 60 men with AGA found that 6 months of supplementation resulted in increased hair density, including count and diameter (level of evidence: 2b).[41]

The high quality of studies examining complex nutraceuticals containing marine proteins stand apart from other CAM therapies for hair loss. Marine proteins appear to be safe and effective in industry-sponsored studies. However, they contain proprietary formulations that are largely unregulated and costly. Commercial supplements, including nutraceuticals, are not covered by insurance and are generally not considered eligible expenses under health savings plans. The authors infrequently recommend marine protein supplements as an adjuvant treatment for AGA. However, it may be appropriate for patients who are highly motivated to treat their hair loss with supplements, are not concerned about cost, and have no history of shellfish allergy.

Botanically Derived 5α-reductase Inhibitors

Inhibition of 5α-reductase prevents conversion of testosterone to dihydrotestosterone (DHT) and is the mechanism underlying the antiandrogen activity of finasteride and dutasteride. DHT contributes to miniaturization of the hair follicle in AGA. Oral 5α-reductase inhibitors are effective in the treatment of male AGA. However, a minority of patients experience sexual and mood side effects. Saw palmetto similarly prevents reduction of testosterone and has been investigated as a naturally sourced treatment for AGA.

Saw palmetto has various antiandrogen effects. It decreases DHT-mediated signal transduction and has inhibitory activity against 5α-reductase isoforms I and II.[43] An open-label study in 100 men with AGA compared daily treatment with oral saw palmetto extract 320 mg daily against oral finasteride 1 mg daily (level of evidence: 2b).[44] After 2 years, both groups experienced improved hair density per investigator assessment. Those on finasteride (n = 50) experienced a 30% greater improvement than those taking saw palmetto. Similar improvement was observed in a smaller study of 26 men with AGA treated with saw palmetto (level of evidence: 2b).[45] Neither study reported sexual or mood side effects from saw palmetto.

Saw palmetto is also an ingredient in multiple nutraceuticals. A RCT examined the effect of treatment with a daily complex nutraceutical containing saw palmetto extract in 40 women with AGA over 6 months (level of evidence: 2b).[46] Those taking the nutraceutical (n = 26) had an average of 6.61 greater frontotemporal terminal hairs than the placebo group. However, the complex supplement had multiple ingredients, precluding direct evaluation of saw palmetto.

Saw palmetto extract is inferior to finasteride in the treatment of AGA. The authors do not recommend saw palmetto for the treatment of AGA. Pumpkin seed oil has also been investigated as a naturally derived 5α-reductase inhibitor and showed positive results in a single study (level of evidence: 2b).[47] Botanically derived 5α-reductase inhibitors may be considered in patients uninterested in finasteride or dutasteride. Patients with reproductive potential should be counseled on the teratogenic effects of 5α-reductase inhibitors in male fetuses.

Caffeine

Caffeine is a naturally occurring and widely consumed stimulant. Topical caffeine-containing preparations have been evaluated in the treatment of hair loss, including gels, creams, and shampoos. In vitro studies demonstrate the action of caffeine on hair growth may be multimodal. Caffeine inhibits phosphodiesterase, increasing cellular cyclic adenosine monophosphate (cAMP).[48,49] Increased cAMP is thought to increase cellular metabolism and induce dermal papilla cell proliferation.[50] Application of caffeine solution to human follicular models results in increased hair density, diameter, and decreases androgen-mediated follicular miniaturization (level of evidence: 5).[49]

An open-label RCT comparing topical caffeine 0.2% twice daily with topical minoxidil 5% twice daily in 215 men with AGA reported that caffeine was noninferior to minoxidil based on investigator assessment of photography and trichoscopy (level of evidence: 2b).[51] A similar study evaluating combined topical caffeine 2.5% and minoxidil 2.5% daily against topical minoxidil 2.5% alone in 60 men with AGA found that the combined treatment group had superior hair density after 6 months of use (level of evidence: 2b).[52] Smaller studies have evaluated the use of topical solutions and shampoos with caffeine and found similar positive results (level of evidence: 4).[53,54]

There are few RCTs that support the use of caffeine as a treatment for AGA. More studies are needed for a true determination of efficacy. Topical caffeine is not an appropriate monotherapy for AGA, and the authors do not routinely recommend topical caffeine for the treatment of AGA.

ESSENTIAL OILS

Essential oils are aromatic plant-derived compounds. The use of aromatic oils for medicinal purposes dates back to early civilizations.[55] Concentrated aldehydes, ketones, phenols, and monoterpenes are responsible for the chemical volatility of essential oils.[55] Topical application of essential oils has been described in the treatment of both AGA and alopecia areata (AA).

An RCT comparing daily application of topical rosemary lotion (3.7 mg/mL *Salvia rosmarinus* oil extract) or topical minoxidil 2% in 100 AGA patients reported a significant increase in hair density in both groups as measured by investigator microphotographic assessment at 6 months (level of evidence: 2b) (Fig. 11.1).[56]

There was no significant density difference between the treated groups. Scalp itch was reported in both groups but was more prevalent among those using minoxidil. The authors suggest that rosemary oil can improve microcirculation to enhance hair growth, but this was not mechanistically examined. Others have argued that essential oils may reduce scalp inflammation impeding hair growth through antifungal activity. Tea-tree oil has activity against *Malassezia*, but quality studies are needed (level of evidence: 5).[57] Essential oils have also been evaluated in the treatment of AA.

An RCT of 84 patients with AA compared response to daily topical application of an essential oil mixture including thyme (*Thymus spp.*, 3.8 mg/mL), rosemary (*Salvia rosmarinus*, 5.0 mg/mL), lavender (*Lavandula agustifolia*, 4.7/mL mg), and cedarwood (*Cedrus atlantica*, 4.1/mL mg) constituted in jojoba and grapeseed oil against jojoba and grapeseed oil alone (level of evidence: 2b) (Fig. 11.2).[58] Of those using essential oils, 44% had regrowth per investigator assessment of photography, which was significantly greater than the 15% improvement seen in the control group. The small study size and variable course of AA makes generalization difficult.

Essential oils are generally considered safe. However, allergic contact dermatitis has been reported and may

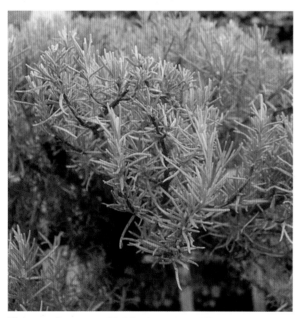

Fig. 11.1 Rosemary *"Salvia rosmarinus."* The purported medicinal benefits of rosemary oil have been written about since ancient times. Two small studies demonstrated that rosemary was beneficial for hair growth, but further large-scale trials are needed. (Photo courtesy Victoria R. Johnson and the Biology Department at The College of St. Benedict & St. John's University in Collegeville, Minnesota; Photographed at the University of Minnesota Landscape Arboretum).

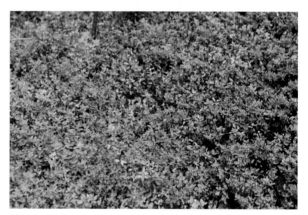

Fig. 11.2 Thyme *"Thymus spp."* Thymol is a phenol compound found in thyme essential oils with antiseptic properties. Thymol is a common ingredient in commercial mouthwashes. A single study investigated thyme as a treatment for pattern hair loss, but the study design prevents conclusions regarding efficacy. Further studies are needed. (Photo courtesy Victoria R. Johnson and the Biology Department at The College of St. Benedict & St. John's University in Collegeville, Minnesota; Photographed at the University of Minnesota Landscape Arboretum).

be reflective of the method by which the oil is processed.[59,60] Oils derived from the compression and steam distillation of plants are considered "true" essential oils and are generally safe.[55] Essential oils extracted with the aid of chemical solvents pose multiple safety risks. Neither the oil extraction method nor its advertising is regulated in the United States. Essential oils are not an appropriate monotherapy for hair loss and may worsen folliculitis or seborrheic disease. More studies are needed to determine the suitability of essential oils as a treatment for alopecia, but they may be pleasant adjuvants for some patients.

SCALP MASSAGE

Mechanical force can induce a variety of tissue-dependent effects on molecular signaling. Repetitive compressive force upregulates Wnt signaling in bone, while potassium channels in the atrium exhibit response to stretch (level of evidence: 5).[61,62] Scalp skin exhibits similar mechanosensitivity. Cultured human dermal papilla cells exposed to 72 hours of unidirectional stretch demonstrated increased expression of anagen-associated noggin, SMAD4, IL-6 signal transducer, and BMP4 (level of evidence: 5).[63] These in vitro findings have prompted clinical investigation of scalp massage as a treatment for hair loss.

A split-scalp study evaluated the effect of standardized scalp massage on hair growth in nine men without hair disorders (level of evidence: 4).[63] Participants used a motorized massage device on a single temporal scalp location for 4 minutes daily. Throughout the 24-week study, there was no significant difference in hair density, hair thickness, or hair growth rate between the massage area and the control area. However, there was an increase in hair thickness in the massage area from baseline to 24 weeks. In a study of 319 patients with self-reported AGA who self-administered 10-minute global scalp massages for 10 weeks, 37.3% reported stabilization of hair loss, and 31.7% reported slight or significant hair regrowth (level of evidence: 4).[64] However, the study had numerous limitations, including subject self-grading.

Scalp massage may promote hair growth through mechanisms partially shared with other stimulation-based therapies including platelet-rich plasma treatment (PRP) and microneedling. The use of scalp-massage devices, including hydromassage, may be helpful in reducing adherent scalp scale (e.g., pityriasis amiantacea)

for those with AGA and concomitant scalp disorders. However, there is insufficient evidence to recommend scalp massage in the treatment of AGA.

PSYCHOSOCIAL INTERVENTIONS

Hair is an important component of self-identity for many. It can be a marker of cultural identity, health, status, personality, religion, and gender expression. The importance of hair may be best highlighted by the psychological distress that can occur with its loss. Those with hair loss are more likely to experience depression, anxiety, and poor self-image (level of evidence: 2b).[65-68] There is growing evidence to suggest that the negative psychosocial burden associated with hair loss can compound over the course of a person's life (level of evidence: 3b).[69] A high incidence of psychological morbidity secondary to alopecia is particularly evident in women, adolescents, and transgender people (level of evidence: 3b).[70-72]

Many patients with alopecia are highly motivated to seek treatment. A single study reported that those with AA would pay 13% to 22% of their monthly income for effective treatment (level of evidence: 4).[73] The increasing popularity of PRP, which is costly and usually paid for out-of-pocket, underscores a similar strong desire to treat among those with AGA.

A majority of the hair-loss literature describes medical treatments. A thorough history, examination, and initiation of evidence-based medical treatment is the cornerstone of alopecia treatment (Pearl 11.3). However, patients with hair loss may also benefit from therapy aimed at addressing the psychological burden of the disease. This section covers the limited but promising evidence for these interventions.

Psychotherapy

The primary aim of any psychotherapy is to improve a person's mental health and wellbeing. Patients with hair loss may have associated feelings of anxiety and depression with variable effect on quality of life.[71,74] There is strong evidence supporting the use of talk therapy,

> **PEARL 11.3:** Many patients will not disclose use of hair supplements. Be sure to ask about supplementation as part of a thorough history.

including cognitive behavioral therapy (CBT), in the treatment of general anxiety and depression.[75] Talk therapy administered by a licensed mental health professional has very few side effects but can be costly without insurance.[76] The evidence for psychotherapy in the treatment of mental health disorders secondary to alopecia is limited.

A cross-sectional survey of 1083 patients with AA reported that almost one-third of patients pursued psychotherapy and nearly one-third attended patient support groups.[77] Most patients (78.1%) surveyed reported dissatisfaction with the medical treatment of their AA. An earlier case series reported patients with alopecia universalis who underwent weekly 30-minute relaxation therapy sessions for 2 months (n = 6) had improved self-image (level of evidence: 4).[78]

Although talk therapy has not been directly studied in AGA, it has been studied in polycystic ovarian syndrome (PCOS). An RCT examined the effectiveness of group talk therapy in 52 women with PCOS (level of evidence: 2b).[79] More than half of the participants (59.6%) reported female pattern hair loss. Those who underwent eight 90-minute group CBT sessions had significantly improved self-esteem and improved body image.

Integration of professional counseling into outpatient visits has been described in patients with AA. A single prospective cohort study in 20 patients with AA reported that all of those who underwent 30-minute behavioral counseling sessions after their outpatient dermatology visits (n = 10) felt their medical care was improved (level of evidence: 2b).[80] Almost all (90%) found the sessions were important in addressing psychosocial issues related to AA. The authors reported that the counseling sessions did not disrupt clinical treatment. This early study lends support to an integrated model of medical and psychological care for patients with alopecia.

Psychotherapy may be a useful adjuvant therapy for patients who have associated depression, anxiety, and low self-esteem. However, the degree of psychoemotional burden secondary to hair loss varies among patients, and there is limited literature to guide practice. The authors recommend dermatologists use clinical judgment and actively engage patients with alopecia in making a shared decision regarding mental-health referral (Pearl 11.4). Referrals should only be placed to licensed mental-health providers.

> **PEARL 11.4:** Patients who are distressed by their hair loss and see a mental health professional for the psychosocial burden of their alopecia report higher satisfaction with their medical care. Consider referring patients with hair loss who are distressed to a licensed mental-health provider.

Patient Support Groups

There are several well-established patient support groups for those with alopecia (Table 11.1). They serve various purposes, including patient education, shared community, research funding, increased public awareness, and political advocacy. Many groups engage patient members through social media and have been embraced by patients and physicians alike.[81,82] Studies examining the role and psychological effect of alopecia support groups are limited to expert opinion summaries and cross-sectional surveys. Benefits reported by patients include increased sense of control over their disease, decreased isolation, increased self-acceptance, and improved education facilitating informed discussions during medical visits (level of evidence: 4).[81,83,84] Patients with alopecia also responded favorably to shared clinical encounters in a single pilot study (level of evidence: 4).[85] Group medical visits may represent an opportunity for patients with hair loss to build community, share information, and receive timely expert care. Ultimately, patient support groups are an excellent resource for patients with hair loss.

Scalp Photography

The successful treatment of hair loss can improve psychosocial outcomes in patients experiencing distress secondary to alopecia.[68] However, the slow rate of hair regrowth can make objective assessment of interval change difficult for patients (Pearl 11.5). Prior studies have demonstrated that there is usually discordance between patient and physician assessment of alopecia

> **PEARL 11.5:** The slow rate of hair growth can make it difficult for patients to appreciate interval hair density changes after starting alopecia treatment. Standardized scalp photos document interval change, facilitating objective discussion during clinical visits.

TABLE 11.1	**Patient Support Groups for Specific Hair-Loss Conditions in the United States**		
Organization	**Condition**	**Website**	**QR Code to Website**
Cicatricial Alopecia Research Foundation (CARF)	Cicatricial (scarring) alopecias	www.carfintl.org	
National Alopecia Areata Foundation (NAAF)	Alopecia areata	www.naaf.org	
TLC Foundation for Body-Focused Repetitive Behaviors	Trichotillomania	www.bfrb.org	

severity.[86-88] A limited number of studies have suggested standardized scalp photography may be a helpful tool to aid patients in objective evaluation of treatment response and may offer therapeutic benefit.[88-90]

A retrospective study of 2999 patients with AGA and AA found those who viewed trichoscopy photos at clinical visits had improved treatment adherence and were less likely to be lost to follow up (level of evidence: 2b).[89] A similar study reported that patients who underwent education regarding the utility of scalp photography, including phototrichogram, found photography useful (level of evidence: 2b).[90] A study of 119 patients with AGA and cicatricial alopecia found that standardized scalp photography improved congruence between patient and physician grading of alopecia severity (level of evidence: 4).[88] Patients also reported that discussing photography with the treatment team lessened self-perceived alopecia severity, decreased alopecia-associated anxiety, and improved motivation to continue treatment.

Many alopecia treatments require a 6-month treatment duration before results are evident, making assessment difficult to appreciate. Scalp photography is a low-cost technique that can guide objective discussion of alopecia severity during clinical encounters. Although further research is needed to definitively determine the effect of scalp photography on alopecia-associated anxiety and self-image, early studies indicate a positive psychosocial effect. The authors routinely obtain standardized scalp photography for all patients with alopecia (Video 11.1).

CONCLUSION

Limited medical treatment options for hair loss and increasing consumer preference for naturally sourced products make CAM therapies increasingly used by those with alopecia. Despite representing a multibillion-dollar sector of the health and wellness market, CAMs face minimal regulation. CAMs are generally considered safe but pose certain safety risks. Quality evidence to support the use of CAM therapies in alopecia is lacking. However, many patients desire CAM therapy and may be reluctant to discuss it with their physician. Physicians should inquire about CAM therapies as part of a thorough patient history. Patients with alopecia who wish to forgo traditional therapies in favor of CAMs should be counseled that CAMs are not considered an appropriate monotherapy for alopecia and can be directed toward efficacious treatments that may be similarly perceived as "natural," including PRP, microneedling, and photobiomodulation. Many of the diverse CAM therapies used for hair loss have demonstrated early potential, and further research is needed.

EVIDENCE SUMMARY

- Complementary and alternative medicines including vitamins, minerals, botanically derived products, and behavioral interventions have been investigated as adjuvant treatments for androgenetic alopecia. There is a lack of evidence to support the use of any complementary and alternative medicine as a monotherapy for androgenetic alopecia (strength of recommendation: B).
- Patients with androgenetic alopecia who have a serum ferritin less than 40 ng/mL should undergo repletion with an oral slow-release ferrous iron supplement for at least 3 to 6 months before laboratory reevaluation (strength of recommendation: C).
- Biotin supplementation is touted as a beneficial treatment for those with androgenetic alopecia. However, there is limited evidence to support its use in otherwise healthy androgenetic alopecia patients. Biotin supplementation can invalidate laboratory assays, posing an increased risk for medical error. The amount of biotin produced by symbiont intestinal bacteria exceeds the recommended dietary intake, making supplementation unnecessary in most cases (strength of recommendation: D).
- Marine supplements contain proteins derived from marine invertebrates and sharks. There are several quality industry-sponsored trials that demonstrate a beneficial effect of marine supplements in androgenetic alopecia. However, the identity of many ingredients in such supplements is shrouded by propriety claims, the products are expensive, and there are no head-to-head studies comparing marine supplements with conventional therapies. Marine supplements can be considered by those with androgenetic alopecia (strength of recommendation: C).
- The psychosocial burden of alopecia varies among patients but can be severe. Patients experiencing psychosocial distress from hair loss may benefit from seeing a licensed mental-health professional, joining a patient support group, and standardized scalp photography (strength of recommendation: C).

REFERENCES

1. Institute of Medicine (US) Committee on the Use of Complementary and Alternative Medicine by the American Public. *Complementary and Alternative Medicine in the United States.* Washington (DC): National Academies Press (US); 2005.
2. Hosking AM, Juhasz M, Atanaskova Mesinkovska N. Complementary and alternative treatments for alopecia: a comprehensive review. *Skin Appendage Disord.* 2019; 5(2):72-89. doi:10.1159/000492035.
3. Trüeb RM. *Nutrition for Healthy Hair: Guide to Understanding and Proper Practice.* Springer International Publishing, Switzerland; 2020. doi:10.1007/978-3-030-59920-1.
4. White A, Boon H, Alraek T, et al. Reducing the risk of complementary and alternative medicine (CAM): challenges and priorities. *Eur J Integr Med.* 2014;6(4): 404-408. doi:10.1016/j.eujim.2013.09.006.
5. Robinson A, McGrail MR. Disclosure of CAM use to medical practitioners: a review of qualitative and quantitative studies. *Complement Ther Med.* 2004;12(2-3):90-98. doi:10.1016/j.ctim.2004.09.006.
6. Andersen MR, Sweet E, Lowe KA, Standish LJ, Drescher CW, Goff BA. Dangerous combinations: ingestible CAM supplement use during chemotherapy in patients with ovarian cancer. *J Altern Complement Med.* 2013;19(8): 714-720. doi:10.1089/acm.2012.0295.
7. Sweet E, Dowd F, Zhou M, Standish LJ, Andersen MR. The use of complementary and alternative medicine supplements of potential concern during breast cancer chemotherapy. *Evid Based Complement Alternat Med.* 2016; 2016:4382687. doi:10.1155/2016/4382687.
8. Ehleringer JR, Covarrubias Avalos S, Tipple BJ, Valenzuela LO, Cerling TE. Stable isotopes in hair reveal dietary protein sources with links to socioeconomic status and health. *Proc Natl Acad Sci USA.* 2020;117(33):20044-20051. doi:10.1073/pnas.1914087117.
9. Pathoulas JT, Bellefeuille G, Lofgreen SJ, et al. Unknown safety profile of ingredients in hair supplements: a call to action for improved patient safety. *J Am Acad Dermatol.* 2020;83(3):e213-e214. doi:10.1016/j.jaad.2020.05.033.
10. Finner AM. Nutrition and hair. *Dermatol Clin.* 2013; 31(1):167-172. doi:10.1016/j.det.2012.08.015.
11. Garg S, Sangwan A. Dietary protein deficit and deregulated autophagy: a new clinico-diagnostic perspective in pathogenesis of early aging, skin, and hair disorders. *Indian Dermatol Online J.* 2019;10(2):115-124. doi:10.4103/idoj.IDOJ_123_18.
12. Fortes C, Mastroeni S, Mannooranparampil TJ, Ribuffo M. The combination of overweight and smoking increases the severity of androgenetic alopecia. *Int J Dermatol.* 2017;56(8):862-867. doi:10.1111/ijd.13652.
13. Institute of Medicine. *Dietary Reference Intakes: The Essential Guide to Nutrient Requirements.* Washington, DC: The National Academies Press; 2006. Available at: https://doi.org/10.17226/11537.
14. Wu G. Dietary protein intake and human health. *Food Funct.* 2016;7(3):1251-1265. doi:10.1039/c5fo01530h.
15. Gehring W, Gloor M. Use of the phototrichogram to assess the stimulation of hair growth – an in vitro study of

women with androgenetic alopecia. *Z Hautkr.* 2000;75:419-423.

16. Hertel H, Gollnick H, Matthies C, Baumann I, Orfanos CE. Niedrig dosierte Retinol-und L-Cystin-Kombination bessern die Alopezie vom diffusen Typ nach peroraler Langzeitapplikation [Low dosage retinol and L-cystine combination improve alopecia of the diffuse type following long-term oral administration]. *Hautarzt.* 1989;40(8):490-495. German.

17. Morganti P, Fabrizi P, James B, Bruno C. Effect of gelatin-cystine and Serenoa repens extract on free radicals level and hair growth. *J Appl Cosmetol.* 1998;16:57-64.

18. Whitting DA. *Hair Growth and Disorders.* (Blume-Peytavi U, Tosti A, Trüeb RM, eds.). Berlin Heidelberg: Springer; 2008. doi:10.1007/978-3-540-46911-7.

19. Trost LB, Bergfeld WF, Calogeras E. The diagnosis and treatment of iron deficiency and its potential relationship to hair loss. *J Am Acad Dermatol.* 2006;54(5):824-844. doi:10.1016/j.jaad.2005.11.1104.

20. Ohyama M. Characterization and isolation of stem cell-enriched human hair follicle bulge cells. *J Clin Invest.* 2005;116(1):249-260. doi:10.1172/JCI26043.

21. Centers for Disease Control and Prevention (CDC). Iron deficiency–United States, 1999-2000. *MMWR Morb Mortal Wkly Rep.* 2002;51(40):897-899.

22. Guyatt GH, Oxman AD, Ali M, Willan A, McIlroy W, Patterson C. Laboratory diagnosis of iron-deficiency anemia: an overview. *J Gen Intern Med.* 1992;7(2):145-153. doi:10.1007/BF02598003.

23. Kantor J, Kessler LJ, Brooks DG, Cotsarelis G. Decreased serum ferritin is associated with alopecia in women. *J Invest Dermatol.* 2003;121(5):985-988. doi:10.1046/j.1523-1747.2003.12540.x.

24. Rushton DH, Ramsay ID, James KC, Norris MJ, Gilkes JJH. Biochemical and trichological characterization of diffuse alopecia in women. *Br J Dermatol.* 1990;123(2):187-197. doi:10.1111/j.1365-2133.1990.tb01846.x.

25. Aydingöz IE, Ferhanoğlu B, Güney O. Does tissue iron status have a role in female alopecia? *J Eur Acad Dermatol Venerol.* 1999;13(1):65-67. doi:10.1111/j.1468-3083.1999.tb00849.x.

26. Sinclair R. There is no clear association between low serum ferritin and chronic diffuse telogen hair loss. *Br J Dermatol.* 2002;147(5):982-984. doi:10.1046/j.1365-2133.2002.04997.x.

27. Saper R, Rash R. Zinc: an essential micronutrient. *Am Fam Physician.* 2009;79(9):768-772.

28. Kil MS, Kim CW, Kim SS. Analysis of serum zinc and copper concentrations in hair loss. *Ann Dermatol.* 2013;25(4):405. doi:10.5021/ad.2013.25.4.405.

29. Siavash M, Tavakoli F, Mokhtari F. Comparing the effects of zinc sulfate, calcium pantothenate, their combination and minoxidil solution regimens on controlling hair loss

in women: a randomized controlled trial. *J Res Pharm Pract.* 2017;6(2):89. doi:10.4103/jrpp.JRPP_17_17.

30. Berger RS, Fu JL, Smiles KA, et al. The effects of minoxidil, 1% pyrithione zinc and a combination of both on hair density: a randomized controlled trial. *Br J Dermatol.* 2003;149(2):354-362. doi:10.1046/j.1365-2133.2003.05435.x.

31. Prasad S, Marks DH, Burns LJ, et al. Patch testing and contact allergen avoidance in patients with lichen planopilaris and/or frontal fibrosing alopecia: a cohort study. *J Am Acad Dermatol.* 2020;83(2):659-661. doi:10.1016/j.jaad.2020.01.026.

32. Almohanna HM, Ahmed AA, Tsatalis JP, Tosti A. The role of vitamins and minerals in hair loss: a review. *Dermatol Ther (Heidelb).* 2019;9(1):51-70. doi:10.1007/s13555-018-0278-6.

33. Schulpis KH, Georgala S, Papakonstantinou ED, Michas T, Karikas GA. The effect of isotretinoin on biotinidase activity. *Skin Pharmacol Appl Skin Physiol.* 1999;12(1-2):28-33. doi:10.1159/000029843.

34. Schulpis KH, Karikas GA, Tjamouranis J, Regoutas S, Tsakiris S. Low serum biotinidase activity in children with valproic acid monotherapy. *Epilepsia.* 2001;42(10):1359-1362. doi:10.1046/j.1528-1157.2001.47000.x.

35. Lipner SR. Rethinking biotin therapy for hair, nail, and skin disorders. *J Am Acad Dermatol.* 2018;78(6):1236-1238. doi:10.1016/j.jaad.2018.02.018.

36. John JJ, Lipner SR. Consumer perception of biotin supplementation. *J Cutan Med Surg.* 2019;23(6):613-616. doi:10.1177/1203475419871046.

37. Walth CB, Wessman LL, Wipf A, Carina A, Hordinsky MK, Farah RS. Response to: "Rethinking biotin therapy for hair, nail, and skin disorders." *J Am Acad Dermatol.* 2018;79(6):e121-e124. doi:10.1016/j.jaad.2018.07.055.

38. Dickinson A, Shao A, Boyon N, Franco JC. Use of dietary supplements by cardiologists, dermatologists and orthopedists: report of a survey. *Nutr J.* 2011;10(1):20. doi:10.1186/1475-2891-10-20.

39. U.S. Food and Drug Administration. *The FDA Warns that Biotin May Interfere with Lab Tests: FDA Safety Communication.* Issued November 28, 2017, updated November 5, 2019. 2018. Available at: https://www.fda.gov/medical-devices/safety-communications/fda-warns-biotin-may-interfere-lab-tests-fda-safety-communication. Accessed March 27, 2021.

40. Ablon G, Dayan S. A randomized, double-blind, placebo-controlled, multi-center, extension trial evaluating the efficacy of a new oral supplement in women with self-perceived thinning hair. *J Clin Aesthet Dermatol.* 2015;8(12):8.

41. Ablon G. A 6-month, randomized, double-blind, placebo-controlled study evaluating the ability of a marine complex supplement to promote hair growth in men with thinning hair. *J Cosmet Dermatol.* 2016;15(4):358-366. doi:10.1111/jocd.12265.

42. Rizer R, Stephens T, Herndon J, Sperber B, Murphy J, Ablon G. A marine protein-based dietary supplement for subclinical hair thinning/loss: results of a multisite, double-blind, placebo-controlled clinical trial. *Int J Trichol.* 2015;7(4):156. doi:10.4103/0974-7753.171573.

43. Chatterjee S, Agrawala SK. An effective phytotherapy. *Nat Prod Radiance.* 2003;2(6):4.

44. Rossi A, Mari E, Scarnò M, et al. Comparitive effectiveness and finasteride vs serenoa repens in male androgenetic alopecia: a two-year study. *Int J Immunopathol Pharmacol.* 2012;25(4):1167-1173. doi:10.1177/039463201202500435.

45. Prager N, Bickett K, French N, Marcovici G. A randomized, double-blind, placebo-controlled trial to determine the effectiveness of botanically derived inhibitors of 5-alpha-reductase in the treatment of androgenetic alopecia [published correction appears in J Altern Complement Med. 2006 Mar;12(2):199]. *J Altern Complement Med.* 2002;8(2):143-152. doi:10.1089/acm.2002.8.143.

46. Ablon G, Kogan S. A six-month, randomized, double-blind, placebo-controlled study evaluating the safety and efficacy of a nutraceutical supplement for promoting hair growth in women with self-perceived thinning hair. *J Drugs Dermatol.* 2018;17(5):558-565.

47. Cho YH, Lee SY, Jeong DW, et al. Effect of pumpkin seed oil on hair growth in men with androgenetic alopecia: a randomized, double-blind, placebo-controlled trial. *Evid Based Complement Alternat Med.* 2014;2014:549721. doi:10.1155/2014/549721.

48. Fischer TW, Hipler UC, Elsner P. Effect of caffeine and testosterone on the proliferation of human hair follicles in vitro: Caffeine and testosterone. *Int J Dermatol.* 2007;46(1):27-35. doi:10.1111/j.1365-4632.2007.03119.x.

49. Fischer TW, Herczeg-Lisztes E, Funk W, Zillikens D, Bíró T, Paus R. Differential effects of caffeine on hair shaft elongation, matrix and outer root sheath keratinocyte proliferation, and transforming growth factor-β2/insulin-like growth factor-1-mediated regulation of the hair cycle in male and female human hair follicles in vitro. *Br J Dermatol.* 2014;171(5):1031-1043. doi:10.1111/bjd.13114.

50. Park S, Kang W, Choi D, Son B, Park T. Nonanal stimulates growth factors via cyclic adenosine monophosphate (cAMP) signaling in human hair follicle dermal papilla cells. *Int J Mol Sci.* 2020;21(21):8054. doi:10.3390/ijms21218054.

51. Dhurat R, Chitallia J, May TW, et al. An open-label randomized multicenter study assessing the noninferiority of a caffeine-based topical liquid 0.2% versus minoxidil 5% solution in male androgenetic alopecia. *Skin Pharmacol Physiol.* 2017;30(6):298-305. doi:10.1159/000481141.

52. Golpour M, Rabbani H, Farzin D, Azizi F. Comparing the effectiveness of local solution of minoxidil and caffeine 2.5% with local solution of minoxidil 2.5% in treatment of androgenetic alopecia. *J Mazandaran Univ Med Sci.* 2013;23(106):30-36.

53. Bussoletti C, Tolaini MV, Celleno' L. Use of a caffeine shampoo for the treatment of male androgenetic alopecia. *J Appl Cosmetology.* 2010;4(28):153.

54. Pazoki-Toroudi H. The efficacy and safety of minoxidil 5% combination with azelaic acid 1/5% and caffeine 1% solution on male pattern hair loss (abstract). *J Invest Dermatol.* 2013;133:S84.

55. PDQ Integrative, Alternative, and Complementary Therapies Editorial Board. *Aromatherapy With Essential Oils (PDQ): Health Professional Version.* Bethesda (MD): National Cancer Institute (US): National Cancer Institute; 2022.

56. Panahi Y, Taghizadeh M, Marzony ET, Sahebkar A. Rosemary oil vs minoxidil 2% for the treatment of androgenetic alopecia: a randomized comparative trial. *Skinmed.* 2015;13(1):15-21.

57. Hammer KA, Carson CF, Riley TV. In vitro activities of ketoconazole, econazole, miconazole, and melaleuca alternifolia (tea tree) oil against malassezia species. *Antimicrob Agents Chemother.* 2000;44(2):467-469. doi:10.1128/AAC.44.2.467-469.2000.

58. Hay IC, Jamieson M, Ormerod AD, Randomized Trial of Aromatherapy. Successful Treatment for Alopecia Areata. *Arch Dermatol.* 1998;134:(11):1349–1352. doi:10.1001/archderm.134.11.1349.

59. Lakshmi C, Srinivas CR. Allergic contact dermatitis following aromatherapy with valiya narayana thailam-an ayurvedic oil presenting as exfoliative dermatitis. *Contact Dermatitis.* 2009;61(5):297-298. doi:10.1111/j.1600-0536.2009.01627.x.

60. Trattner A, David M, Lazarov A. Occupational contact dermatitis due to essential oils. *Contact Dermatitis.* 2008;58(5):282-284. doi:10.1111/j.1600-0536.2007.01275.x.

61. Chen X, Guo J, Yuan Y, et al. Cyclic compression stimulates osteoblast differentiation via activation of the Wnt/β-catenin signaling pathway. *Mol Med Rep.* 2017;15(5):2890-2896. doi:10.3892/mmr.2017.6327.

62. Van Wagoner DR. Mechanosensitive gating of atrial ATP-sensitive potassium channels. *Circ Res.* 1993;72(5):973-983. doi:10.1161/01.RES.72.5.973.

63. Koyama T, Kobayashi K, Hama T, Murakami K, Ogawa R. Standardized scalp massage results in increased hair thickness by inducing stretching forces to dermal papilla cells in the subcutaneous tissue. *Eplasty.* 2016;16:e8.

64. English RS, Barazesh JM. Self-assessments of standardized scalp massages for androgenic alopecia: survey results. *Dermatol Ther (Heidelb).* 2019;9(1):167-178. doi:10.1007/s13555-019-0281-6.

65. Guo F, Yu Q, Liu Z, et al. Evaluation of life quality, anxiety, and depression in patients with skin diseases.

Medicine. 2020;99(44):e22983. doi:10.1097/MD. 0000000000022983.

66. Montgomery K, White C, Thompson A. A mixed methods survey of social anxiety, anxiety, depression and wig use in alopecia. *BMJ Open.* 2017;7(4):e015468. doi:10.1136/bmjopen-2016-015468.

67. Hadshiew IM, Foitzik K, Arck PC, Paus R. Burden of hair loss: stress and the underestimated psychosocial impact of telogen effluvium and androgenetic alopecia. *J Invest Dermatol.* 2004;123(3):455-457. doi:10.1111/j.0022-202X. 2004.23237.x.

68. Alfonso M, Richter-Appelt H, Tosti A, Viera MS, García M. The psychosocial impact of hair loss among men: a multinational European study. *Curr Med Res Opin.* 2005;21(11):1829-1836. doi:10.1185/030079905X61820.

69. Burns LJ, Flanagan KE, Pathoulas JT, Ellison A, Mesinkovska N, Senna MM. Patient perspectives of the cumulative life course impairment of alopecia areata. *Clin Exp Dermatol.* Published online March 23, 2021:935-936. doi:10.1111/ced.14597.

70. Teichgräber F, Jacob L, Koyanagi A, Shin JI, Seiringer P, Kostev K. Association between skin disorders and depression in children and adolescents: a retrospective case-control study. *J Affect Disord.* 2021;282:939-944. doi:10.1016/j.jad.2021.01.002.

71. Kozicka K, Łukasik A, Jaworek A, et al. The level of stress and the assessment of selected clinical parameters in patients with androgenetic alopecia. *Pol Merkur Lekarski.* 2020;48(288):427-430.

72. Yeung H, Luk KM, Chen SC, Ginsberg BA, Katz KA. Dermatologic care for lesbian, gay, bisexual, and transgender persons. *J Am Acad Dermatol.* 2019;80(3):591-602. doi:10.1016/j.jaad.2018.02.045.

73. Okhovat JP, Grogan T, Duan L, Goh C. Willingness to pay and quality of life in alopecia areata. *J Am Acad Dermatol.* 2017;77(6):1183-1184. doi:10.1016/j.jaad.2017.07.023.

74. Alirezaei P, Ahmadpanah M, Rezanejad A, Soltanian A, Sadeghi Bahmani D, Brand S. Compared to controls, individuals with lichen planopilaris have more depression, a lower self-esteem, and a lower quality of life. *Neuropsychobiology.* 2019;78(2):95-103. doi:10.1159/000499135.

75. Beck JS. *Cognitive Behavior Therapy, Second Edition: Basics and Beyond.* 2nd ed. New York: The Guilford Press; 2011.

76. Harth W, Gieler U, Kusnir D, Tausk FA: *Clinical Management in Psychodermatology.* Berlin Heidelberg: Springer; 2009. doi:10.1007/978-3-540-34719-4.

77. Hussain ST, Mostaghimi A, Barr PJ, Brown JR, Joyce C, Huang KP. Utilization of mental health resources and complementary and alternative therapies for alopecia areata: a U.S. Survey. *Int J Trichol.* 2017;9:160-164.

78. Teshima H, Sogawa H, Mizobe K, Kuroki N, Nakagawa T. Application of psychoimmunotherapy in patients with alopecia universalis. *Psychother Psychosom.* 1991;56(4): 235-241. doi:10.1159/000288561.

79. Moradi F, Ghadiri-Anari A, Dehghani A, Reza Vaziri S, Enjezab B. The effectiveness of counseling based on acceptance and commitment therapy on body image and self-esteem in polycystic ovary syndrome: An RCT. *Int J Reprod Biomed.* 2020;18:243-252. doi:10.18502/ijrm.v13i4.6887.

80. Gorbatenko-Roth K, Hodges JS, Lifson D, et al. Integrating colocated behavioral health care into a dermatology clinic: a prospective randomized controlled treatment pilot study in patients with alopecia areata. *J Am Acad Dermatol.* 2021;84(5):1487-1489. doi:10.1016/j.jaad.2020.07.070.

81. Rolstad T, Zimmerman G. Patient advocacy groups. *Dermatol Clin.* 2000;18(2):277-285. doi:10.1016/S0733-8635 (05)70173-X.

82. Prickitt J, McMichael AJ, Gallagher L, Kalabokes V, Boeck C. Helping patients cope with chronic alopecia areata. *Dermatol Nurs.* 2004;16(3):237-241.

83. Aschenbeck KA, McFarland SL, Hordinsky MK, Lindgren BR, Farah RS. Importance of group therapeutic support for family members of children with alopecia areata: a cross-sectional survey study. *Pediatr Dermatol.* 2017;34(4): 427-432. doi:10.1111/pde.13176.

84. Iliffe LL, Thompson AR. Investigating the beneficial experiences of online peer support for those affected by alopecia: an interpretative phenomenological analysis using online interviews. *Br J Dermatol.* 2019;181(5): 992-998. doi:10.1111/bjd.17998.

85. Senna MM, Marks DH, Smith GP. Shared medical appointments for female pattern hair loss. *J Am Acad Dermatol.* 2021;84(1):180-182. doi:10.1016/j.jaad.2020.04.066.

86. Biondo S, Goble D, Sinclair R. Women who present with female pattern hair loss tend to underestimate the severity of their hair loss. *Br J Dermatol.* 2004;150(4):750-752. doi:10.1046/j.0007-0963.2003.05809.x.

87. Tosti A, Bellavista S, Longo S, Pazzaglia M. Tendency to underestimate the severity of androgenetic alopecia. *Br J Dermatol.* 2005;152(6):1362-1363. doi:10.1111/ j.1365-2133.2005.06595.x.

88. Pathoulas JT, Flanagan KE, Walker CJ, Wiss IMP, Azimi E, Senna MM. Evaluation of standardized scalp photography on patient perception of hair loss severity, anxiety, and treatment. *J Am Acad Dermatol.* 2021;85(6): 1604-1641. doi:10.1016/j.jaad.2020.12.059.

89. Lee S, Lee H, Lee C, Lee WS. Photographic assessment improves adherence to recommended follow-up in patients with androgenetic alopecia and alopecia areata: a retrospective cohort study. *Indian J Dermatol Venereol Leprol.* 2019;85(4):431. doi:10.4103/ijdvl.IJDVL_696_18.

90. Park SY, Lee WS. Impact of phototrichogram education on satisfaction of patients with androgenetic alopecia in clinical practice. *J Dermatol.* 2014;41(8):773-774. doi:10.1111/1346-8138.12548.

SECTION 4

Procedural Treatments for Hair Loss

12

Platelet-Rich Plasma

Geraldine C. Ranasinghe and Shilpi Khetarpal

KEY POINTS

- Androgenetic alopecia is the most common form of hair loss and is characterized by progressive reduction and miniaturization of terminal hair follicles on the scalp.
- Although androgenetic alopecia is benign in nature and often considered part of the normal aging process, it is a familiar cosmetic concern encountered by dermatologists, as it negatively affects patient quality of life.
- Developing a therapeutic regimen for patients is often challenging as treatment options are limited, often not well tolerated by all patients, and may result in suboptimal treatment outcomes.

- Platelet-rich plasma is a relatively novel therapeutic option and appears to be effective for the treatment of androgenetic alopecia in some patients.
- Platelet-rich plasma is likely most effective as an adjuvant therapy in combination with other treatments, such as topical minoxidil.
- Adverse events of platelet-rich plasma are typically self-limited and include pain at injection sites, swelling, bruising, and, occasionally, mild headache.
- In this chapter, we will discuss the use of platelet-rich plasma as an adjuvant therapy for the treatment of androgenetic alopecia.

INTRODUCTION

Androgenetic alopecia (AGA) is the most common form of hair loss. It is characterized by progressive reduction and miniaturization of terminal hair follicles on the scalp. Caucasian men are a notably vulnerable population, with 50% of Caucasian men experiencing AGA by age 50.[1] In women, AGA is referred to as female pattern hair loss (FPHL). FPHL may occur at any age with varying degrees of severity and becomes clinically detectable in about 3% of women by 29 years of age, 13% by 49 years, 19% by 69 years, and 25% among those over 69 years. The prevalence of FPHL has been shown to be lower among women of Asian descent.[2] AGA typically occurs over many years but can progress more rapidly for some younger men with a strong family history. In addition to genetics, the presence of high levels of circulating androgens, specifically dihydrotestosterone (DHT), the end product of 5α-reductase enzymatic action on testosterone, contributes to this disease process. The typical distribution of hair loss in males with AGA involves the frontotemporal hairline and the vertex of the scalp, while women most often experience a widened hair part with relative sparing of the frontal hairline. These areas are the androgen-dependent areas on the scalp.

Although this condition is benign in nature and often considered part of the normal aging process, it is a familiar cosmetic concern encountered by dermatologists as it frequently poses significant psychological distress for patients.[3,4] Currently, the only FDA approved therapies for AGA are topical minoxidil for both men and women and oral finasteride for men only. Unfortunately, many patients report mixed outcomes and are either disappointed with treatment response or experience adverse drug events related to these agents.

Surgical hair transplantation is an option for a select number of patients; however, the invasive nature and financial commitment may be a significant limitation for most patients. Several studies evaluating various oral, topical, and minimally invasive alternative treatment options for AGA have been published. Off-label antiandrogenetic therapies such as oral dutasteride, oral spironolactone, topical ketoconazole, and topical finasteride have been shown to improve hair density with significant reduction in serum DHT concentrations.[5-8] Additionally, minimally invasive treatment options including oral minoxidil, low level light laser, transdermal drug delivery via microneedling, and platelet-rich plasma therapy (PRP) have demonstrated promising results in randomized trials during the 2000s.[9-11] In this chapter, we will discuss the pathophysiology and clinical features of AGA and the use of PRP for the treatment of AGA.

PATHOPHYSIOLOGY OF ANDROGENETIC ALOPECIA

Elevated androgen levels in genetically susceptible individuals serve as a crucial predisposing factor for AGA. The key androgen involved in this pathway is DHT, which is the end product of testosterone acted upon by the enzyme 5α-reductase. There are three forms of this enzyme, with the two most notable being type 1 and type 2. Type 1 is found in the sebaceous glands and liver, and type 2 is found in the liver, prostate, and the scalp, beard, and chest hair follicles.[12] Interactions between DHT and androgen receptors in scalp hair follicles results in shortening of the anagen phase, leading to follicular miniaturization and an increase in vellus hairs. In men, this occurs most commonly over the frontal hairline and vertex of the scalp, leading to the characteristic male patterned hair loss (MPHL).[12] Conversely, in FPHL, some but not all patients may have elevated circulating androgens. Compared with men, the androgen receptors are fewer in number and the conversion of testosterone to estrogen in the scalp hair follicles occurs via increased activity of the cytochrome P-450-aromatase enzyme. It is the differences in the quantities of these key enzymes that are hypothesized to account for the diffuse central thinning along the hair part in FPHL rather than discrete areas of hair thinning seen in MPHL.[13]

CLINICAL FEATURES OF ANDROGENETIC ALOPECIA

MPHL characteristically involves the frontotemporal and vertex regions of the scalp. Findings are classified

into stages using the Hamilton-Norwood scale. Patients are categorized on a scale of II to VII based on severity of recession[12] (Fig. 12.1). In contrast, FPHL typically presents with diffuse central thinning of the crown with maintenance of the frontal hairline, often referred to as the "Christmas tree" pattern. The central part width can be compared with the occipital part width and severity is assessed using the Sinclair scale[12] (Fig. 12.2).

MECHANISM OF ACTION OF PLATELET-RICH PLASMA FOR TREATMENT OF ANDROGENETIC ALOPECIA

The dermal papillae (DP) are not only the site of stem cells but also home to the highest concentration of androgen receptors and nutrients that stimulate growth of the hair shaft. It is here that the platelet derived growth factors, chemokines, and cytokines work together to induce hair growth in AGA via the wingless (Wnt)/β-catenin, extracellular signaling regulated kinase (ERK), and protein kinase B (Akt) signaling pathways.[14]

When DHT binds to androgen receptors found in the DP, this inhibits the Wnt/β-catenin pathway. Inhibition of this pathway results in hair remaining in the telogen phase, instead of activating into the growth phase of anagen.[14] PRP has been shown to stimulate the Wnt/β-catenin pathway by inhibiting GSK-3b, the enzyme responsible for β-catenin degradation. β-catenin is involved in gene expression responsible for hair cell differentiation from stem cells. As such, accumulation of β-catenin promotes folliculoneogenesis. Additionally, activation of the Wnt/β-catenin pathway has been shown to accelerate the transition of hair cycling from telogen to anagen and prolong the anagen phase.[14-16]

The activated platelets degranulate upon injection and release platelet-derived growth factor (PDGF), transforming growth factor (TGF)β-1, TGFβ-2, vascular endothelial derived growth factor (VEGF), basic fibroblastic growth factor, endothelial growth factor, and insulin-like growth factors from alpha granules, which initiates a cascade of events. Once bound to their transmembrane receptor, these growth factors halt miniaturization of hair follicles and induce gene expression by stimulating ERK and Akt pathways responsible for cell proliferation within dermal papillae, angiogenesis, and collagen synthesis (level of evidence: 5).[14,17,18] The resultant increased blood flow, oxygen, and nutrients not only support new hair growth, but also provide a

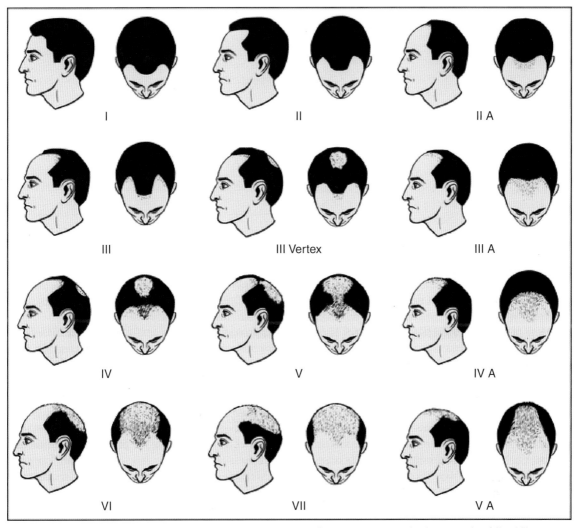

Fig. 12.1 Hamilton-Norwood male pattern baldness scale. Patients are categorized on a scale of II to VII based on severity of recession. Typically, men experience gradually recessing temporal hairlines. In Noorwood Class A (right), there is a predominant front to back progression of hair loss. (From (Norwood, O.T.), (Hair Transplant Surgery), (1st edn), 1973. Courtesy of Charles C Thomas Publisher Ltd., Springfield, Illinois.)

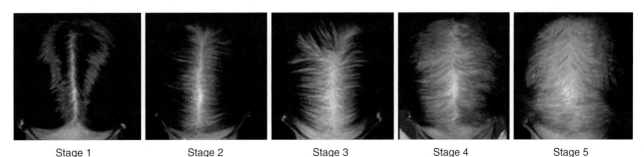

| Stage 1 | Stage 2 | Stage 3 | Stage 4 | Stage 5 |

Fig. 12.2 Sinclair classification of female pattern hair loss. (Courtesy Sinclair R, Torkamani N, Jones L. Androgenetic alopecia: new insights into the pathogenesis and mechanism of hair loss. *F1000Res*. 2015;4:585. doi:10.12688/f1000research.6401.1)

microenvironment that nourishes miniaturized hair follicles. Additionally, in mouse models, DHT has been shown to prevent hair growth by inhibiting insulin-like growth factor 1, a growth factor that is found in PRP.[14] Thus PRP's mechanism of action makes it a viable therapeutic option for the treatment of AGA, as it directly replenishes factors lost or decreased in AGA and activates pathways involved in folliculoneogenesis.

Histologic evaluation of biopsies from PRP-treated scalps demonstrated increased epidermal thickness and number of hair follicles compared with baseline after three monthly sessions of PRP (level of evidence: 2b).[19,20] These studies measured Ki67$^+$ activity of basal keratinocytes as a measure of cell proliferation and demonstrated an increase in activity within the epidermis and hair follicular bulge cells compared with baseline. In support of the angiogenic potential of PRP, an increase in vasculature surrounding hair follicles compared with baseline was seen as well.[19,20]

TREATMENT TECHNIQUES AND BEST PRACTICES

PRP is an autologous concentrate of platelets obtained by centrifuging patients' own venous blood. In the authors' clinical practice, a single-spin centrifuge method is used to produce PRP, with a mean increase in platelet concentration of three- to-six fold the mean concentration of peripheral blood, and only minimal increase in granulocytes and inflammatory cells (Pearl 12.1). The platelet-rich supernatant is then injected as 0.2 cc subdermal depo bolus injections into androgen-dependent areas of the scalp.[2] The injector should be mindful to space injections among the thinning areas, specifically along the hairline, hair part, and vertex of the scalp (Pearl 12.2). Upon injection into the scalp, the platelets are activated and act upon the hair follicle as mentioned previously. The patient should be educated on expected and transient side effects, including pain at injection sites, swelling, bruising, and, occasionally, mild

> **PEARL 12.1:** In the authors' clinical practice, a single-spin centrifuge method is used to produce platelet-rich plasma, with a mean increase in platelet concentration of three- to-six fold the mean concentration of peripheral blood, and only minimal increase in granulocytes and inflammatory cells.

> **PEARL 12.2:** The platelet-rich supernatant is injected as 0.2 cc subdermal depo bolus injections into androgen-dependent areas of the scalp. The injector should be mindful to space injections among the thinning areas, specifically along the hairline, hair part, and vertex of the scalp.

> **PEARL 12.3:** The patient should be educated on expected and transient side effects including pain at injection sites, swelling, bruising, and, occasionally, mild headache. Side effects can be managed by application of ice and administration of acetaminophen.

headache. Side effects can be managed by application of ice and administration of acetaminophen (Pearl 12.3).

Although there is no universally accepted protocol in terms of treatment timing, the authors perform monthly sessions for the first 3 months followed by every 3 months for the first year (six total treatment sessions in first year: months 1, 2, 3, 6, 9, and 12)[2] (Figs. 12.3-12.5).

PLATELET-RICH PLASMA AS AN ADJUVANT THERAPY FOR TREATMENT OF ANDROGENETIC ALOPECIA

Uebel et al. were among the first to describe the use of PRP as a treatment for hair loss. This group demonstrated an increase in the yield of follicular units treated with PRP as a technique to enhance results of hair transplantation.[21] Over 10 years later, more studies have demonstrated PRP to be a suitable adjuvant therapy in the treatment of AGA.[22-24] In the authors' practice, the initial approach to patients with AGA involves starting with first-line agents such as minoxidil 5% foam and/or oral antiandrogenetic agents (i.e., finasteride for men and spironolactone for women). If clinical outcomes do not meet the satisfaction of compliant patients after 6 months of therapy, or if the patient is experiencing undesirable adverse drug events, a discussion about alternative therapies is warranted. It is at this point that we recommend discussing the addition of PRP to the patient's current hair loss regimen, with an emphasis on continuing topical and/or oral antiandrogen therapies, as PRP does not directly influence the hormonal component of AGA. Smaller case reports and the authors' personal experience is that a combination of treatment

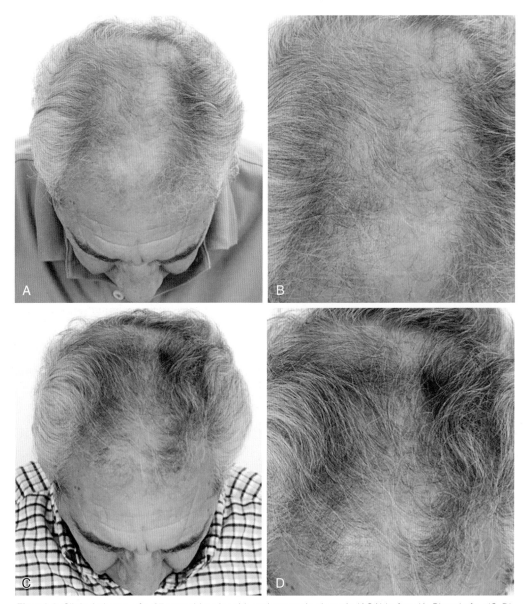

Fig. 12.3 Clinical photos of a 67-year-old male with androgenetic alopecia (AGA) before (A–B) and after (C–D) four platelet-rich plasma (PRP) sessions in the authors' clinic. All sessions were 6 months apart.

with autologous PRP, antiandrogenic therapies, and topical minoxidil ensures the most favorable outcome for a majority of patients, as these agents have a cumulative effect on the miniaturized hair follicles within the dermal papilla.[22-24]

This is further supported by a study of 78 patients by Ferrando et al. in which regularly administered PRP coupled with pharmacologic treatments resulted in successful clinical outcomes for patients with AGA (level of evidence: 4).[25] In this study, a total of 19 men and 59 women had been on topical minoxidil and/or oral finasteride for more than a year without improvement in hair regrowth. PRP was prepared using a single spin method, and patients received injections in

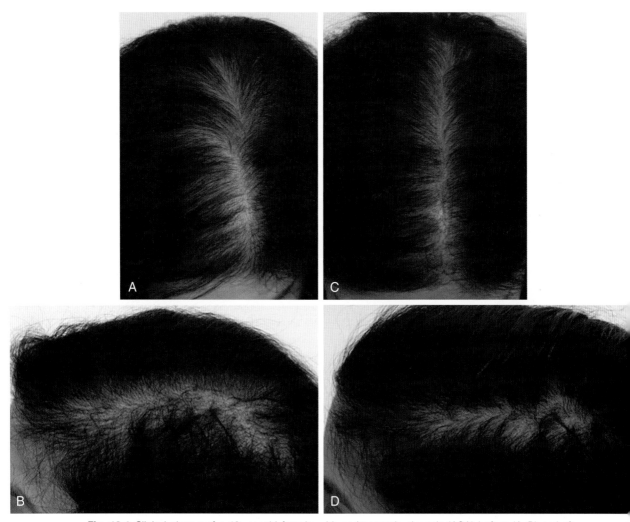

Fig. 12.4 Clinical photos of a 42-year-old female with androgenetic alopecia (AGA) before (A–B) and after (C–D) three platelet-rich plasma (PRP) treatments in the authors' clinic. Photos taken 5 months apart.

three monthly sessions followed by three bimonthly sessions. After the sixth session, 71.4% of men and 73.4% of women demonstrated a decrease of at least one grade or higher of AGA Grades II-IV in the Ebling's scale.[25]

EXPECTED OUTCOMES

The use of PRP for hair restoration in AGA remains a relatively novel therapeutic option. Although somewhat variable, the current overall consensus in the available literature is that PRP is a promising treatment modality

(Table 12.1, see Figs. 12.3-12.5). However, several limitations including a paucity of long-term studies, lack of an established universal protocol for preparation and administration, heterogeneity in study design and measurable outcomes, and small sample sizes make fair and objective comparisons to more established therapeutic options difficult.

A randomized, placebo-controlled and double-blind case study of 12 men and 13 women with AGA studied patients who received a total of three monthly sessions. Patients had PRP injected into one-half of their scalp and placebo injections of saline in the other half.

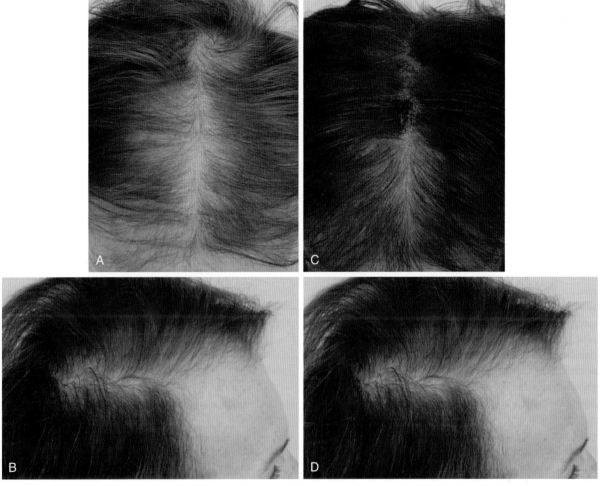

Fig. 12.5 Clinical photos of a 66-year-old female with androgenetic alopecia (AGA) before (A–B) and after (C–D) four platelet-rich plasma (PRP) treatments in the authors' clinic. This patient was also using minoxidil 5% foam prior to PRP treatment.

The results of the study showed that, 6 months after the first treatment with PRP, there was a significant difference in mean anagen, telogen, terminal hairs, and hair density compared with baseline and a significant increase in hair density compared with the saline-injected half (level of evidence: 1b).[26] The clinical benefit was significantly more pronounced in patients who were male, younger than 40 years of age, noticed hair loss after 25 years of age, had a positive family history, or experienced hair loss for greater than 10 years.[26]

Similar findings were seen in a meta-analysis of 13 studies that investigated the use of PRP for treatment of AGA. Although the studies used variable protocols, the preliminary evidence of the meta-analysis suggested that PRP scalp injections can increase the yield of follicular units in the treatment of AGA.[34] This study and others stressed the importance of establishing a standardized treatment protocol (quantity of injections and frequency of treatments) and method to objectively measure treatment success, as the most ideal protocol remains unclear. The commonalities in frequency of treatments between successful studies described by the authors included three treatment sessions in monthly intervals, followed by booster treatment at 6 months, with maximum results observed at 3 months.[34,35] The study with the longest patient follow-up duration of 2 years observed relapse at

Text continued on page 157

TABLE 12.1   Randomized Controlled Trials Evaluating the Effects of Platelet-Rich Plasma in Androgenetic Alopecia and Outcome Study Evaluation

Study, Year	No. of Patients; Males (M), Females (F)	Treatment	Summary of Outcomes	Quality of Assessment	Level of Evidence
Alves, 2016[26]	25 (13 F, 12 M) 22 completed (11 F, 11 M)	Three monthly PRP treatments injected into half of the scalp, saline injections into the contralateral scalp	• Increase in mean anagen hairs, telogen hairs, hair density, and terminal hair density at 3 and 6 months in PRP treated scalp compared with baseline • Increase in hair density in PRP treated scalp compared with control side at 3 and 6 months	• Independent evaluator analyzed both global photographs and phototrichogram • Patients were evaluated in 4 visits: baseline, 2 months, 3 months, 6 months • Evaluator was blinded regarding the treatment and control areas and was not involved in the administration of treatments	1b
Cervelli, 2014[20]	10 M	Three monthly PRP treatments injected into half of the scalp, saline injections into the contralateral scalp	• Increase in hair count and density in PRP injected scalp compared with baseline and control side at 3 months • Increase in epidermal thickness, number of hair follicles, Ki67+ basal keratinocytes and blood vessels around hair follicles on microscopic exam of treated scalp compared with baseline	• Independent evaluator analyzed both global photographs and phototrichogram • Patients were evaluated in 4 visits: baseline, 14 weeks, 6 months, 12 months • Evaluator was blinded regarding the treatment and control areas and was not involved in the administration of treatments	1b

| Gentile, 2015[19] | 23 M | Three monthly PRP treatments injected into half of the scalp, saline injections into the contralateral scalp | • Increase in hair count, hair density, and terminal hair density in PRP injected scalp compared with baseline and control side at 3 months
 • Increase in epidermal thickness, number of follicles, Ki67+ basal keratinocytes and blood vessels around hair follicles on microscopic exam of treated scalp compared with baseline | • Independent evaluator analyzed both global photographs and phototrichogram
 • Patients were evaluated in 6 visits: baseline, 2 months, 6 months, 12 months, 16 months, 24 months.
 • Evaluator was blinded regarding the treatment and control areas and was not involved in the administration of treatments | 1b |

(Continued)

TABLE 12.1 **Randomized Controlled Trials Evaluating the Effects of Platelet Rich Plasma in Androgenetic Alopecia and Outcome Study Evaluation—cont'd**

Study, Year	No. of Patients; Males (M), Females (F)	Treatment	Summary of Outcomes	Quality of Assessment	Level of Evidence
Gentile, 2017[17]	24 M	• Eighteen participants received three monthly nonactivated PRP treatments injected into half the scalp and saline injected into contralateral scalp • Six participants randomized to receive a single treatment of calcium activated PRP prepared by one of two different systems	• Increase in hair count and hair density in area treated with nonactivated PRP compared with control area by TrichoScan analysis at 3 months • Increase in epidermal thickness, number of follicles, Ki67+ basal keratinocytes, and improved vascularization on microscopic exam of nonactivated PRP treated scalp compared with baseline at 3 months • Increase in hair density and follicular unit density in subjects receiving PRP generated from the Arthex Angel System at 6 months compared with baseline	• Independent evaluator analyzed both global photographs and phototrichogram • Patients were evaluated at 2 visits: baseline and 12 weeks after final injections administered • Evaluator was blinded regarding the treatment and control areas and was not involved in the administration of treatments	1b

Study	Subjects	Methods	Results	Evaluation	Level of evidence
Hausauer, 2018[27]	40 (30 M, 10 F) 39 completed (29 M and 10 F)	Subjects randomized into one of two groups: • Group 1: Three monthly PRP treatments with booster treatment after 3 months • Group 2: Two PRP treatments spaced 3 months apart	• Significant increase in hair count at 3 months seen in Group 1 compared with baseline • Significant increase in hair count in both groups at 6 months compared with baseline • Significantly higher mean percent change in Group 1 compared with Group 2 at 6 months • Increase in hair shaft caliber in both groups at 3 and 6 months compared with baseline (no significant difference between treatment groups) • Satisfaction scores higher in Group 1 compared with Group 2	• Authors evaluated patients via folliscope and global photography • Patients were evaluated at three visits: baseline, 3 months, 6 months	1b
Kachhawa, 2017[28]	50 M (44 completed)	Six PRP treatments separated by 21 days injected into the androgen dependent areas of the left scalp, saline injections into androgen dependent areas of the right scalp	Increase in overall hair density, quality, and thickness noted in images and on trichoscopy after treatment on left side of scalp compared with baseline	• Patient were evaluated at all 6 visits using global photography, TrichoScan and hair pull test • The same two physicians performed hair pull tests in a standardized manner at each visit	1c

(Continued)

TABLE 12.1 **Randomized Controlled Trials Evaluating the Effects of Platelet Rich Plasma in Androgenetic Alopecia and Outcome Study Evaluation—cont'd**

Study, Year	No. of Patients; Males (M), Females (F)	Treatment	Summary of Outcomes	Quality of Assessment	Level of Evidence
Mapar, 2016[29]	19 M (17 completed)	Two 2.5 × 2.5 cm square-shaped areas at least 3 cm apart on the scalp chosen; one spot injected with PRP and one with saline; two injections 1 month apart	No change in terminal hair count or vellus hair count in the experimental square compared with the control square at 6 months	• Authors evaluated patients using magnifying glass • Patients were evaluated at three visits: 1 month, 3 months, and 6 months after first treatment	1c
Puig, 2016[30]	26 F	Subjects randomized to receive either one treatment of PRP or one injection of saline into the central scalp	• No statistical difference in hair count or hair mass index between experimental and control groups • More subjects in experimental group reported substantial improvement in hair loss, rate of hair loss, hair thickness, ease of managing hair, and coarser/heavier hair	• Independent evaluator analyzed both global photography and hair max index using Cohen hair check system • Patients evaluated at baseline and at 26 weeks +/- 1 week • Evaluator was blinded regarding the treatment and control areas and was not involved in the administration of treatments	1b

(Continued)

Study	Subjects	Treatment	Outcomes	Level
Rodrigues, 2018[31]	26 M	Subjects randomly assigned to receive either four treatments of PRP or saline injections every 15 days	• Increase in hair count, density, and the percentage of anagen hairs in PRP group compared with control and baseline after treatment • No change in terminal/vellus hair ratio between the PRP and control group	1b • Authors evaluated patients using Tricho-Scan • Patients evaluated at three visits: baseline, 15 days after last treatment, and 3 months after last treatment • Authors were blinded regarding the treatment and control areas
Tawfik, 2018[32]	30 F	Four weekly PRP treatments injected into select area of the scalp, saline injected into another selected area of the scalp	• Increase in hair density and thickness in PRP treated area compared with control area and baseline by physician assessment of photographs and folliscope at 6 months • Decrease in number of subjects with positive pull test in the PRP treated area compared with control area at 6 months	1b • Independent evaluator analyzed both global photographs and photoトリchodogram • Hair pull test performed at every session and at 6-month follow up by the same clinician • Patients were evaluated at two visits: baseline and 6 months after last treatment • Evaluator was blinded regarding the treatment and control areas and was not involved in the administration of treatments

TABLE 12.1 Randomized Controlled Trials Evaluating the Effects of Platelet Rich Plasma in Androgenetic Alopecia and Outcome Study Evaluation—cont'd

Study, Year	No. of Patients; Males (M), Females (F)	Treatment	Summary of Outcomes	Quality of Assessment	Level of Evidence
Dubin, 2020[33]	30 F (28 completed)	Subjects randomly assigned to receive either three treatments of PRP or saline injections at weeks 0, 4, and 8	• Increase in hair density and caliber in PRP treated area compared with baseline and control at week 8, with sustained improvement at week 24	• Independent evaluator analyzed both global photographs and folliscope • Patients were evaluated in three visits: baseline, 8 weeks, and 24 weeks • Evaluator was blinded regarding the treatment and control areas	1b

AGA, Androgenetic alopecia; *F*, female; *M*, male; *PRP*, platelet-rich plasma.
Adapted from Semsarzadeh N, Khetarpal S. Platelet-rich plasma and stem cells for hair growth: a review of the literature. *Aesthet Surg J.* 2019.

around 1 year after the last treatment and thus recommended a regular ongoing maintenance regimen to prevent loss of newly formed regrowth.[34]

In an effort to determine an optimal protocol and address the issue of discrepancies in frequency and intervals between PRP treatments in treating AGA, Hausauer et al. conducted a prospective, randomized, single-blinded trial over a 6-month period of patients with moderate AGA (level of evidence: 1b).[27] Forty patients received PRP injections after one of two treatment protocols: three monthly sessions with a 3-month booster (Group 1) or two sessions spaced by 3-month intervals (Group 2). At 6 months, both groups demonstrated a statistically significant increase in average hair counts. However, patients expressed higher satisfaction rates with improvements occurring faster, as early as 3 months, in Group 1 compared with Group 2.[27] This study further aided in three monthly sessions at the initiation of treatment to produce an optimal outcome. Although few in number, there are trials showing failure of PRP in treatment of AGA. In a single-blind trial, Mapar et al. looked at two scalp sites in 17 men with severe AGA (level of evidence: 1c).[29] One scalp site was injected with PRP; the second site served as the control and was injected with normal saline. Injections were administered in two sessions 1 month apart. The results did not reveal a significant difference among the terminal or vellus hair counts 6 months after the first treatment in either the PRP or saline injection sites.[29] The authors acknowledged that their low number of subjects, all of whom presented with a prolonged course of advanced stages of AGA (stage IV-VI Norwood hairloss scale), and low number of PRP injection sessions were likely contributing factors to the poor outcomes.[29] Similarly, a study by Puig et al. demonstrated no significant difference in hair count when evaluating the efficacy of PRP for treatment of female AGA; however, lack of more than one treatment procedure and a small study population are likely contributory factors (level of evidence: 1b).[30]

Overall, it is important to educate patients that, while ideal protocols are yet to be determined, the data suggests that some patients respond to PRP with notable improvement. Setting realistic expectations and informing patients that PRP is not efficacious in all patients is paramount. Additionally, PRP's low side-effect profile further supports this as a therapeutic option worth pursuing.

EFFICACY OF PLATELET RICH PLASMA IN COMBINATION WITH MICRONEEDLING

A more recently studied topic is the use of microneedling as a therapeutic modality of transdermal drug delivery for treatment of AGA. There are various microneedling devices on the market available for both consumers and medical offices to purchase. Microneedling for AGA is most commonly carried out using a dermaroller, which typically contains 192 titanium-alloy coated needles and comes in variable sizes; 1.5 to 2 mm is the preferred treatment depth for AGA.[36,37] The procedure involves multiple repetitive, multidirectional passes along the scalp with the dermaroller until pinpoint bleeding is achieved. Those who favor the use of microneedling state that this method allows for much greater dermal entry points for topical medications such as minoxidil or PRP to be absorbed into surrounding tissue and act more closely upon the hair follicle while bypassing the thick epidermis of the scalp. However, with more cutaneous entry points in the scalp, this welcomes an increased opportunity for infections, hypersensitivity reactions, or even foreign body granulomatous reactions to topicals applied to the open channels, which may remain open for up to 24 hours post procedure. More case-controlled studies evaluating protocols and adverse effects and investigations with objective measurements evaluating hair density are needed to further support the utility of this therapeutic option.

Albeit few, there are case reports of PRP injections used in conjunction with microneedling for the treatment of AGA. Smaller randomized controlled studies have shown both PRP with microneedling and a combination of 5% topical minoxidil twice daily with PRP injections and microneedling are well tolerated, safe, and exhibit significant improvement in both patient and physician assessment of hair growth (level of evidence: 1b).[37-40] Higher powered studies are required, as the optimal protocol for the combination of techniques remains to be determined.

VARIATIONS IN PLATELET-RICH PLASMA FORMULATIONS FOR TREATMENT OF ANDROGENETIC ALOPECIA

As stated earlier, components of PRP have been shown to upregulate angiogenesis and improve blood flow within the DP. To enhance the angiogenesis effect of PRP,

CD34+ hematopoietic stem cells, which have been shown to promote angiogenesis in ischemic conditions, were added to autologous PRP preparations, as levels have been shown to decrease with age.[41] Patients received two sessions of CD34+ cell-containing PRP 3 months apart. Overall, results showed a significant increase in the mean number of hairs and thickness compared with baseline values at 3 and 6 months.[41] Further studies comparing CD34+ cell-containing PRP and pure PRP are needed to determine whether there is a true benefit of this supplementation.

Another potential avenue for enhancing the therapeutic effects of PRP is ensuring that there is a high concentration of growth factors within the PRP preparation. In a small pilot study of 10 patients with AGA, Siah et al. quantified growth-factor concentrations within PRP preparations for each patient (level of evidence: 4).[42] The clinical results demonstrated increased hair density in patients whose PRP preparations had higher growth-factor concentrations of glial cell line-derived neurotrophic factor (GDNF). Findings of this study suggest the discrepancy in hair growth among PRP treated individuals may be caused by variability in growth factor concentrations present in their PRP samples.[42] Future studies evaluating standardization of growth factors within PRP preparations is necessary, as this may increase rates of predictable and favorable outcomes for patients.

EVIDENCE SUMMARY

- Platelet-rich plasma therapy is a promising adjuvant treatment modality for androgenetic alopecia (strength of recommendation: B).
- Monthly sessions for the first 3 months followed by treatments every 3 months for the first year have demonstrated increased hair density and hair caliber with sustained optimal clinical outcomes in patients with androgenetic alopecia (strength of recommendation: D).
- The clinical benefit of platelet-rich plasma may be more pronounced in patients who are male, younger than 40 years of age, began noticing hair loss after 25 years of age, have a positive family history of hair loss, or experienced hair loss for greater than 10 years (strength of recommendation: B).
- Platelet-rich plasma's low side-effect profile further supports this as a therapeutic option worth pursuing in combination with antiandrogenic therapies and

topical minoxidil. This ensures the most favorable outcome for the majority of patients, as these agents have a cumulative effect on the miniaturized hair follicles within the dermal papillae (strength of recommendation: D).

REFERENCES

1. Sinclair R. Clinical review: male pattern androgenetic alopecia. *BMJ.* 1998;317:865-869.
2. Conic RR, Khetarpal S, Bergfeld W. Treatment of female pattern hair loss with combination therapy. *Semin Cutan Med Surg.* 2018;37(4):247-253.
3. Camacho FM, García-Hernández M. Psychological features of androgenetic alopecia. *J Eur Acad Dermatol Venereol.* 2002;16(5):476-480.
4. Cash TF, Price VH, Savin RC. Psychological effects of androgenetic alopecia on women: comparisons with balding men and with female control subjects. *J Am Acad Dermatol.* 1993;29(4):568-575.
5. Amory JK, Wang C, Swerdloff RS, et al. The effect of 5alpha-reductase inhibition with dutasteride and finasteride on semen parameters and serum hormones in healthy men. *J Clin Endocrinol Metab.* 2007;92(5):1659-1665.
6. Olsen EA, Hordinsky M, Whiting D, et al. The importance of dual 5alpha-reductase inhibition in the treatment of male pattern hair loss: results of a randomized placebo-controlled study of dutasteride versus finasteride. Dutasteride Alopecia Research Team. *J Am Acad Dermatol.* 2006;55(6):1014.
7. Fields JR, Vonu PM, Monir RL, Schoch JJ. Topical ketoconazole for the treatment of androgenetic alopecia: a systematic review. *Dermatol Ther.* 2020;33(1):e13202.
8. Lee SW, Juhasz M, Mobasher P, Ekelem C, Mesinkovska NA. A systematic review of topical finasteride in the treatment of androgenetic alopecia in men and women. *J Drugs Dermatol.* 2018;17(4):457-463.
9. Sinclair RD. Female pattern hair loss: a pilot study investigating combination therapy with low-dose oral minoxidil and spironolactone. *Int J Dermatol.* 2018;57:104-109.
10. Leavitt M, Charles G, Heyman E, Michaels D. HairMax LaserComb laser phototherapy device in the treatment of male androgenetic alopecia: a randomized, double-blind, sham device-controlled, multicentre trial. *Clin Drug Investig.* 2009;29(5):283-292.
11. Jimenez JJ, Wikramanayake TC, Bergfeld W, et al. Efficacy and safety of a low-level laser device in the treatment of male and female pattern hair loss: a multicenter, randomized, sham device-controlled, double-blind study. *Am J Clin Dermatol.* 2014;15(2):115.
12. Bolognia J, Schaffer J, Cerroni L. *Dermatology.* 4th ed. Philadelphia, PA: Elsevier Saunders; 2017.

13. Sawaya ME, Price VH. Different levels of 5alpha-reductase type I and II, aromatase, and androgen receptor in hair follicles of women and men with androgenetic alopecia. *J Invest Dermatol.* 1997;109(3):296-300.

14. Gupta AK, Carviel J. A mechanistic model of platelet-rich plasma treatment for androgenetic alopecia. *Dermatol Surg.* 2016;42(12):1335-1339. doi:10.1097/DSS.0000000000000901.

15. Kwack MH, Sung YK, Chung EJ, et al. Dihydrotestosteroneinducible dickkopf 1 from balding dermal papilla cells causes apoptosis in follicular keratinocytes. *J Invest Dermatol.* 2008;128:262-269.

16. Chesire DR, Isaacs WB. Ligand-dependent inhibition of beta-catenin/ TCF signaling by androgen receptor. *Oncogene.* 2002;21:8453-8469.

17. Gentile P, Cole JP, Cole MA, et al. Evaluation of not-activated and activated PRP in hair loss treatment: role of growth factor and cytokine concentrations obtained by different collection systems. *Int J Mol Sci.* 2017;18(2):408. doi:10.3390/ijms18020408.

18. York K, Meah N, Bhoyrul B, Sinclair R. A review of the treatment of male pattern hair loss. *Expert Opin Pharmacother.* 2020;21(5):603-612. doi:10.1080/14656566.2020.1721463.

19. Gentile P, Garcovich S, Bielli A, et al. The Effect of platelet rich plasma in hair regrowth: a randomized placebo-controlled trial. *Stem Cells Transl Med.* 2015;4:1317-1323.

20. Cervelli V, Garcovich S, Bielli A, et al. The effect of autologous activated platelet rich plasma (AA-PRP) injection on pattern hair loss: clinical and histomorphometric evaluation. *Biomed Res Int.* 2014;2014:760709. doi:10.1155/2014/760709.

21. Uebel CO, da Silva JB, Cantarelli D, Martins P. The role of platelet plasma growth factors in male pattern baldness surgery. *Plast Reconstr Surg.* 2006;118(6):1458-1466; discussion 1467.

22. Alves R, Grimalt R. Platelet-rich plasma in combination with 5% minoxidil topical solution and 1 mg oral finasteride for the treatment of androgenetic alopecia: a randomized placebo-controlled, double-blind, half-head study. *Dermatol Surg.* 2018;44(1):126–130. doi:10.1097/DSS.0000000000001198.

23. Anitua E, Pino A, Jaen P, Navarro MR. Platelet rich plasma for the management of hair loss: better alone or in combination? *J Cosmet Dermatol.* 2019;18(2):483-486.

24. Juhasz M, Sukhedeo K, Lo Sicco K, Shapiro J. Stratifying clinical response to adjuvant platelet-rich plasma in patients with androgenetic alopecia. *Br J Dermatol.* 2020;183(3):580-582.

25. Ferrando J, García-García SC, González-de-Cossío AC, Bou L, Navarra E. A proposal of an effective platelet-rich plasma protocol for the treatment of androgenetic alopecia.

26. Alves R, Grimalt R. Randomized placebo-controlled, double-blind, half-head study to assess the efficacy of platelet-rich plasma on the treatment of androgenetic alopecia. *Dermatol Surg.* 2016;42(4):491-497. doi:10.1097/DSS.0000000000000665.

27. Hausauer AK, Jones DH. Evaluating the efficacy of different platelet-rich plasma regimens for management of androgenetic alopecia: a single-center, blinded, randomized clinical trial. *Dermatol Surg.* 2018;44(9):1191-1200.

28. Kachhawa D, Vats G, Sonare D, Rao P, Khuraiya S, Kataiya R. A spilt head study of efficacy of placebo versus platelet-rich plasma injections in the treatment of androgenic alopecia. *J Cutan Aesthet Surg.* 2017;10(2):86–89. doi:10.4103/JCAS.JCAS_50_16.

29. Mapar MA, Shahriari S, Haghighizadeh MH. Efficacy of platelet-rich plasma in the treatment of androgenetic (male-patterned) alopecia: a pilot randomized controlled trial. *J Cosmet Laser Ther.* 2016;18(8):452-455.

30. Puig CJ, Reese R, Peters M. Double-blind, placebo-controlled pilot study on the use of platelet-rich plasma in women with female androgenetic alopecia. *Dermatol Surg.* 2016;42(11):1243-1247. doi:10.1097/DSS.0000000000000883.

31. Rodrigues BL, Montalvão SAL, Cancela RBB, et al. Treatment of male pattern alopecia with platelet-rich plasma: a double-blind controlled study with analysis of platelet number and growth factor levels. *J Am Acad Dermatol.* 2019;80(3):694-700.

32. Tawfik AA, Osman MAR. The effect of autologous activated platelet-rich plasma injection on female pattern hair loss: a randomized placebo-controlled study. *J Cosmet Dermatol.* 2018;17(1):47-53.

33. Dubin DP, Lin MJ, Leight HM, et al. The effect of platelet-rich plasma on female androgenetic alopecia: a randomized controlled trial. *J Am Acad Dermatol.* 2020;83(5):1294-1297. doi:10.1016/j.jaad.2020.06.1021.

34. Gupta AK, Carviel JL. Meta-analysis of efficacy of platelet-rich plasma therapy for androgenetic alopecia. *J Dermatolog Treat.* 2017;28(1):55-58.

35. Gkini MA, Kouskoukis AE, Tripsianis G, et al. Study of platelet-rich plasma injections in the treatment of androgenetic alopecia through an one-year period. *J Cutan Aesthetic Surg.* 2014;7:213-219.

36. Jha AK, Vinay K. Androgenetic alopecia and microneedling: every needling is not microneedling. *J Am Acad Dermatol.* 2019;81(2):e43-e44.

37. Ramadan WM, Hassan AM, Ismail MA, El Attar YA. Evaluation of adding platelet-rich plasma to combined medical therapy in androgenetic alopecia. *J Cosmet Dermatol.* 2021;20(5):1427-1434. doi:10.1111/jocd.13935.

Int J Trichology. 2017;9(4):165-170. doi:10.4103/ijt.ijt_27_17.

38. Jha AK, Udayan UK, Roy PK, Amar AKJ, Chaudhary RKP. Original article: platelet-rich plasma with microneedling in androgenetic alopecia along with dermoscopic pre- and post-treatment evaluation. *J Cosmet Dermatol.* 2018;17(3):313-318.

39. Shah KB, Shah AN, Solanki RB, Raval RC. A comparative study of microneedling with platelet-rich plasma plus topical minoxidil (5%) and topical minoxidil (5%) alone in androgenetic alopecia. *Int J Trichology.* 2017;9(1): 14-18. doi:10.4103/ijt.ijt_75_16.

40. Jha AK, Vinay K, Zeeshan M, Roy PK, Chaudhary RKP, Priya A. Platelet-rich plasma and microneedling improves hair growth in patients of androgenetic alopecia when used as an adjuvant to minoxidil [published online ahead of print, 2019 Jan 28]. *J Cosmet Dermatol.* 2019. doi:10.1111/jocd.12864.

41. Kang JS, Zheng Z, Choi MJ, Lee SH, Kim DY, Cho SB. The effect of CD34+ cell-containing autologous platelet-rich plasma injection on pattern hair loss: a preliminary study. *J Eur Acad Dermatol Venereol.* 2014;28(1):72-79. doi:10.1111/jdv.12062.

42. Siah TW, Guo H, Chu T, et al. Growth factor concentrations in platelet-rich plasma for androgenetic alopecia: an intra-subject, randomized, blinded, placebo-controlled, pilot study. *Exp Dermatol.* 2020;29(3):334-340.

13

Stem Cell–Based Therapies

Bianca Y. Kang and Murad Alam

KEY POINTS

- Stem cells are a potential therapeutic option for the treatment of androgenetic alopecia and other forms of hair loss. However, serious adverse events have been previously reported from the use of stem cells for non dermatologic applications. As such, stem cell therapy is subject to strict regulation by the US Food and Drug Administration.
- Adipose tissue is a readily accessible and abundant source of multipotent adipose-derived stem cells and

may be processed into stromal vascular fraction. The regenerative effects of stromal vascular fraction are primarily attributed to paracrine signaling between stem cells and hair follicles and the secretion of anti-inflammatory and antiandrogen molecules.
- Other stem cell–derived therapies include adipose-derived stem cell–conditioned medium, exosomes, and small molecules that induce lactate production within hair follicle stem cells.

BACKGROUND, DEFINITIONS, AND HISTORY

The possible applications of regenerative therapies span every field of medicine and have the potential to significantly improve patient outcomes. The treatment of hair loss is particularly well suited for stem cell–based interventions. Accessible treatment sites allow for minimally invasive or noninvasive approaches, select regenerative therapies require only a modest amount of additional training or equipment, and procedures can be performed on an outpatient basis. Additionally, autologous stem cell–containing regenerative substances are readily harvestable by lipoaspiration or surgical resection (Pearl 13.1).

Adipose tissue is an abundant and accessible source of adipose-derived stem cells (ADSCs), a type of mesenchymal stem cell (MSC). These multipotent stem cells can self-renew and also have the capacity to differentiate into other cell types, including adipocytes, keratinocytes, chondrocytes, osteocytes, osteoblasts, vascular and endothelial lineages, hematopoietic cells, hepatocytes, cardiomyocytes, and neurons, depending on culture conditions (Fig. 13.1) (level of evidence: 5).[1-3]

> **PEARL 13.1:** Adipose tissue is rich in multipotent adipose-derived stem cells. These cells may be concentrated by processing adipose into stromal vascular fraction.

ADSCs may be concentrated by processing adipose tissue either chemically or mechanically into stromal vascular fraction (SVF), which is the substance that remains after removal of adipocytes and connective tissue (Pearl 13.2).[3] In addition to ADSCs, SVF contains other stem cells (e.g., hematopoietic stem cells, pericytes), progenitor cells (e.g., adipocyte progenitors), mature cells (e.g., endothelial cells, erythrocytes, immune cells, smooth muscle cells, fibroblasts), and an abundance of growth factors and other secreted molecules (Fig. 13.2).

In the twenty-first century, there has been growing interest in the use of stem cells and stem cell–based modalities for the treatment of various types of alopecia, with a particular focus on androgenetic alopecia (AGA) and alopecia areata (AA). White adipose tissue (WAT) in the dermis is closely associated with hair follicles (Fig. 13.3). The dermal WAT remodels in concert with the hair cycle,

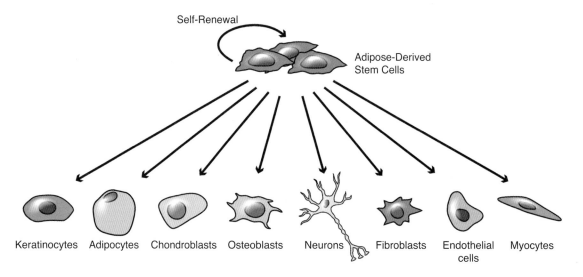

Fig. 13.1 Adipose-derived stem cells (ADSCs) are multipotent mesenchymal stem cells (MSCs). These multipotent stem cells can self-renew and also have the capacity to differentiate into other cell types, depending on culture conditions. (Courtesy of Sheila Macomber.)

PEARL 13.2: Stromal vascular fraction contains stem cells, progenitor cells, mature cells, growth factors, and other secreted molecules. The potential applications of stromal vascular fraction and other stem cell–based therapies are broad and span specialties other than dermatology.

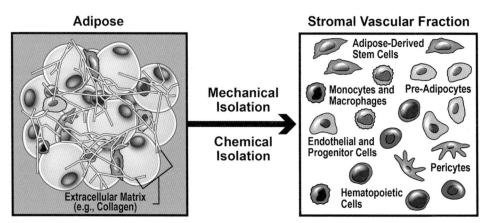

Fig. 13.2 Adipose tissue may be processed into stromal vascular fraction (SVF) by enzymatically or nonenzymatically removing adipocytes and connective tissue, leading to a higher concentration of adipose-derived stem cells (ADSCs) in SVF than found in unprocessed adipose. SVF contains other stem cells (e.g., ADSCs, hematopoietic stem cells, pericytes), progenitor cells (e.g., adipocyte progenitors), mature cells (e.g., endothelial cells, erythrocytes, immune cells, smooth muscle cells, fibroblasts), and an abundance of growth factors and other secreted molecules. (Courtesy of Sheila Macomber.)

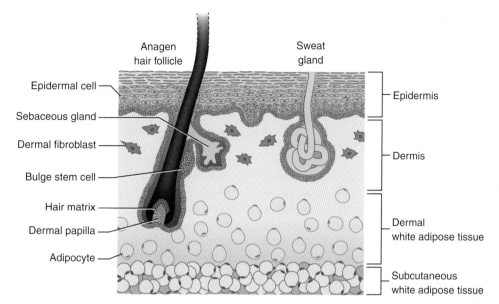

Fig. 13.3 White adipose tissue (WAT) in the dermis is closely associated with hair follicles and remodels with the hair cycle (i.e., thickening around follicles during anagen and thinning during the transition from catagen to telogen). This is related to reciprocal signaling between dermal WAT and the dermal papillae. (Courtesy of Sheila Macomber.)

PEARL 13.3: The dermal white adipose tissue rapidly cycles in concert with the hair cycle, and paracrine signaling between the white adipose tissue and dermal papillae appears to be important in regulation of normal hair growth.

PEARL 13.4: The regenerative function of stem cell–based therapies such as stromal vascular fraction in the treatment of alopecia is largely attributed to paracrine signaling between stem cells and hair follicles, as stem cells secrete growth factors that stimulate hair growth, reduce inflammation, and have antiandrogen effects.

---

thickening around follicles during anagen, and thinning by approximately 50% during the transition from catagen to telogen (level of evidence: 5) (Pearl 13.3).[4,5] This synchronous cycling of dermal fat and hair growth is related at least in part to reciprocal signaling between dermal WAT and the dermal papillae and is likely altered in alopecia and other conditions affecting hair growth (e.g., lipodystrophy, obesity).

As a result, adipocyte progenitors and ADSCs contained within SVF may be particularly important in the treatment of alopecia. Although precise mechanisms are not understood, the regenerative potential of SVF is theorized to arise primarily from paracrine signaling that stimulates regeneration of the host tissue (i.e., hair follicles) and secretion of anti-inflammatory and antiandrogen molecules (level of evidence: 5).[6,7] SVF cells secrete platelet derived growth factor (PDGF) and insulin-like growth factor 1 (IGF-1) and express leptin,

adiponectin, bone morphogenic protein, and other molecules that regulate hair growth (level of evidence: 5) (Pearl 13.4).[5] Neovascularization and direct tissue formation from differentiation of individual SVF cells (e.g., differentiation into follicular progenitor cells and adipocytes) may also play a role (level of evidence: 5).[8]

The objective of this chapter is to discuss the use of SVF in the treatment of AGA and other nonscarring alopecias. Additional stem cell–based therapies, including ADSC-conditioned medium (ADSC-CM), exosomes, and small molecules that promote activation of hair follicle stem cells, will also be briefly discussed.

INDICATIONS AND PATIENT SELECTION

At the time of this publication, there are no clinical practice guidelines for the use of SVF or other stem cell

> **PEARL 13.5:** Patients with early androgenetic alopecia may benefit more from regenerative therapies than those with severe hair loss.

therapies in treating alopecia. As a result of scarce high-quality clinical studies, it remains unclear which types of alopecia may respond best to SVF. The majority of ongoing and published clinical trials treat patients with AGA or AA, but studies are limited by sample size, heterogeneity in reported outcomes, and differing treatment techniques (level of evidence: 2b).[8,9] As with most interventional therapies for AGA, patients with early hair loss may benefit more than those with severe hair loss (level of evidence: 5) (Pearl 13.5).[10] SVF is not a first-line therapy for AGA, so patient education should focus on the role of less invasive techniques with robust efficacy and safety evidence, such as finasteride, topical minoxidil, or platelet-rich plasma (PRP) (level of evidence: 1a).[11] SVF injections are likely not appropriate for patients who are risk averse or who are not candidates for liposuction (e.g., in patients with severe cardiovascular disease or severe coagulation disorders or in pregnant patients) (level of evidence: 5).[12]

It should be noted that, at the time of this publication in the United States, the use of SVF and other stem cell therapies should be restricted to US Food and Drug Administration (FDA)-supervised clinical trials. The FDA has released warnings regarding stem cell therapies, stating they are "concerned that some patients seeking cures and remedies are vulnerable to stem cell treatments that are illegal and potentially harmful." As of August 2017, the FDA announced increased regulation enforcement and stem cell clinic oversight. This was largely prompted by several notable adverse events that were related to stem cell injection, including bilateral blindness after intravitreal injection of autologous ADSCs by a nurse practitioner without MD or FDA oversight and development of an aggressive spinal cord tumor in a patient who received multiple intrathecal stem cell injections. The FDA urges patients to only undergo stem cell therapy if the treatment is FDA-approved or being studied as part of an FDA-supervised clinical trial with an Investigational New Drug Application (IND). Currently, the only FDA-approved stem cell–based products are hematopoietic progenitor cells indicated for use in patients with hematopoietic disorders.[13] The FDA warns that they may take

"administrative and judicial actions" against unapproved use of stem cell products if stem cells are "processed in ways that are more than minimally manipulated."

EXPECTED OUTCOMES

Ideally, patients with AGA who are treated with SVF will experience improvement in hair density and hair diameter. The increases in hair density and diameter should be apparent within approximately 6 months and may range from 14%-23% and 11%-24%, respectively.[8,9] The proportion of anagen hairs may also increase. Although hair growth may improve after a single treatment, these effects may not persist.[10] Similar to PRP injections, two to three treatments of SVF at approximately 1-month intervals may lead to more noticeable and sustained outcomes.[9]

The degree and duration of improvement is likely dependent on multiple factors, including patient age, etiology and severity of hair loss, and use of adjunctive therapies.[8] Treatment technique is also likely to be important, although sufficiently powered, high-quality clinical trials are required to further elucidate best practices for optimizing outcomes (Pearl 13.6). Current evidence suggests that SVF with low-density ADSCs (0.5×10^6 ADSCs/cm^2) may be more beneficial than SVF with high-density ADSCs (1×10^6 ADSCs/cm^2).[10] Also, combination therapy (e.g., SVF with finasteride or topical minoxidil) is likely more effective than SVF alone.[9]

TREATMENT TECHNIQUE AND BEST PRACTICES

The treatment techniques described here are intended to be neither comprehensive nor prescriptive, but rather to offer a succinct review of currently available literature. The treating physician should exercise good judgment to care for each patient individually. SVF should be used in an FDA-supervised clinical trial setting, with strict adherence to the trial's study protocol.

> **PEARL 13.6:** Current evidence suggests that treatment with stromal vascular fraction may lead to increased hair density and hair diameter after approximately 6 months. High-powered, randomized, controlled clinical trials are needed to identify ideal candidates and treatment techniques for stromal vascular fraction.

Pretreatment Considerations

The procedure should be performed by a board-certified physician with sufficient education and training in liposuction and skin surgery such as dermatology or plastic surgery. At present, because SVF is not FDA-approved for the treatment of alopecia, this treatment should be under the purview of an FDA-supervised clinical trial with an IND.[14] Also, as a result of the investigative nature of stem cell therapies, obtaining informed consent is extremely important. The International Society for Stem Cell Research (ISSCR) provides professional standards for consent for stem cell–based interventions but does also urge that such treatments be performed only with FDA oversight.[15]

The preoperative evaluation should include a thorough past medical history, including a history of poor wound healing or abnormal scarring, bleeding abnormalities, immunosuppression, severe infection, prior reactions to surgery and anesthesia, and treatments that the patient has used or is currently using for hair loss.[12] The patient's medication list should be reviewed, including for medications that affect coagulation or metabolism of local anesthesia. Laboratory studies depend on provider preferences and institution and clinical trial-specific regulations and may include a complete blood count, coagulation studies, and, in women with childbearing potential, a urine pregnancy test. A physical examination should assess for evidence of poor healing or abnormal scarring and evaluate sites appropriate for liposuction, such as the lateral thigh and abdoment.

On the day of treatment, which may take place in an ambulatory setting, photographs of treatment sites should be obtained and used to monitor patient response moving forward. Baseline vital signs should be measured and documented. An oral anxiolytic, sedative, or analgesic may be appropriate, depending on the comfort level of the patient and provider.[12] Parenteral anxiety and pain medications should be used with caution or avoided completely if possible, and general anesthesia is not recommended.

Tumescent Liposuction

Tumescent liposuction is typically performed to harvest adipose tissue from which the SVF will be isolated (Fig. 13.4).[9] The American Society for Dermatologic Surgery (ASDS) and the American Academy of Dermatology (AAD) provide clinical practice guidelines for liposuction (level of evidence: 5).[12,16]

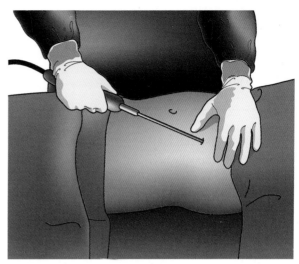

Fig. 13.4 Adipose tissue, an abundant source of adipose-derived stem cells, may be harvested via tumescent liposuction. (Courtesy of Sheila Macomber.)

The physician should supervise mixing of tumescent local anesthesia solutions so that the maximum lidocaine dose is 35 to 55 mg/kg and that the concentration of lidocaine ranges from 0.05 to 0.1%. The total dose of epinephrine should typically not exceed 50 μg/kg, and the concentration should be 0.25 to 1.5 mg/L.

The cannula diameter should be no larger than 4 to 4.5 mm. The amount of supernatant fat removed should not exceed 4 L in a single session, though this may be irrelevant if fat is harvested only for SVF and not for body-contouring purposes, as only small amounts of fat are needed for the former.[12,16] Depending on the isolation technique and whether adipose will also be used for other purposes (e.g., culture, or biochemical or cellular analyses, based on the study protocol), the amount of fat required may range from 30 to 500 mL (level of evidence: 4).[17,18] The desired amount of aspirated fat should be aseptically transferred to the appropriate container, which may be a sterile centrifuge tube, syringe, or bag, depending on requirements of the subsequent SVF isolation technique.

Isolation of SVF

SVF may be isolated through enzymatic (chemical) or nonenzymatic (mechanical) techniques, both of which can be performed at the bedside (Pearl 13.7).[18,19] The isolation protocol may significantly vary based on the device being investigated.

> **PEARL 13.7:** Stromal vascular fraction may be isolated via either enzymatic (chemical) or non enzymatic (mechanical) processing of adipose tissue. Enzymatic methods are more expensive and time-consuming, produce higher concentrations of stem cells, and are subject to stricter regulation.

Enzymatic (Chemical) Isolation Methods

SVF has conventionally been isolated via enzymatic digestion of adipose tissue, and this technique is also commonly used in the laboratory setting to isolate stem cells for bench research. Isolation procedures vary greatly based on types and concentrations of enzyme(s) used, number of washing steps, centrifugation parameters, and addition of optional steps, such as erythrocyte lysis. In general, adipose tissue is first washed with an aqueous salt solution such as Lactated Ringer's or phosphate-buffered saline, then digested with one or more proteolytic enzymes, typically collagenase type I and/or II, trypsin, or dispase (level of evidence: 5).[19] Digestion is then performed in a heated shaker for 30 to 120 minutes (level of evidence: 5).[20] Centrifugation separates the processed sample into several layers: the oil layer, adipocyte layer, aqueous layer, and the SVF pellet (Fig. 13.5).[20]

Nonenzymatic (Mechanical) Isolation Methods

Nonenzymatic isolation relies on mechanical forces to concentrate SVF. Often, this involves washing and shaking or vibrating the adipose tissue, followed by centrifugation.[20] Some device protocols involve fractionation of condensed lipoaspirate by pushing the sample back and forth through two syringes connected by a fractionator.

Comparison of Enzymatic Versus Nonenzymatic Isolation

Enzymatic and nonenzymatic isolation methods both have unique advantages and disadvantages (Table 13.1). The former is more costly and time consuming, with an additional 30 to 120 minutes required for enzymatic digestion. Enzymatic processing of stem cells is also considered nonminimal manipulation and thus subject to stricter regulation by the FDA.[21]

Without enzymatic digestion, many stem cells and progenitor cells remain trapped between adipocytes, and this results in lower cell counts in mechanically isolated SVF. Although nucleated cell counts in enzymatically isolated SVF have been reported to range between

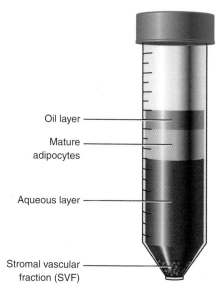

Oil layer

Mature adipocytes

Aqueous layer

Stromal vascular fraction (SVF)

Fig. 13.5 Stromal vascular fraction (SVF) is conventionally isolated via enzymatic digestion of adipose tissue with collagenase, trypsin, or dispase. Centrifugation then separates the processed sample into several layers (from top to bottom): the oil layer, adipocyte layer, aqueous layer, and the SVF pellet. (Courtesy of Sheila Macomber.)

100,000 to 1,300,000 cells/cc of processed lipoaspirate, cell counts in mechanically isolated SVF are typically between 10,000 and 240,000 cells/cc.[20] Mechanically isolated SVF also contains more connective tissue fragments and peripheral blood cells. However, other factors such as patient age, site of fat extraction, patient medical history, and current medications may also affect the quality of SVF Additional clinical research is necessary to determine the ideal concentration of SVF cells for the treatment of hair loss. A randomized, controlled trial of SVF for AGA suggested that lower concentrations may be more beneficial than higher concentrations.[10]

Injection of SVF

After isolation, SVF may be reconstituted into autologous fat, PRP, or saline. The reconstitution technique and desired SVF dose per injection site determines the injection volume, usually 0.1 to 0.15 cc of reconstituted SVF. The treatment site is cleaned, then the SVF is injected (e.g., with a 25-30 gauge needle) into the subcutaneous fat layer of the scalp. Injections should be focused on androgen-dependent areas of the scalp, such as the hair line, hair part, and vertex, depending on the severity of AGA and whether the hair loss is of the male or female

TABLE 13.1   Comparison of Enzymatic Versus Nonenzymatic Stromal Vascular Fraction (SVF) Isolation Methods

	Enzymatic (Chemical) Isolation of SVF	Nonenzymatic (Mechanical) Isolation of SVF
Summary of Technique	Adipose tissue is washed, digested with proteolytic enzyme(s) (e.g., collagenase, trypsin, dispase), then centrifuged.	Relies on mechanical forces to concentrate SVF cells (e.g., centrifugation, fractionation).
Cell Yield	Higher concentration of SVF cells (100,000 to 1,300,000 nucleated cells/cc of lipoaspirate processed).	Lower concentration of SVF cells (10,000 to 240,000 nucleated cells/cc of lipoaspirate processed). More tissue, connective tissue, and peripheral blood cells.
Regulation	Considered nonminimal manipulation. Subject to stricter regulation.	May be considered as minimal manipulation and subject to less strict regulation.
Cost	More expensive.	Less expensive.
Time	More time consuming, largely as a result of the additional 30 to 120 minutes required for enzymatic digestion.	Faster, with some protocols requiring less than 15 minutes.

pattern. The spacing between injections varies by study protocol and may range from one injection every 1 cm^2 to one every 2 cm^2 (level of evidence: 2b).[10,22] Bleeding at injection sites should be controlled by applying pressure with sterile gauze. Methods to control injection-related discomfort include distraction, ice, topical lidocaine, and oral medications such as analgesics or anxiolytics.

Post-Treatment Care

Patients who have been medicated should be monitored for any medication-related effects, and, if appropriate, should have a ride home arranged. The provider may obtain and document postprocedure vital signs. Cannula insertion and SVF injection sites are usually left open, and patients should be instructed on wound care (e.g., gentle cleansing and use of clean and dry dressings, if indicated). The majority of surgeons recommend wearing compression garments for 1 to 4 weeks after the procedure.[12] Most patients are ambulatory after the procedure and should be encouraged to resume normal activity as they are comfortable.

PREVENTION AND MANAGEMENT OF ADVERSE EVENTS

There have been no prior reports of serious adverse events associated with SVF injection into the scalp for the treatment of nonscarring alopecia.[9] Adverse events

tend to be mild, self-limited, and localized. At cannula insertion and SVF injection sites, patients often experience pain or discomfort, erythema, itching, bruising, or edema.[9,12] Ice, compression, topical anesthetic, and, if appropriate, oral pain medication may be helpful to reduce these symptoms. Especially at liposuction sites, the patient may experience drainage of blood-tinged fluid, and there is also a risk of scarring or hyperpigmentation. Compression garments, binders, and tape at the sites of liposuction may help minimize postoperative pain, bruising, and fluid collections.[12,16]

As with any procedure involving skin breakage, there is a small risk of bleeding or infection. The risk of these adverse events is patient-specific, and it may be prudent to avoid treating patients with a history of bleeding abnormality, immunosuppression, active herpes infection, or serious infection related to prior surgical procedures.

FUTURE DIRECTIONS: ADDITIONAL STEM CELL–BASED THERAPIES

Adipose-Derived Stem Cell–Conditioned Medium

Because the regenerative potential of ADSCs is largely attributed to secretion of cytokines, some research has investigated the utility of ADSC-conditioned medium (ADSC-CM) for the treatment of alopecia. ADSC-CM

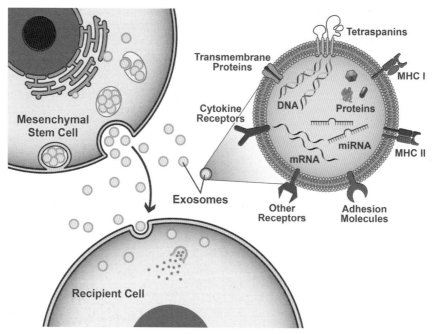

Fig. 13.6 Mesenchymal stem cell–derived exosomes are membrane-bound vesicles that contain various proteins and DNA, messenger RNA (mRNA), and microRNA (miRNA). Exosomes may be useful for the treatment of alopecia. *MHC,* Major histocompatibility complex. (Courtesy of Sheila Macomber.)

is an acellular medium that contains secreted molecules (e.g., growth factors) from stem cells and may have similar effects on alopecia as SVF.

First, ADSCs are isolated, then cultured and expanded, often under hypoxic conditions, which is believed to increase the production of molecules that promote hair growth, including PDGF, vascular endothelial growth factor (VEGF), and hepatocyte growth factor (HGF) (level of evidence: 5).[23,24] After culture, the sample is passed through a filter to remove cells and any debris. The resulting ADSC-CM may be freeze dried then later reconstituted in saline solution and injected into the scalp.

Animal studies and several small clinical studies have found that treatment with ADSC-CM improved hair density and hair thickness (level of evidence: 5).[23-25]

Stem Cell–Derived Exosomes

Mesenchymal stem cell–derived exosomes are another novel acellular product based on use of growth factors and cytokines secreted by stem cells to promote hair growth. Exosomes are involved in paracrine signaling and are membrane-bound vesicles that contain various proteins and DNA, messenger RNA (mRNA), and microRNA (miRNA) (Fig. 13.6).[26]

Stem cells, which may be dermal papilla cells and outer root sheath cells, are first isolated and cultured. Next, the supernatant is centrifuged, ultrafiltered, then ultracentrifuged to isolate pelleted exosomes, which may be frozen until use (level of evidence: 5).[26]

In vitro studies have found that exosomes stimulate proliferation of dermal papilla cells and induce secretion of VEGF and IGF-1, and studies in mice have found increased telogen to anagen conversion (level of evidence: 5).[26,27] A pilot study in 20 humans reported increased hair density and thickness after 12 weeks of treatment with exosomes (level of evidence: 4) (Pearl 13.8).[28]

PEARL 13.8: Adipose-derived stem cell–conditioned medium and stem cell–derived exosomes are acellular techniques intended to improve hair growth through growth factors secreted by stem cells.

> **PEARL 13.9:** Topical application of small molecules that promote lactate production within hair follicle stem cells may induce hair growth.

Small Molecules to Promote Lactate Dehydrogenase Activity

Rather than injecting stem cells or substances produced by these cells, it may also be possible to stimulate existing hair follicle stem cells in the scalp through the application of small molecules. Specifically, some research has investigated the use of UK-5099 and RCGD423, molecules that promote hair follicle lactate production, which is theorized to accelerate entry of hairs into anagen (level of evidence: 5).[29] Unlike SVF, ADSC-CM, and exosomes, these medications may be administered topically (Pearl 13.9).

Summary of Additional Stem Cell–Based Therapies

Advantages of ADSC-CM, exosomes, and small molecules include that these products do not contain stem cells, which allows for easier and less costly storage. Acellular products may additionally be safer than injection of undifferentiated stem cells as a result of theoretically lower risk of immunogenicity and tumor formation. Controlled production in the laboratory also makes standardization and manipulation of desirable growth factors or small molecules possible, which may lead to decreased variability in outcomes.

EVIDENCE SUMMARY

- Stromal vascular fraction may be an effective adjuvant treatment for androgenetic alopecia (strength of recommendation: D).
- Injection of stromal vascular fraction into androgen-dependent areas of the scalp leads to improvement in hair density and hair thickness in some patients with androgenetic alopecia (strength of recommendation: D). Additional research is required to better understand ideal candidate selection and the most effective treatment techniques.
- Stromal vascular fraction may be more effective in patients with early hair loss versus severe hair loss, and there may be additional benefit when stromal vascular fraction is used in combination with first-line

androgenetic alopecia therapies, including minoxidil or finasteride (strength of recommendation: D).
- There are currently no reported serious adverse events associated with injection of stromal vascular fraction for the treatment of androgenetic alopecia. Adverse events tend to be mild, self-limited, and localized to injection sites (e.g., pain or discomfort, erythema, itching, bruising, or edema), and ice, compression, and topical anesthetic may be helpful to reduce these symptoms (strength of recommendation: C).
- Outside of dermatology, stem cell therapies have been associated with serious adverse events, including blindness and malignancy. At present, because stromal vascular fraction is not approved by the US Food and Drug Administration for the treatment of alopecia, patients should undergo this treatment only as part of an Food and Drug Administration–supervised clinical trial with an Investigational New Drug Application (strength of recommendation: C).

REFERENCES

1. Schäffler A, Büchler C. Concise review: adipose tissue-derived stromal cells—basic and clinical implications for novel cell-based therapies. *Stem Cells.* 2007;25(4):818-827. doi:10.1634/stemcells.2006-0589.
2. Du Y, Roh DS, Funderburgh ML, et al. Adipose-derived stem cells differentiate to keratocytes in vitro. *Mol Vis.* 2010;16:2680-2689.
3. Bourin P, Bunnell BA, Casteilla L, et al. Stromal cells from the adipose tissue-derived stromal vascular fraction and culture expanded adipose tissue-derived stromal/stem cells: a joint statement of the International Federation for Adipose Therapeutics and Science (IFATS) and the International Society for Cellular Therapy (ISCT). *Cytotherapy.* 2013;15(6):641-648. doi:10.1016/j.jcyt.2013.02.006.
4. Guerrero-Juarez CF, Plikus MV. Emerging nonmetabolic functions of skin fat. *Nat Rev Endocrinol.* 2018;14(3):163-173. doi:10.1038/nrendo.2017.162.
5. Schmidt B, Horsley V. Unraveling hair follicle-adipocyte communication. *Exp Dermatol.* 2012;21(11):827-830. doi:10.1111/exd.12001.
6. Guo J, Nguyen A, Banyard DA, et al. Stromal vascular fraction: a regenerative reality? Part 2: Mechanisms of regenerative action. *J Plast Reconstr Aesthet Surg.* 2016;69(2):180-188. doi:10.1016/j.bjps.2015.10.014.
7. Epstein GK, Epstein JS. Mesenchymal stem cells and stromal vascular fraction for hair loss: current status. *Facial Plast Surg Clin N Am.* 2018;26(4):503-511. doi:10.1016/j.fsc.2018.06.010.

8. Stefanis AJ, Groh T, Arenbergerova M, Arenberger P, Bauer PO. Stromal vascular fraction and its role in the management of alopecia: a review. *J Clin Aesthetic Dermatol.* 2019;12(11):35-44.

9. Kang BY, Li AW, Lee MH, et al. The safety and efficacy of autologous adipose-derived stromal vascular fraction for nonscarring alopecia: a systematic review. *Arch Dermatol Res.* 2022;314(4):349-356. doi:10.1007/s00403-021-02238-7.

10. Kuka G, Epstein J, Aronowitz J, et al. Cell enriched autologous fat grafts to follicular niche improves hair regrowth in early androgenetic alopecia. *Aesthet Surg J.* 2020;40(6):NP328-NP339. doi:10.1093/asj/sjaa037.

11. Gupta AK, Mays RR, Dotzert MS, Versteeg SG, Shear NH, Piguet V. Efficacy of non-surgical treatments for androgenetic alopecia: a systematic review and network meta-analysis. *J Eur Acad Dermatol Venereol.* 2018;32(12): 2112-2125. doi:10.1111/jdv.15081.

12. Svedman KJ, Coldiron B, Coleman WP, et al. ASDS guidelines of care for tumescent liposuction. *Dermatol Surg Off Publ Am Soc Dermatol Surg Al.* 2006;32(5): 709-716. doi:10.1111/j.1524-4725.2006.32159.x.

13. U.S. Food & Drug Administration. *Approved Cellular and Gene Therapy Products.* FDA; October 26, 2021. Accessed November 17, 2021. Available at: https://www.fda.gov/vaccines-blood-biologics/cellular-gene-therapy-products/approved-cellular-and-gene-therapy-products.

14. U.S. Food & Drug Administration. *FDA Warns About Stem Cell Therapies.* FDA; September 3, 2020. Accessed November 17, 2021. Available at: https://www.fda.gov/consumers/consumer-updates/fda-warns-about-stem-cell-therapies.

15. Sugarman J, Barker RA, Charo RA. A professional standard for informed consent for stem cell therapies. *JAMA.* 2019;322(17):1651-1652. doi:10.1001/jama.2019.11290.

16. Coleman WP, Glogau RG, Klein JA, et al. Guidelines of care for liposuction. *J Am Acad Dermatol.* 2001;45(3): 438-447. doi:10.1067/mjd.2001.117045.

17. Stevens HP, Donners S, de Bruijn J. Introducing platelet-rich stroma: Platelet-Rich Plasma (PRP) and Stromal Vascular Fraction (SVF) Combined for the Treatment of Androgenetic Alopecia. *Aesthet Surg J.* 2018;38(8): 811-822. doi:10.1093/asj/sjy029.

18. Aronowitz JA, Ellenhorn JDI. Adipose stromal vascular fraction isolation: a head-to-head comparison of four commercial cell separation systems. *Plast Reconstr Surg.* 2013;132(6):932e. doi:10.1097/PRS.0b013e3182a80652.

19. Oberbauer E, Steffenhagen C, Wurzer C, Gabriel C, Redl H, Wolbank S. Enzymatic and non-enzymatic isolation systems for adipose tissue-derived cells: current state of the art. *Cell Regen.* 2015;4(1):7. doi:10.1186/s13619-015-0020-0.

20. Aronowitz JA, Lockhart RA, Hakakian CS. Mechanical versus enzymatic isolation of stromal vascular fraction cells from adipose tissue. *Springerplus.* 2015;4:713. doi:10.1186/s40064-015-1509-2.

21. U.S. Food and Drug Administration. *Regulatory Considerations for Human Cells, Tissues, and Cellular and Tissue-Based Products: Minimal Manipulation and Homologous Use.* FDA; July 21, 2020. Accessed November 19, 2021. Available at: https://www.fda.gov/regulatory-information/search-fda-guidance-documents/regulatory-considerations-human-cells-tissues-and-cellular-and-tissue-based-products-minimal.

22. Kim SJ, Kim MJ, Lee YJ, et al. Innovative method of alopecia treatment by autologous adipose-derived SVF. *Stem Cell Res Ther.* 2021;12(1):486. doi:10.1186/s13287-021-02557-6.

23. Park BS, Kim WS, Choi JS, et al. Hair growth stimulated by conditioned medium of adipose-derived stem cells is enhanced by hypoxia: evidence of increased growth factor secretion. *Biomed Res Tokyo Jpn.* 2010;31(1):27-34. doi:10.2220/biomedres.31.27.

24. Narita K, Fukuoka H, Sekiyama T, Suga H, Harii K. Sequential scalp assessment in hair regeneration therapy using an adipose-derived stem cell–conditioned medium. *Dermatol Surg.* 2020;46(6):819-825. doi:10.1097/DSS.0000000000002128.

25. Shin H, Ryu HH, Kwon O, Park BS, Jo SJ. Clinical use of conditioned media of adipose tissue-derived stem cells in female pattern hair loss: a retrospective case series study. *Int J Dermatol.* 2015;54(6):730-735. doi:10.1111/ijd.12650.

26. Zhou L, Wang H, Jing J, Yu L, Wu X, Lu Z. Regulation of hair follicle development by exosomes derived from dermal papilla cells. *Biochem Biophys Res Commun.* 2018;500(2):325-332. doi:10.1016/j.bbrc.2018.04.067.

27. Nestor MS, Ablon G, Gade A, Han H, Fischer DL. Treatment options for androgenetic alopecia: Efficacy, side effects, compliance, financial considerations, and ethics. *J Cosmet Dermatol.* 2021;20(12):3759-3781. doi:10.1111/jocd.14537.

28. Huh CH. Exosome for hair regeneration: from bench to bedside. *J Am Acad Dermatol.* 2019;81(4):AB62. doi:10.1016/j.jaad.2019.06.256.

29. Flores A, Schell J, Krall AS, et al. Lactate dehydrogenase activity drives hair follicle stem cell activation. *Nat Cell Biol.* 2017;19(9):1017-1026. doi:10.1038/ncb3575.

14

Hair Transplantation

Marc R. Avram

KEY POINTS

- Hair transplantation consistently creates natural-appearing hair for men and women with hair loss. Indications for hair transplantation include male and female pattern hair loss, inactive inflammatory scalp dermatoses, and reconstruction of hairlines lost to trauma or surgery.
- Realistic expectations of what hair transplant can and cannot achieve is key to patient satisfaction. Successful combination treatment with medical therapy allows the greatest long-term density, as hair transplantation does not alter ongoing male and female pattern hair loss.

- Appropriate candidate selection is key to the success of the procedure.
- Both follicular unit extraction and elliptical donor harvesting (follicular unit transplantation) are state-of-the-art donor harvesting techniques and should be discussed with patients to determine which technique is most appropriate.
- Medical and surgical complications due to hair transplantation are rare.

BACKGROUND

Hair transplantation is based on the theory of donor dominance, first introduced in modern medical journals in 1959 (level of evidence: 4).[1] It has been clinically demonstrated that hair will grow for as long as it was genetically programmed to grow based on where it was harvested from, not where it was placed. In practice, this allows physicians to harvest a patient's own hair from their occipital scalp and place it into thinning areas in the frontal scalp, which increase in size in both male and female pattern hair loss (MPHL/FPHL).

From the 1960s to the early 1990s, hair transplantation was a scientific success but often a cosmetic failure with tufts of unnatural "plugs." Since the mid-1990s, the procedure has been both a scientific and cosmetic success. The reason for this was the advent of the individual follicular unit graft as opposed to the previous multiple follicular unit "pluggy" graft. Although medical therapy

can be successful for treating hair loss, it is not always effective, and hair transplantation is an outpatient surgery performed under local anesthesia that can help restore hair for men and women with hair loss. For dermatologists, hair transplant surgery offers an option to help restore hair for their patients. Awareness of the procedure and how it is performed allows physicians to counsel patients in their practice.

INDICATIONS AND PATIENT SELECTION

Hair transplantation can be performed on any man or woman of any ethnicity or age who is an appropriate candidate for the procedure. Most patients undergoing the procedure still have pigmented terminal hair follicles and want greater density in the thinning regions. Therefore, to achieve maximum long-term density, patients need a combination of successful medical therapy and surgical hair restoration. Patients undergoing concurrent successful medical therapy to halt further hair loss will perceive the greatest cosmetic effect from a transplant surgery.

Hair transplantation can treat MPHL and FPHL, inactive inflammatory scalp dermatoses, and reconstruct hairlines lost to trauma or surgery. There are no clear guidelines regarding how long active inflammation on the scalp needs to be dormant prior to performing a transplant, but most dermatologic surgeons wait for 6 to 18 months. Hair transplantation should not be pursued in patients with alopecia areata (AA), active inflammatory scalp dermatosis, or active infections.

As with all procedures, a consult is essential to establish candidate selection. MPHL and FPHL are ongoing conditions. There are physical criteria to establish whether a patient is a good candidate, and the density and caliber of a patient's donor hair are key physical attributes for selection. Patients with high density and thick caliber hair follicles are excellent candidates for a hair transplant. Patients with reduced donor density and fine caliber follicles can undergo the procedure but will have less perceived density. Patients with stable hair loss patterns after successful medical therapy, good donor density, and thick caliber hair follicles are ideal candidates for the procedure (Table 14.1).

Patients with continuing hair loss who have failed or declined medical therapy must be aware that the net perceived density from a hair transplant is equal to the number of hair follicles transplanted minus the ongoing loss of hair (Pearl 14.1).

EXPECTED OUTCOMES

Hair is one of the few physical characteristics that we can readily control. The length, color, and style of our hair are a reflection of our personality, how we see ourselves, and how we want the world to perceive us. Hair frames our face. If the frame thins or disappears over time, it changes our physical appearance. Our face is the same and unchanged, yet we appear different physically

> **PEARL 14.1:** Realistic expectations are key to success for the procedure. The net perceived density from a hair transplant is equal to the number of hair follicles transplanted minus the ongoing loss of hair.

to the world and to ourselves. In addition, MPHL and FPHL progress slowly over years at different rates and to different extents but always inexorably altering the frame of hair. For men, hairlines recede and disappear. For women, hairlines become "see through," limiting hair styling options.

Hair transplantation allows patients to restore the frame of hair around their face. In the present day, all patients should expect consistently natural appearing transplanted hair (Figs. 14.1 and 14.2). The reason for this has been the evolution away from 2 to 4 mm "plugs," each containing 20 to 40 hair follicles, and toward transplanting individual follicular units. Although a transplant will consistently create natural-appearing transplant hair, it does not stop ongoing MPHL and FPHL. Over time, the increased density from a transplant can be lost. In fact, depending on the stage of hair loss when a transplant is performed, a patient can eventually have less hair than before the transplant.

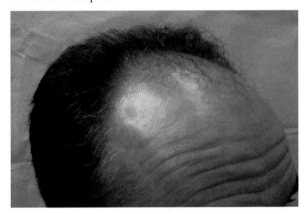

Fig. 14.1 Before hair transplant.

TABLE 14.1 **Candidate Selection for Hair Transplantation**	
Good Candidate	**Relatively Poor Candidate**
Stable hair loss pattern by successful medical therapy	Ongoing hair loss
Good donor density (>80 follicular units per cm²)	Low donor density (<50 follicular units per cm²)
Thick caliber hair	Fine-caliber hair
Realistic expectations	Unrealistic expectations - should not have the procedure

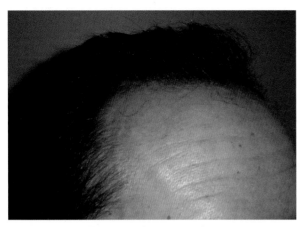

Fig. 14.2 After 1460 grafts.

> **PEARL 14.2:** The number of procedures needed depends on the rate of ongoing hair loss. The majority of patients are satisfied after one or two hair transplant surgeries.

The number of procedures needed depends on the rate of ongoing hair loss. Patients with stable hair loss patterns via successful medical therapy may only require one surgery to achieve their cosmetic goals. For patients who continue to lose hair, subsequent procedures may be desired. Most patients will be happy after one or two procedures. A minority will have more than two procedures to combat ongoing hair loss over years or simply to create the maximum density from their existing donor hair (Pearl 14.2).

TREATMENT TECHNIQUES AND BEST PRACTICES

Hair transplantation is performed as an outpatient procedure under local anesthesia. After a consultation in the author's practice, patients are encouraged to contact the office with any other questions or concerns regarding the procedure. Patients who understand what the procedure can and cannot accomplish are most likely to be happy with their results.

Once patients schedule their procedure, they are sent preoperative and postoperative instructions and written consent. Patients are encouraged to call the office and ask any questions regarding instructions or the consent. This will help make the procedure easier for patients.

The preoperative instructions encourage patients to wear comfortable, loose-fitting clothing and to bring their phone or tablet to listen to music, podcasts, or movies. In addition, the patient should eat before the procedure and bring any food or snacks they may want during the procedure. Patients often associate surgery with not eating on the day of the procedure, and a patient who comes to the office having not eaten may become hungry or dehydrated over the several hours that it takes to perform the procedure. Patients should let their care provider know if they would like a bathroom break, need to check a work email, or simply want to stretch for a few minutes. The author has found that these preoperative instructions are critical to making the procedure comfortable for the patient, which, in turn, allows the surgical team to work efficiently.

On the day of the procedure, the author spends 20 to 30 minutes reviewing the preoperative and postoperative instructions and written consent. The area to be transplanted is marked and shown to the patient in a mirror so that everyone knows where the procedure will and will not be performed. Photographs are taken. Photographs are often important for follow up 1 year later, as a transplant grows in so gradually and naturally over many months that patients may not be sure what did and did not grow. After reviewing instructions, signing consent, marking off the area to transplant, and photographing the area, the patient is brought to the procedure room and introduced to all staff members that will be working on them that day.

Donor Harvesting

The first step in the procedure is to obtain the donor hair follicles that will be transplanted. The mid occipital scalp is the donor region for both men and women, as it is the area most likely to have the greatest density of hair in the occipital scalp and to thin the least in the future. Transplanted hair will grow for as long as it was genetically programmed to grow from the donor region. For most patients, this results in transplanted hair growing for years to decades.

There are two techniques to donor harvesting: (1) elliptical donor harvesting (follicular unit transplantation [FUT]); and (2) follicular unit extraction (FUE) (Table 14.2). Both options are reviewed during the consult. Both techniques are state-of-the-art and can obtain large numbers of follicular units from the transplant to the recipient area (Pearl 14.3).

TABLE 14.2	**Comparison of Techniques for Donor Harvesting**	
	Elliptical Donor Harvesting	**Follicular Unit Extraction**
Method of Harvest	Trim 1 mm to 1 cm wide donor region in the midoccipital scalp. This must be camouflaged by existing hair if greater than 1 cm in length.	Trim entire occipital scalp to 1 mm for maximum donor harvesting of individual follicular units.
Scarring	Linear scar 8 to 18 cm in length if hair is trimmed short.	Pinpoint 0.9 mm scars, which are minimally visible even with close-trimmed hair.
Patient Selection	Preferred technique for most women and some men who never intend to wear their occipital hair closely trimmed.	Preferred technique for patients with closely cropped hair in the occipital scalp or who may want to in the future. For patients who prefer a minimally invasive procedure.

> **PEARL 14.3:** Elliptical donor harvesting and follicular unit extraction are both state-of-the-art donor harvesting techniques.

Elliptical Donor Harvesting

Elliptical donor harvesting, also known as follicular unit transplantation, has been performed for more than two decades (level of evidence: 2b).[2] Technically, it follows the same rules as any cutaneous excision. One difference is the need for minimal transaction (damage) of hair follicles as the ellipse is obtained. This is accomplished using a surgical blade and "scoring" an incision just through the dermis. The ellipse is then retracted at 90 degrees to the incision by skin hooks that allow the tissue to be opened down to the level of the subcutaneous tissue with minimal trauma to hair follicles (level of evidence: 4) (Fig. 14.3).[3]

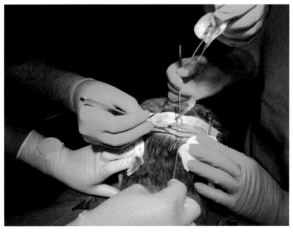

Fig. 14.3 Retraction at 90 degrees with skin hooks to minimize transection of hair follicles.

To obtain the ellipse, the patient's hair above the ellipse is lifted and held in place by paper tape, and the area where the ellipse will be obtained is trimmed to 1 mm, about 1.5 cm wide in length, using a trimmer. This allows for hair, when released, to cover the staples so that the donor region is not visible the next day. The patient lies on the surgical table in the prone position and is anesthetized with 1% lidocaine with epinephrine. Before removing the ellipse, chlorhexidine gluconate (Hibiclens) is applied, and the team wears sterile gloves and follows sterile technique for the ellipse removal. The length and width of the ellipse depend on the amount of donor hair desired for the procedure. On average, a patient has 80 follicular units/cm[2], so the physician is able to extrapolate how many grafts they need for the area to be transplanted in each patient. To leave a minimal scar, minimal tension is desired on the donor ellipse; therefore, a longer rather than wider ellipse is preferred. Typically, the author's practice will harvest no greater than 1 cm in width and up to 15-18 cm in length. Once the ellipse is removed, it is closed with either staples, running sutures, or interrupted sutures and left in place for 7 to 10 days (Fig. 14.4). After the ellipse is obtained, a trained surgical staff divides the strip into even smaller slivers, then finally into individual follicular units. This is done under magnification, and ergonomics are vital for success, as it does take an hour for an experienced surgical assistant to separate 400 grafts from the ellipse (Fig. 14.5). Therefore, it will take 1 to 2 hours for two or three assistants to separate 1000 to 1500 follicular units (level of evidence: 4).[4] If the surgical assistant is not comfortable, with good lighting, good magnification, and a chair and countertop appropriate for comfortable sitting, this will become a challenging experience. Once the follicular units are separated from the ellipse, they

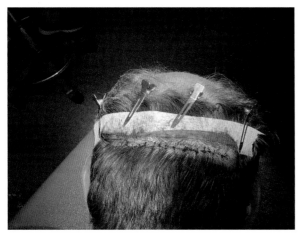

Fig. 14.4 Sutures placed in donor ellipse will be removed in 7 to 10 days.

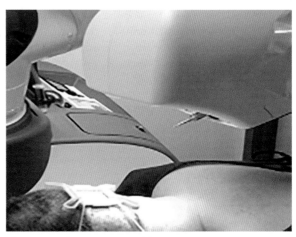

Fig. 14.6 Robotic removal of follicular units using a 0.9-mm punch.

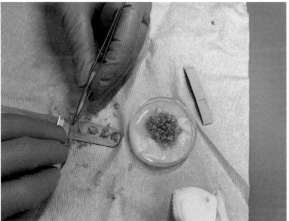

Fig. 14.5 Dissecting donor ellipse into individual follicular units.

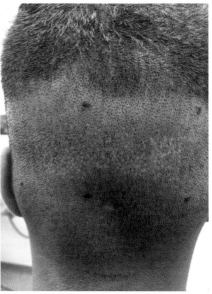

Fig. 14.7 Pinpoint white scars from previous follicular unit extraction procedure. (From Avram MR, Rogers N, Watkins S. Side-effects from follicular unit extraction in hair transplantation. *J Cutan Aesthet Surg.* 2014; 7:177-179.)

are placed in a holding solution until they are transplanted into the frontal scalp.

Follicular Unit Extraction

Follicular unit extraction has also been performed for the last two decades as an alternate method for donor harvesting (level of evidence: 5).[5] It is based on the principal of direct removal of each follicular unit from the posterior scalp. There are various methods of removing follicular units: individual 0.8 to 1 mm punch biopsies, a variety of mechanical devices that assist removal of follicular units, and robotic systems that allow independent removal of follicular units (level of evidence: 5)

(Fig. 14.6).[6] The chief advantage of FUE is that there is no linear scar, and, in fact, not a single suture required in the entire procedure. There are pinpoint white scars, but these are so small that they are of no practical consequence for most patients (level of evidence: 5) (Fig. 14.7).[7] This is appealing to a large number of patients and has made it a popular donor harvesting method. Once the follicular units are removed, they are placed in holding solution, then transplanted into the frontal scalp the same way they would after being divided through a donor ellipse.

Ellipse Versus Follicular Unit Extraction – Which Technique is Superior?

Patients will often ask, "Which is a better donor harvesting technique?" Both are state-of-the-art and can create consistently natural appearing transplanted hair for patients. During the consult, the pros and cons of each are reviewed. For most patients, the technique appropriate for them quickly becomes clear. The overwhelming majority of women will opt for an ellipse, as there is a minimal chance that they will ever choose to closely cut their hair to millimeters in length, exposing a donor scar. In addition, the length of their hair will camouflage the staples the day of the procedure and the scar long-term. On the other hand, a man who wears his hair short and may opt for FUE because the pinpoint scars are less visible than a linear scar from and ellipse. Currently, FUE is a more popular modality overall, but FUT is an excelletion option for many patients, as well.

Recipient Site Placement

Once the donor hairs are harvested, patients are encouraged to stretch, take a bathroom break, and have a drink before placement of the grafts begins.

The recipient areas are anesthetized with 1% lidocaine with epinephrine. In addition, 0.25% bupivacaine with epinephrine is used for longer-acting anesthesia. Some physicians perform supraorbital and supratrochlear nerve blocks in addition to local anesthesia.

The grafts are removed from their holding solution and placed using microvascular forceps (Fig. 14.8). Standard surgical forceps used for an excision in dermatologic surgery will not be adequate to place individual follicular units. Microvascular forceps are used to pick up individual follicular units by their perifollicular tissue without crushing follicles and place them into the recipient area by trained staff, one at a time. Once the last follicular unit is placed into the recipient areas, a dressing is placed overnight to protect the grafts as they heal. The dressing consists of non adherent Telfa pads with emollient over the recipient site, and the donor

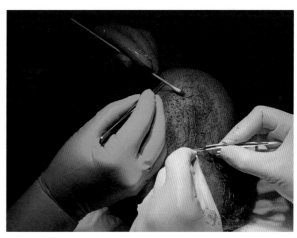

Fig. 14.8 Placing grafts with microvascular forceps.

region is held in place by Kerlix. No tape is applied to the scalp.

Postoperative Wound Care

Patients are sent home with the dressing and told they may resume normal activities immediately. We tell them not to perform heavy, sweaty exercise for 5 to 7 days while the donor area heals, whether performed through FUT or FUE. Most patients opt to take prednisone 40 mg daily for 3 days to prevent frontal edema in the scalp. Regarding pain medications, the majority are comfortable with acetaminophen 500 mg (Extra Strength Tylenol) every 6 to 8 hours for 24 hours. The author prescribes acetaminophen with codeine (Tylenol with codeine), as well, in case patients require a stronger medication for pain control on the first day. Patients are instructed that they should have no discomfort after the first day postoperatively and, if they do, to let the office know.

The day after the procedure, the dressing is removed by the patient at home. Patients should be instructed not to pick the scabs in the recipient areas, but instead let them fall off over 6 to 10 days via daily showers. The only wound care required is to put an emollient over the donor area for 7 days. After 7 days, patients may resume normal sports activities. The hemorrhagic follicular scabbing in the frontal scalp disappears in 6 to 10 days, then the grafts enter the telogen stage for 3 to 6 months. Patients are told not to expect any clear cosmetic difference from the surgery for 9 to 14 months after the procedure.

PREVENTION AND MANAGEMENT OF ADVERSE EVENTS

As with all procedures, complications may arise with hair transplant surgery (level of evidence: 5) (Table 14.3).[8] Fortunately, the rate of medical and surgical complications is low. This is mostly a result of the excellent blood supply to the scalp, which makes the rate of infections extremely low. There are no well-designed studies confirming the rate of infection, but there is consensus that the rate is less than 1%.

The most common adverse event and complication in hair transplant surgery is iatrogenic, caused by poor technique, planning of the procedure and anticipation of future hair loss. This section will review medical, surgical, and iatrogenic complications.

Common Side Effects

Some changes in the skin are expected after each procedure; these are not complications but part of postsurgical wound healing. Patients should be aware of these changes. Most procedures involve restoring hair to the frontal half of the scalp. This makes the biggest cosmetic effect for men and women. The lymphatic drainage in the frontal scalp drains to the forehead. Therefore, 24 hours after a procedure, patients should expect edema in the frontal scalp. This peaks at 48 hours postprocedure and resolves 4-5 days after the procedure. It can sometimes result in periorbital edema and bruising around the eyes. The frontal edema can be avoided by using a short course of steroids. Typically, 40 mg daily for 3 days will prevent edema.

Patients may also experience pruritus in both the donor and recipient areas as a result of normal wound healing. This typically resolves in 5-10 days. If a patient is uncomfortable, a course of a moderate topical steroid solution for 4-5 days will resolve these symptoms. Folliculitis may occur in both the recipient and donor regions for days or weeks after the procedure. It may be triggered by heavy emollients used for wound healing and close-trimmed hair or placed grafts creating irritation in the skin. Most cases resolve with a 7-10 day course of a topical antibiotic. Rarely, oral antibiotics are used for folliculitis. Telogen effluvium (TE) may occur, as well, post hair transplant. This is more likely to occur in patients such as women with diffuse thinning of their hair. Although upsetting, this telogen is temporary and the lost hair will regrow with transplanted hair in 8-12 months.

Rare Side Effects

Elliptical donor harvesting can result in broad or hypertrophic scars (Fig. 14.9). This can spontaneously occur in any patient or, more often, result from too much tension on the wound. This risk can be mitigated by harvesting longer, more narrow ellipses, therefore reducing tension on the wound. It is unclear how wide

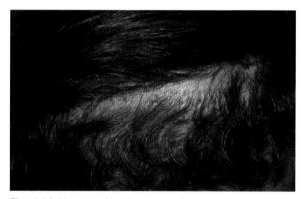

Fig. 14.9 Hypertrophic donor scar from too broad a donor ellipse.

TABLE 14.3	Side Effects Associated With Hair Transplantation	
Common Side Effects With Hair Transplantation	**Rare Side Effects With Hair Transplantation**	**Physician-Created, Long-Term Side Effects**
• Folliculitis • Pruritis • Edema	• Infection • Numbness or paresthesia in donor or recipient region • Arteriovenous malformation • Hiccups • Poor donor scar	• Low frontal hairline • Straight frontal hairline • Distribution of transplanted hair that does not look natural with future hair loss • Cosmetic "donut" bald skin around transplanted hair in vertex of the scalp

an ellipse can safely be harvested without increasing the risk of hypertrophic or broad scars. Most physicians believe that a range from 0.7-1.2 cm is safe.

If an undesirable scar occurs, it can be improved but not eliminated. Pulsed dye laser, nonablative fractional lasers, and ablative fractional lasers can all help improve the scar. In addition, scalp micropigmentation may be an excellent option to camouflage certain scars.

Other unusual side effects include persistent numbness or pain in the donor or recipient regions and necrosis from excessive tension on the donor scar, over-harvesting of follicular units, or dense-packing the recipient region. An arteriovenous malformation can rarely occur in the donor region and should be removed by a vascular surgeon.

Iatrogenic Adverse Outcomes

Disappointing density from a procedure can occur. There are a variety of reasons for this. Poor technique, such as transecting hair follicles during donor harvesting, allowing grafts to desiccate before they are placed, or causing damage during placement of grafts in recipient sites, may lead to hair density that is lower than desired.

Patients may not follow postsurgical wound care instructions or limitations on physical activities, resulting in lost hair. More commonly, patients either had unrealistic expectations regarding density from a procedure or continued losing hair throughout the postsurgical period. This is why the consult is vital for the success of the surgical procedure. Donor density, caliber of hair follicle, and success of medical therapy will help determine realistic expectations regarding density from a procedure. Patients with fine-caliber hair will have a thin natural coverage from a transplant, while those with thick, curly hair will have a greater perceived density from a procedure with an equal number of grafts transplanted.

Patients with long-term stable hair loss patterns as a result of successful medical therapy will more likely see a clear increase in density. Patients with ongoing hair loss may see no clear increase in density after a transplant. A patient will be happy if they understand that, without the procedure, their hair would be even thinner. Patients who understand the effect of ongoing hair loss, caliber of follicles transplanted, and limits in donor density are often happy with their procedure. Patients who do not understand the effect of ongoing hair loss and the need for successful medical therapy may be disappointed with the perceived density from a procedure.

The majority of complications occur as a result of poor planning of the hair transplant surgery. The technical aspect of skillfully harvesting donor hair and placing them into recipient sites is essential, but so is the knowledge that a transplant will not stop the ongoing nature of MPHL and FPHL. Understanding the ongoing nature of pattern hair loss is vital to appropriate short- and long-term planning for a procedure. Common mistakes that can occur include placing the frontal hairline too low for a patient, often mimicking the patient's hairline before they began losing their hair. The problem with this approach is that, as the hair loss continues, there will be a further recession of not only the frontal hairline but also of the temporal and posterior hairlines in men. A natural hairline for the frontal, temporal, and posterior scalp is best achieved by assuming future hair loss whether or not a patient is on successful medical therapy; they may stop their medical therapy in the future. A receded frontal hairline will look natural short and long term whether or not patients continue to lose their hair (level of evidence: 5).[9]

Another challenge is transplanting the vertex for male patients. Over time, the enlarging area of bald skin in the vertex is a challenge for planning a transplant. If a region is transplanted, and then, over the years, the area of hair loss expands, a "donut" of bald skin surrounding transplanted hair may emerge and appear unnatural. This is avoided in general by not transplanting the vertex at all or, if transplanted, with thinner density than the frontal scalp. The maximum cosmetic and safety effect is achieved for men by transplanting the frontal half of the scalp. This allows maximum cosmetic effect with minimal long-term cosmetic risk. Ongoing hair loss may thin the region of a transplant, but it will look natural.

Women do not have the challenge of shifting hairlines as their hair continues to thin. FPHL has stable, intact hairlines. The chief cosmetic complaint is often a see-through frontal hairline. Transplanting a large number of follicular units in the frontal half of the scalp will produce greater density with low long-term cosmetic risk because all hairlines are intact.

FUTURE DIRECTIONS

For the entire 21st century, patients have been able to obtain consistently natural appearing transplanted hair. Current challenges include how to (1) more to efficiently move large numbers of hair follicles from the occipital scalp to the frontal scalp, (2) maintain existing pigmented terminal hair follicles for maximum long-term density, and (3) overcome the rate-limiting step of the procedure – the limited donor hairs available to transplant. Future evolution of the procedure will address each of these challenges.

Robotics will continue to evolve, reducing the need to train surgical assistants while also reducing the length of the procedure. Platelet-rich plasma (PRP) and low-level light are important additions to help maintain existing hair for patients, and even more effective therapies in the future will address this as well. These therapies will allow maximum long-term density and, if given early, will reduce the need for surgery. Finally, cloning of follicles will occur. This will allow physicians to completely restore lost hair nonsurgically and retire surgical hair transplantation as previously performed.

EVIDENCE SUMMARY

- Hair transplantation is an effective treatment for male and female pattern hair loss, inactive inflammatory scalp dermatoses, and reconstruction of hairlines lost to trauma or surgery (strength of recommendation: B).
- Hair transplantation is a lengthy procedure. Ensuring a positive surgical experience is critical to patient and staff satisfaction. Patients should be encouraged to ask questions, eat snacks, and take breaks when needed. Staff should be provided with ergonomic workstations and adequate support (strength of recommendation: D).
- Elliptical donor harvesting results in a linear scar at the donor site and is preferred for most women and some men who do not intend to wear their occipital hair closely trimmed. Follicular unit extraction leaves pinpoint scars at the donor site and is a better option for patients who plan to wear their hair closely cropped on the occipital scalp or who are interested in a less invasive procedure (strength of recommendation: C).
- The majority of patients are satisfied after one to two transplant surgeries. Patients undergoing concurrent medical therapy to halt further hair loss will perceive the greatest cosmetic effect from hair transplant (strength of recommendation: B).

REFERENCES

1. Orentreich N. Autografts in alopecias and other selected dermatologic conditions. *Ann N Y Acad Sci.* 1959.83(3): 463-479. doi:10.1111/j.1749-6632.1960.tb40920.x.
2. Limmer BL. Elliptical donor stereoscopically assisted micrografting as an approach to further refinement in hair transplantation. *J Dermatol Surg Oncol.* 1994.20(12): 789-793. doi:10.1111/j.1524-4725.1994.tb03706.x.
3. Pathomvanich D. Donor harvesting: a new approach to minimize transection of hair follicles. *Dermatol Surg.* 2000.26(4):345-348. doi:10.1046/j.1524-4725.2000. 99226.x.
4. Avram MR. Polarized light-emitting diode magnification for optimal recipient site creation during hair transplant. *Dermatol Surg.* 2005. 31(9 Pt 1.:1127; discussion1127. doi:10.1097/00042728-200509000-00007.
5. Jiménez-Acosta F, Ponce-Rodríguez I. Follicular unit extraction for hair transplantation: an update. *Actas Dermosifiliogr.* 2017.108(6):532-537. doi:10.1016/j.ad.2017.02.015.
6. Harris JA. Follicular unit extraction. *Facial Plast Surg Clin North Am.* 2013.21(3):375-384. doi:10.1016/j. fsc.2013.05.002.
7. Avram MR, Rogers N, Watkins S. Side-effects from follicular unit extraction in hair transplantation. *J Cutan Aesthet Surg.* 2014.7(3):179. doi:10.4103/0974-2077.146681.
8. Nadimi S. Complications with hair transplantation. *Facial Plast Surg Clin North Am.* 2020.28(2):225-235. doi:10.1016/j.fsc.2020.01.003.
9. Shapiro R, Shapiro P. Hairline design and frontal hairline restoration. *Facial Plast Surg Clin North Am.* 2013.21(3): 351-362. doi:10.1016/j.fsc.2013.06.001.

15

Lasers, Lights, and LEDs

Frances Walocko, Bianca Y. Kang, Yu-Feng Chang, Jeffrey S. Dover, and Murad Alam

KEY POINTS

- Several laser and light-based therapies, including low-level laser/light therapy, excimer laser, monochromatic excimer light, narrowband ultraviolet B phototherapy, and fractional laser, have been studied for the treatment of androgenetic alopecia. Most research has focused on low-level laser/light therapy, also known as photobiomodulation. Evidence for other energy-based modalities is limited.
- There are a variety of low-level laser/light therapy devices cleared by the U.S. Food and Drug Administration that are available for home use, including combs, bands, caps, and helmets, as well as hoods for in-office use. Current evidence suggests that low-level laser/light therapy is safe and effective for the treatment of mild to moderate androgenetic alopecia in men and women, Fitzpatrick skin types I to IV.

- Less frequent treatments and shorter total weekly treatment duration (<60 minutes per week) may lead to improved hair growth compared with more frequent use and longer treatment times. In general, devices are used two to four times per week, with individual treatment session durations ranging from 90 seconds to 35 minutes. Recommended treatment protocols vary based on the particular technology, wavelength, and specific manufacturer.
- The efficacy of laser and light treatments may be increased when used in combination with other therapies such as topical minoxidil. Additional research is needed to better understand the most effective treatment techniques and to identify ideal treatment candidates.

BACKGROUND, DEFINITIONS, AND HISTORY

Hair loss affects a significant proportion of the population. The most common type of hair loss is androgenetic alopecia (AGA), a nonscarring alopecia that affects at least 50% of males 40 years and older and 75% of females 65 years and older. The extent of hair loss as a result of AGA is generally less in women than in men.[1,2] Other forms of nonscarring alopecia include alopecia areata (AA) and telogen effluvium (TE), and these are distinguished from scarring alopecias by preservation of the hair follicles and potential for hair regrowth. Certain infections (e.g., tinea capitis), medications, hormonal imbalances, hair styling techniques,

genetic conditions, and anxiety or stress can also lead to hair loss, and some treatment overlap exists between AGA and other causes of alopecia. The objective of this chapter is to discuss the efficacy and safety of laser and light devices for the treatment of alopecia, with a focus on AGA.

AGA is driven by increased activity of androgen hormones, leading to a shorter anagen (growth) phase and follicular miniaturization (see Fig. 4.1).[3] Men with AGA experience a gradual thinning of hair on the crown and frontal scalp, while females tend to experience thinning along the central part-line. There are various scales that are available to grade the severity of AGA, commonly the Norwood-Hamilton scale (see Fig. 12.1) for male-pattern hair loss (MPHL) and the Savin (Fig. 15.1) and

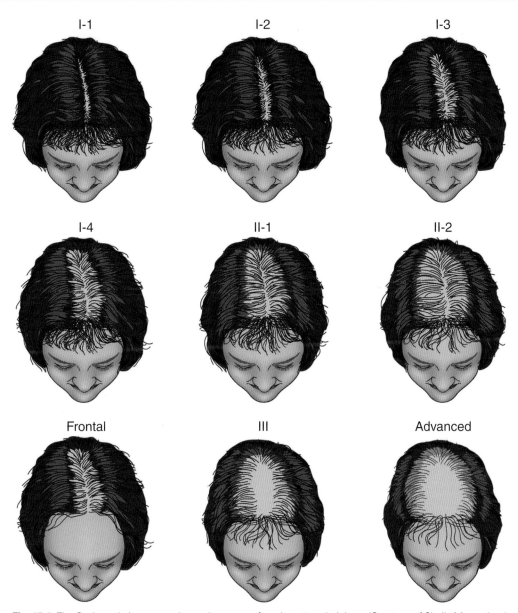

I-1 I-2 I-3

I-4 II-1 II-2

Frontal III Advanced

Fig. 15.1 The Savin scale is commonly used to assess female-pattern hair loss. (Courtesy of Sheila Macomber.)

Sinclair scales (see Fig. 12.2) for female-pattern hair loss (FPHL).

Numerous treatment modalities are used for AGA, including topical therapies, oral medications and supplements, injections, laser and light devices, and surgical interventions. Currently, the only U.S Food and Drug Administration (FDA)-approved treatments for AGA are oral finasteride and topical minoxidil (Rogaine) (level of evidence: 1a) (Pearl 15.1).[4]

Note that "clearance" merely confirms that devices are found to be substantially equivalent to approved "predicate" devices through the FDA Premarket Notification 510(k) process and does not denote "approval," which requires a device be found to be safe and effective

PEARL 15.1: At present, the only U.S. Food and Drug Administration–approved treatments for androgenetic alopecia are topical minoxidil and oral finasteride, and these are typically first line. Energy-based modalities such as low-level laser/light therapy are usually considered alternative or adjunctive treatments, especially in patients who are interested in avoiding surgical measures.

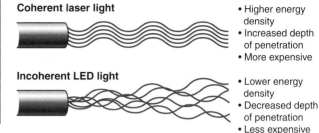

Coherent laser light

- Higher energy density
- Increased depth of penetration
- More expensive

Incoherent LED light

- Lower energy density
- Decreased depth of penetration
- Less expensive

Fig. 15.2 Low-level laser/light therapy (LLLT, or photobiomodulation) may use coherent (i.e., lasers) and/or noncoherent light sources (i.e., filtered lamps or light-emitting diodes [LEDs]). Coherent light sources have a higher energy density and increased depth of penetration but are more expensive compared with noncoherent sources. (Courtesy of Sheila Macomber.)

through the FDA's Premarket Approval (PMA) application or Humanitarian Device Exemption (HDE) pathway. Further, representing a device as officially FDA-approved when it is only cleared is considered misleading and constitutes misbranding (21 CFR 807.97), which is a prohibited act under 21 U.S.C. 331(b).[5,6] Because LLLT devices are both medical devices and electronic radiation-emitting products, these devices must comply with two independent sets of regulations: medical device regulations and radiation safety regulations.[5,6]

Laser and Light Devices

Several laser and light-based interventions have been used to treat alopecia in clinical and experimental studies. These include LLLT (level of evidence: 1a), excimer laser (level of evidence: 1a), monochromatic excimer light (level of evidence: 1a), narrowband ultraviolet B phototherapy (NBUVB) (level of evidence: 3b), and fractional lasers, such as erbium-glass, erbium-doped yttrium aluminium garnet (Er: YAG), and CO_2 (level of evidence: 3b).[4,7,8] Among these, the best studied for the treatment of AGA is LLLT.

Low-Level Laser and Light Therapy

LLLT, also known as photobiomodulation, was first discovered as a treatment for hair loss by Endre Mester in the 1960s while he was experimenting with a low-power ruby laser to treat cancer in mice (level of evidence: 5).[9] Mester noted paradoxical hair growth on areas of skin treated with laser therapy. After this experiment, lasers at low-power settings were further explored as a treatment for hair loss (Pearl 15.2). In the 2020s, LLLT

PEARL 15.2: Low-level laser/light therapy devices may use coherent light sources (lasers) or noncoherent light sources (lamps or light-emitting diodes [LEDs]), or both.

involves using coherent (i.e., lasers) or noncoherent light sources (i.e., filtered lamps or light-emitting diodes [LEDs]) that emit red or near infrared light at lower energy densities compared with other laser therapies (Fig. 15.2).[10] These laser and light sources can be used separately or in combination. Wavelengths typically range between 640 to 680 nanometers (nm) (Fig. 15.3) and power output per diode is less than or equal to 5 milliwatts (mW).

The precise mechanism of action of LLLT is not fully understood. Various theories exist (Pearl 15.3). LLLT is believed to result in increased production of nitric oxide and adenosine triphosphate (ATP) in addition to modulation of reactive oxygen species (ROS) in hair follicle and perifollicular cells (level of evidence: 5).[11,12] These activated cells may then help promote reentry of hairs from telogen into anagen, thereby increasing the duration of anagen.[11] LLLT has additionally been demonstrated to cause vasodilation, which may increase blood flow to the hair follicle and further promote growth.[11]

There is debate regarding whether lasers or LEDs are more effective in stimulating hair growth (Pearl 15.4). Initial studies used low-power ruby (694 nm) and helium-neon (633 nm) lasers to stimulate hair follicles. However, LEDs emitting light at similar wavelengths have also shown comparable hair regrowth in clinical studies. Medical-grade laser diodes that emit wavelengths of 630 to 680 nm are the most commonly used energy source in LLLT devices. LEDs deliver less energy than their laser counterparts and do not penetrate as deeply, but they are less costly and easier to manufacture.

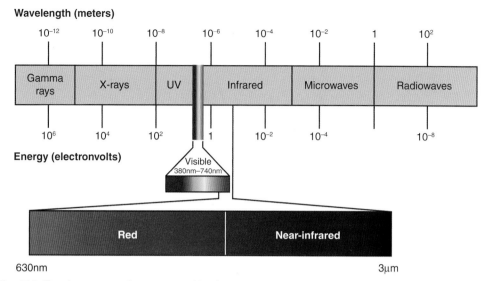

Wavelength (meters)

Fig. 15.3 The electromagnetic spectrum with a focus on visible red light and near-infrared radiation. (Courtesy of Sheila Macomber.)

PEARL 15.3: Proposed mechanisms of action of low-level laser/light therapy in stimulating hair growth include increased production of nitric oxide and adenosine triphosphate, modulation of reactive oxygen species, and vasodilation.

PEARL 15.4: Additional research is needed to better understand whether coherent (laser) or noncoherent (light-emitting diode [LED]) low-level laser/light therapy is more effective for androgenetic alopecia. Lasers are more commonly used, while LEDs deliver less energy, do not penetrate as deeply, and are less expensive.

PEARL 15.5: Low-level laser/light therapy is the best-studied energy-based device for the treatment of hair loss. Other modalities include excimer laser, monochromatic excimer light, narrowband ultraviolet B phototherapy, and fractional laser. These devices have primarily been studied in alopecia areata. Additional data is required to better understand their safety and efficacy in the treatment of androgenetic alopecia.

Additional Laser and Light Devices

Aside from LLLT, other laser and light devices employed to treat alopecia include excimer laser, NBUVB (including monochromatic excimer light), and fractional lasers.[13] In the context of hair regrowth, excimer laser and NBUVB have been studied primarily for AA. These devices are thought to induce apoptosis of T-cells, which are involved in the pathogenesis of AA.[8] Case reports and case series have demonstrated increased hair growth after treatment, but large, randomized, controlled clinical trials are needed. There is very limited evidence supporting the efficacy of excimer lasers and NBUVB for other forms of alopecia, such as AGA (Pearl 15.5).

Fractional lasers have also been found in a handful of studies to be efficacious for the treatment of hair loss. These lasers work by creating small columns of thermal energy (microthermal zones [MTZs]), thereby promoting dermal remodeling. Fractional lasers may be either ablative or nonablative. Ablative lasers remove the top layer of skin, whereas nonablative lasers leave the epidermis intact (Fig. 15.4). The nonablative fractional 1550-nm erbium-glass laser has been well-studied for treatment of both AGA and AA. Case reports and case series have reported improved hair density, hair thickness, anagen-to-telogen ratio, and hair regrowth (level of evidence: 4).[13-15] On the other hand, ablative fractional lasers, such as CO_2 and

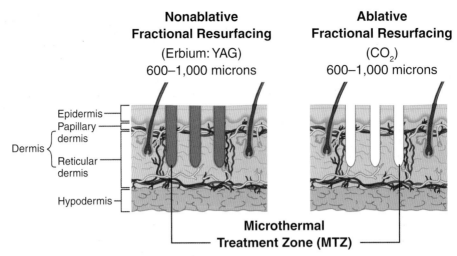

Fig. 15.4 Fractional lasers may be helpful for the treatment of alopecia, and these lasers work by creating small columns of thermal energy (microthermal zones, or MTZs) to promote dermal remodeling. Fractional lasers may be either ablative or nonablative. Nonablative fractional lasers (e.g., erbium-doped yttrium aluminium garnet laser or ER:YAG laser) leave the epidermis intact, while fractional ablative lasers (e.g., CO_2) remove the top layer of skin. (Courtesy of Sheila Macomber.)

Er: YAG, are believed to stimulate hair growth by prolonging the duration of anagen. A controlled clinical trial by Yalici-Armagon et al. of CO_2 lasers to treat patients with AA did not demonstrate any significant improvement in hair count, but hair growth has been reported in various forms of alopecia in small case series (level of evidence: 2b).[16] The ablative fractional 2940-nm Er:YAG laser has induced improved hair regrowth in animal studies, but studies in humans remain lacking (level of evidence: 5).[17]

High-quality research is necessary to better understand the effectiveness of excimer laser, NBUVB, and fractional lasers in treating AGA and to optimize treatment parameters and patient selection. Given that work with these devices is in early stages and that there is a dearth of well-designed clinical studies, these modalities will not be further discussed in this chapter.

INDICATIONS AND PATIENT SELECTION

LLLT is indicated for use in patients with AGA (both male- and female-pattern) and, at present, numerous devices are FDA-cleared (Table 15.1). Improvement in hair growth can be expected in men with Norwood-Hamilton classifications IIa to V, and women with Savin classifications of I-II.[18] LLLT is FDA-cleared for use in patients with Fitzpatrick skin types I to IV (Pearl 15.6). Additional research is required to determine the safety and efficacy of LLLT in darker skin types. There is also limited guidance regarding patient selection based on demographic factors (e.g., age, sex, race, ethnicity), with further research potentially to reveal which patients may benefit the most from LLLT. Aside from AGA, LLLT has also been used to treat patients with other forms of alopecia, such as AA, lichen planopilaris (LPP), central centrifugal cicatricial alopecia (CCCA), and chemotherapy-induced hair loss, but to date there are no randomized controlled clinical trials investigating LLLT for these indications.[8]

Contraindications to LLLT include history of photosensitizing disorder or concomitant use of photosensitizing medications. Pregnancy is also a contraindication, as such patients were excluded from clinical trials of LLLT. The presence of melanocytic nevi or malignant lesions on the scalp is a relative contraindication. Frigo et al. demonstrated melanoma tumor growth in a mouse model when using LLLT to deliver high levels of irradiation, but further research is needed to better understand this potential risk.[19]

TABLE 15.1 List of FDA-Cleared Low-Level Laser/Light Therapy (LLLT) Devices Available in October 2021

Product Name	501(k) Number	Device Type	Wavelength (nm)	Power Output (mW)	Approximate Cost
LED Only					
Celluma RESTORE	K211038	Band	640	1316	$995
REVIAN RED	K211038	Helmet	620 + 660	1.67 mW/cm2	$1,495
Laser Only					
Bosley Revitalizer Flex 164	K181253	Cap	650	820	$1,799
Bosley Revitalizer Flex 272	K192585	Cap	650	1360	$2,799
CapillusPro	K163172	Cap	650	1360	$2,999
CapillusPlus	K163171	Cap	650	1010	$1,999
CapillusUltra	K163170	Cap	650	410	$999
COSMO Diode Laser Cap	K173678	Cap	650	1360	$800
GrivaMax Laser Cap 148	K211192	Cap	650	740	$549
GrivaMax Laser Cap 272 Pro	K211192	Cap	650	1360	$649
HairMax Flip 80 Laser Cap	K180885	Cap	655	800	$899
HairMax LaserBand 41	K142573	Band	655	1230	$549
HairMax LaserBand 82	K142573	Band	655	1230	$799
HairMax PowerFlex Laser Cap 202	K180885	Cap	655	1010	$1,699
HairMax PowerFlex Laser Cap 272	K180885	Cap	655	1360	$1,899
HairMax Ultima 12 LaserComb	K103368	Comb	655		$399
HairMax Ultima 9 Classic LaserComb	K103368	Comb	655		$199
HairPro (272 diode)	K192552	Cap	650	1360	$600
HairPro (81 diode)	K171835	Cap	650	456	$450
iHelmet Hair Growth System	K190467	Helmet	650	800–1000	Inquiry required
illumiflow 148 Laser Cap	K173843	Cap	650	740	$549
illumiflow 272 Laser Cap	K162071	Cap	650	1360	$799
illumiflow 272 Pro Laser Cap	K162071	Cap	650	1360	$999
Kernel Hair Growth System KN-8000B	K200929	Helmet	655	1020	Inquiry required
Kiier 272 Premier	K181878	Cap	650	1360	$925
Kiierr 148 Pro	K181878	Cap	650	740	$595
Laser Hair Growth Cap (Shang Fa Biotechnology)	K192627	Cap	650	400–1400	Inquiry required
NutraStim Laser Hair Comb	K160728	Comb	655		$279
Shapiro MD Laser Hair Regrowth System (272 diode)	K193667	Cap	650	1360	$995
Sunetics Hair Growth Laser	K132646	Hood	650		In office use only
SuperGrow Laser Cap	K181308	Helmet	650	1360	$795
Theradome LH40	K180460	Helmet	678	200	$595
Theradome PRO LH80	K171775	Helmet	678	400	$895
LED + Laser					
Hair Up (Y&J Bio)	K172968	Helmet	655		Inquiry required
iGrow Hair Growth Laser System	K141567	Helmet	655		$599
iRestore Essential	K151662	Helmet	650	255	$695
iRestore Professional	K183417	Helmet	650	1410	$1,195

Devices were identified via search of the FDA 501(k) Premarket Approval (PMA) database using product code OAP (radiation emitting products used to promote hair growth) on October 9, 2021. Devices were excluded from this list if they were not currently available for purchase or in-office use.

> **PEARL 15.6:** Low-level laser/light therapy devices are cleared by the U.S. Food and Drug Administration for treatment of androgenetic alopecia in males and females with Fitzpatrick skin types I to IV. Further research is needed to assess their safety and efficacy in darker skin types and to better understand ideal candidates.

> **PEARL 15.7:** For low-level laser/light therapy, less frequent treatments and shorter total weekly treatment duration (<60 minutes per week) may lead to improved hair growth compared with more frequent use and longer total weekly treatment times. Combination therapy with topical minoxidil may be more effective than monotherapy with either treatment.

EXPECTED OUTCOMES

Systematic reviews and meta-analyses have reported that LLLT represents a potentially effective treatment for AGA, either as monotherapy or in combination with other therapies. Liu et al. identified 11 randomized, controlled trials of LLLT as a treatment for AGA in a total of 667 patients (level of evidence: 1a).[18] All studies included in this meta-analysis found a statistically significant increase in hair density with LLLT compared with sham control (standardized mean difference 1.316 [95% confidence interval CI 0.993–1.639]). There was no difference in hair density between men and women or between LLLT administered through a helmet-type versus comb-type device. A list of devices compared in this meta-analysis is included in Table 15.2. The authors did find that a shorter total weekly treatment duration of less than 60 minutes per week was associated with a significantly greater increase in hair density compared with a longer total treatment time.

Zhou et al. performed a systematic review and meta-analysis of combination treatments for AGA (level of evidence: 1a-).[28] The authors compared global photographic assessment and hair-count increase for combination treatment versus monotherapy. For LLLT with minoxidil solution, three studies were identified that assessed global appearance by photographic assessment, and two studies that assessed change in hair count. All studies reported significant improvement with combination treatment compared with treatment with LLLT alone (Pearl 15.7).

Limitations of existing clinical trials for LLLT include low patient numbers, the sponsoring of trials by industry, and the difficulty inherent in comparing devices with varying treatment parameters (e.g., wavelength, power, energy density) and treatment protocols (e.g., treatment duration and frequency). In many studies, outcome measures are subjective, and follow-up durations are usually short, in the order of months. Additionally, some studies have noted no difference in hair regrowth with LLLT (level of evidence: 5).[29] Highly powered, randomized, controlled clinical trials in the future will ensure better elucidation of treatment efficacy and optimization of device parameters and treatment protocols.

TREATMENT TECHNIQUES AND BEST PRACTICES

For patients with AGA and no other underlying systemic or cutaneous conditions contributing to hair

TABLE 15.2 Low-Level Laser/Light Therapy (LLLT) Devices Compared in a Meta-Analysis by Liu et al.[18]

Device Name	Device Type	Wavelength (nm)	Study
HairMax LaserComb (7-, 9-, and 12-diode)	Comb	655	Leavitt et al. (2009)[20]; Jimenez et al. (2014)[21]
Oaze 3R LLLT device	Helmet	Combined 630, 650, and 660	Kim et al. (2013)[22]
TopHat 655 (iGrow Hair Growth Laser System)	Helmet	655	Lanzafame et al. (2013)[23]; Lanzafame et al. (2014)[24]
CapillusPro	Cap	650	Friedman et al. (2017)[25]
Laser scanner	Band	Combined 655 and 808	Barikbin et al. (2017)[26]
iRestore ID-520	Helmet	Combined 650 and 660	Mai-Yi Fan et al. (2018)[27]

loss, topical minoxidil and, in men, finasteride are typically employed as first-line treatment options given the high level of evidence supporting the efficacy and safety of these medications (level of evidence: 1a).[30] LLLT and platelet-rich plasma injections (level of evidence: 1a) may then be considered as alternative or adjunctive treatments, especially in patients who prefer to avoid or who are not candidates for surgical hair transplant.[31]

LLLT may be performed in the office or at home, depending on patient and provider preferences. LLLT devices include caps, helmets, handheld combs, bands, and hoods. Although caps, helmets, and combs are portable devices that may be used by the patient at home, hoods are overhead panels that require a prescription and are administered in the office. Figs. 15.5-15.8 illustrate examples of various LLLT devices available for home use. It is important to note that numerous LLLT devices are available on the market, but not all have FDA clearance or have been clinically studied. Devices that were FDA-cleared for the treatment of alopecia as of October 2021 are summarized in Table 15.1, along with their respective wavelength, power level, and approximate cost. Costs of portable LLLT devices range from $300 to $400 for

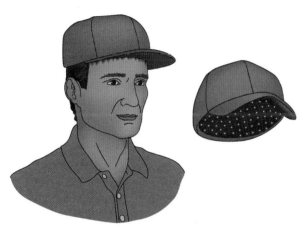

Fig. 15.5 Illustration of a low-level laser/light therapy (LLLT) cap, which may contain lasers and/or light-emitting diodes (LEDs). (Courtesy of Sheila Macomber.)

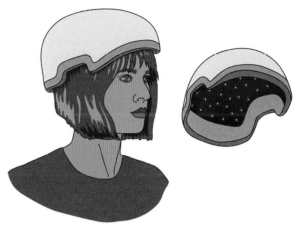

Fig. 15.6 Illustration of a low-level laser/light therapy (LLLT) helmet, which may contain lasers and/or light-emitting diodes (LEDs). (Courtesy of Sheila Macomber.)

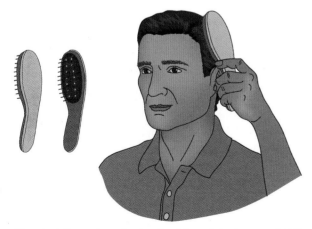

Fig. 15.7 Illustration of a low-level laser/light therapy (LLLT) comb, which may contain lasers and/or light-emitting diodes (LEDs). (Courtesy of Sheila Macomber.)

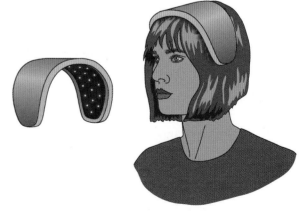

Fig. 15.8 Illustration of a low-level laser/light therapy (LLLT) band, which may contain lasers and/or light-emitting diodes (LEDs). (Courtesy of Sheila Macomber.)

TABLE 15.3 Example of Treatment Protocols for Low-Level Laser/Light Therapy (LLLT) Comb, Band, Cap, and Helmet

Device Type	Example Treatment Protocol
Comb	8 minutes, three treatments per week
Band	1.5-3 minutes, three treatments per week 30 minutes, three treatments per week
Cap	6 minutes, daily 15-30 minutes, three treatments per week
Helmet	10-20 minutes, daily 20-35 minutes, two-four treatments per week

Actual treatment protocol depends on the specific device and manufacturer. Each device should be used according to manufacturer instructions.

combs to more than $1000 for caps or helmets. These devices are typically not covered by insurance.

Treatment protocols are highly variable based on the device and manufacturer. Frequency of treatment ranges from daily use to two or three times per week, and the duration of individual treatments may span from 90 seconds to 35 minutes. Table 15.3 provides examples of treatment protocols for portable laser devices, including combs, caps, and helmets. With consistent use, patients may expect visible improvement after at least 3 to 4 months.

PREVENTION AND MANAGEMENT OF ADVERSE EVENTS

Overall, LLLT is a safe therapy with no severe adverse effects reported in clinical trials. Common adverse effects are usually mild and transient and include scalp irritation and tenderness, headache, erythema, acne, mild sensation changes (e.g., paresthesias), initial TE, and pruritus.[32]

FUTURE DIRECTIONS

Laser and light-based therapies are a promising treatment for AGA and other types of alopecia. Most existing studies investigate LLLT for AGA, and additional research is needed to better understand other treatment options, including excimer laser, NBUVB, and fractional laser, which have primarily been studied in AA.

Laser and light-based interventions are likely most useful when used in conjunction with other effective therapies, including medications such as minoxidil or finasteride, or hair transplantation. Further research is required to optimize treatment protocols, including adjunctive therapies, wavelengths, power output, and treatment frequency and duration, to better understand ideal treatment candidates, and to confirm long-term safety and efficacy.

EVIDENCE SUMMARY

- Low-level laser/light therapy, or photobiomodulation, is effective for the treatment of mild-to-moderate androgenetic alopecia in men and women (strength of recommendation: B). Further research is required to better understand ideal treatment candidates.
- Low-level laser/light therapy is safe to use in Fitzpatrick skin types I to IV (strength of recommendation: B). Additional research is required to determine its safety and efficacy in darker skin types.
- Adverse events related to low-level laser/light therapy are typically mild and self-limited and include scalp irritation and tenderness, headache, erythema, acne, mild sensation changes, transient telogen effluvium, and pruritus (strength of recommendation: B).
- For low-level laser/light therapy, less frequent treatments and shorter total weekly treatment duration (<60 minutes per week) may lead to improved hair growth compared with more frequent use and longer total treatment times (strength of recommendation: C).
- Combination therapy with low-level laser/light therapy and topical minoxidil may be more effective than monotherapy with either treatment (strength of recommendation: C).
- Low-level laser/light therapy is contraindicated in patients with history of photosensitizing disorder and patients who are taking photosensitizing medications (strength of recommendation: B). It is relatively contraindicated in patients with melanocytic nevi or malignant lesions on the scalp (strength of recommendation: D).
- Laser and light-based therapies should not be used in pregnant or lactating women because there is a paucity of safety data in this population (strength of recommendation: D).

REFERENCES

1. Price VH. Androgenetic alopecia in women. *J Investig Dermatol Symp Proc.* 2003;8(1):24-27. doi:10.1046/j.1523-1747.2003.12168.x.

2. Olsen EA, Messenger AG, Shapiro J, et al. Evaluation and treatment of male and female pattern hair loss. *J Am Acad Dermatol.* 2005;52(2) 2):301–311. doi:10.1016/j.jaad.2004.04.008.

3. Whiting DA. Possible mechanisms of miniaturization during androgenetic alopecia or pattern hair loss. *J Am Acad Dermatol.* 2001;45(suppl 3):S81-6. doi:10.1067/mjd.2001.117428.

4. Adil A, Godwin M. The effectiveness of treatments for androgenetic alopecia: a systematic review and meta-analysis. *J Am Acad Dermatol.* 2017;77(1):136–141.e5. doi:10.1016/j.jaad.2017.02.054.

5. *Key Legal Concepts for Cosmetics Industry: Interstate Commerce, Adulterated, and Misbranded.* Available at: https://www.fda.gov/cosmetics/cosmetics-laws-regulations/key-legal-concepts-cosmetics-industry-interstate-commerce-adulterated-and-misbranded. Accessed November 18, 2021.

6. *CFR - Code of Federal Regulations Title 21.* Available at: https://www.accessdata.fda.gov/scripts/cdrh/cfdocs/cfcfr/CFRSearch.cfm?fr=807.97. Accessed November 18, 2021.

7. Lee JH, Eun SH, Kim SH, Ju HJ, Kim GM, Bae JM. Excimer laser/light treatment of alopecia areata: a systematic review and meta-analyses. *Photodermatol Photoimmunol Photomed.* 2020;36(6):460–469. doi:10.1111/phpp.12596.

8. Mlacker S, Aldahan AS, Simmons BJ, et al. A review on laser and light-based therapies for alopecia areata. *J Cosmet Laser Ther.* 2017;19(2):93–99. doi:10.1080/14764172.2016.1248440.

9. Mester E, Spiry T, Szende B, Tota J. Effect of laser rays on wound healing. *Am J Surg.* 1971;122(4):532-535.

10. Avci P, Gupta A, Sadasivam M, et al. Low-level laser (light) therapy (LLLT) in skin: stimulating, healing, restoring. *Semin Cutan Med Surg.* 2013;32(1):41–52.

11. Guo Y, Qu Q, Chen J, Miao Y, Hu Z. Proposed mechanisms of low-level light therapy in the treatment of androgenetic alopecia. *Lasers Med Sci.* 2021;36(4):703–713. doi:10.1007/s10103-020-03159-z.

12. Chung H, Dai T, Sharma SK, Huang YY, Carroll JD, Hamblin MR. The nuts and bolts of low-level laser (light) therapy. *Ann Biomed Eng.* 2012;40(2):516–533. doi:10.1007/s10439-011-0454-7.

13. Perper M, Aldahan AS, Fayne RA, Emerson CP, Nouri K. Efficacy of fractional lasers in treating alopecia: a literature review. *Lasers Med Sci.* 2017;32(8):1919–1925. doi:10.1007/s10103-017-2306-7.

14. Kim WS, Lee HI, Lee JW, et al. Fractional photothermolysis laser treatment of male pattern hair loss. *Dermatol Surg.* 2011;37(1):41–51. doi:10.1111/j.1524-4725.2010.01833.x.

15. Cho S, Choi MJ, Zheng Z, Goo B, Kim DY, Cho SB. Clinical effects of non-ablative and ablative fractional lasers on various hair disorders: a case series of 17 patients. *J Cosmet Laser Ther.* 2013;15(2):74–79. doi:10.3109/14764172.2013.764436.

16. Yalici-Armagan B, Elcin G. The effect of neodymium: yttrium aluminum garnet and fractional carbon dioxide lasers on alopecia areata: a prospective controlled clinical trial. *Dermatol Surg.* 2016;42(4):500–506. doi:10.1097/DSS.0000000000000649.

17. Ke J, Guan H, Li S, Xu L, Zhang L, Yan Y. Erbium: YAG laser (2,940 nm) treatment stimulates hair growth through upregulating Wnt 10b and β-catenin expression in C57BL/6 mice. *Int J Clin Exp Med.* 2015;8(11):20883–20889.

18. Liu KH, Liu D, Chen YT, Chin SY. Comparative effectiveness of low-level laser therapy for adult androgenic alopecia: a system review and meta-analysis of randomized controlled trials. *Lasers Med Sci.* 2019;34(6):1063–1039. doi:10.1007/s10103-019-02723-6.

19. Frigo L, Luppi JSS, Favero GM, et al. The effect of low-level laser irradiation (In-Ga-Al-AsP - 660 nm) on melanoma in vitro and in vivo. *BMC Cancer.* 2009;9:404. doi:10.1186/1471-2407-9-404.

20. Leavitt M, Charles G, Heyman E, Michaels D. HairMax LaserComb laser phototherapy device in the treatment of male androgenetic alopecia: a randomized, double-blind, sham device-controlled, multicentre trial. *Clin Drug Investig.* 2009;29(5):283–292. doi:10.2165/00044011-200929050-00001.

21. Jimenez JJ, Wikramanayake TC, Bergfeld W, et al. Efficacy and safety of a low-level laser device in the treatment of male and female pattern hair loss: a multicenter, randomized, sham device-controlled, double-blind study. *Am J Clin Dermatol.* 2014;15(2):115–127. doi:10.1007/s40257-013-0060-6.

22. Kim H, Choi JW, Kim JY, Shin JW, Lee S-J, Huh C-H. Low-level light therapy for androgenetic alopecia: a 24-week, randomized, double-blind, sham device-controlled multicenter trial. *Dermatol Surg.* 2013;39(8):1411–1420. doi:10.1097/DSS.0000000000001577.

23. Lanzafame RJ, Blanche RR, Bodian AB, Chiacchierini RP, Fernandez-Obregon A, Kazmirek ER. The growth of human scalp hair mediated by visible red light laser and LED sources in males. *Lasers Surg Med.* 2013;45(8):487–495. doi:10.1002/lsm.22173.

24. Lanzafame RJ, Blanche RR, Chiacchierini RP, Kazmirek ER, Sklar JA. The growth of human scalp hair in females

using visible red light laser and LED sources. *Lasers Surg Med.* 2014;46(8):601–607. doi:10.1002/lsm.22277.

25. Friedman S, Schnoor P. Novel Approach to Treating Androgenetic Alopecia in Females With Photobiomodulation (Low-Level Laser Therapy). *Dermatol Surg.* 2017;43(6):856–867.doi:10.1097/DSS.0000000000001114.

26. Barikbin B, Khodamrdi Z, Kholoosi L, et al. Comparison of the effects of 665 nm low level diode Laser Hat versus and a combination of 665 nm and 808nm low level diode Laser Scanner of hair growth in androgenic alopecia. *J Cosmet Laser Ther.* 2017. doi:10.1080/14764172.2017.1326609. Epub ahead of print.

27. Mai-Yi Fan S, Cheng YP, Lee MY, Lin SJ, Chiu HY. Efficacy and safety of a low-level light therapy for androgenetic alopecia: a 24-week, randomized, double-blind, self-comparison, sham device-controlled trial. *Dermatol Surg.* 2018;44(11):1411–1420. doi:10.1097/DSS.0000000000001577.

28. Zhou Y, Chen C, Qu Q, et al. The effectiveness of combination therapies for androgenetic alopecia: a systematic review and meta-analysis. *Dermatol Ther.* 2020;33(4):e13741. doi:10.1111/dth.13741.

29. Avram MR, Rogers NE. The use of low-level light for hair growth: part I. *J Cosmet Laser Ther.* 2009;11(2):110–117. doi:10.1080/14764170902842531.

30. Kanti V, Messenger A, Dobos G, et al. Evidence-based (S3) guideline for the treatment of androgenetic alopecia in women and in men - short version. *J Eur Acad Dermatol Venereol.* 2018;32(1):11–22. doi:10.1111/jdv.14624.

31. Gupta AK, Carviel JL. Meta-analysis of efficacy of platelet-rich plasma therapy for androgenetic alopecia. *J Dermatolog Treat.* 2017;28(1):55–58. doi:10.1080/09546634.2016.1179712.

32. Zarei M, Wikramanayake TC, Falto-Aizpurua L, Schachner LA, Jimenez JJ. Low level laser therapy and hair regrowth: an evidence-based review. *Lasers Med Sci.* 2016;31(2):363–371. doi:10.1007/s10103-015-1818-2.

Emerging Therapies
for Hair Loss

16

Emerging Medications

Fiore Casale, Cristina Nguyen, and Natasha Atanaskova Mesinkovska

KEY POINTS

- Topical prostaglandin analogs may increase vellus and terminal hair density and stimulate hair follicle activity.
- Janus kinase inhibitors demonstrate great success in the treatment of alopecia areata, with potential for androgenetic alopecia.
- Therapies targeting growth-factor regulation offer innovative options with success in androgenetic alopecia.

- Antiandrogen therapy has a long history of investigation for therapeutic use androgenetic alopecia, and new topical therapies show promise.
- Topical estrogen therapy is supported by several studies for the treatment of androgenetic alopecia, but conflicting reports exist.

INTRODUCTION

Androgenetic alopecia (AGA) is a common age-dependent hair-loss disorder affecting more than 60% to 70% of men and women worldwide.[1] The exact pathogenesis of AGA is not well understood, but genetic susceptibility and androgens are pivotal in predisposing individuals to pattern hair loss. There are currently only two pharmacologic treatments that the U.S. Food and Drug Administration (FDA) has approved for AGA: oral finasteride and topical minoxidil. Several new medical treatment modalities and pathways are being explored. Remarkable progress has been made in delineating novel signaling targets implicated in hair growth regulation, including pathways that upregulate key growth factors for germ-cell activation (Wnt mediators), reduce pathologic levels of androgenetic hormones (antiandrogen therapy), and reduce the level of inflammatory mediators (prostaglandins, Janus kinase [JAK] inhibitors). The scope of therapeutic options for AGA is rapidly expanding (Fig. 16.1) with emerging treatments that hold promise for improved results.

INFLAMMATORY PATHWAYS

Prostaglandin Analogs

Prostaglandins (PGs), a lipid-derived prostanoid family generated from arachidonic acid by cyclooxygenase (COX) isoenzymes, are known to variably modulate inflammatory responses.[2] PG production typically increases significantly during acute inflammatory processes prior to leukocyte recruitment and immune cell infiltration. The most commonly bioactive prostaglandins implicated in regulation of the hair cycle with distinguishing effects include PGE_2, $PGF_2\alpha$, PGD_2, and prostacyclin (PGI_2) (Fig. 16.2) (level of evidence: 5).[2] PGE_2 and $PGF_{2\alpha}$ can prolong the anagen phase of the hair cycle, with studies showing that patients with AGA have reduced levels of PGE_2.[3,4] PGE_2 acts as a direct vasodilator and suppressor of T-cell signaling and proliferation and can help reduce inflammation present in AGA. PGF_2 and its analogs stimulate follicular melanocytes and murine hair follicles in both the telogen and anagen phases.[5]

In contrast, AGA scalps have increased levels of PGD_2, a lipid synthesized via the COX and PGD_2

1. *Inflammatory pathway*
    Prostaglandin analogs
    Janus kinase inhibitors

2. *Growth factor regulation*
    Wnt pathway mediators
    Topical growth factors
    Adenosine
    Caffeine
    Botulinum toxin

3. *Hormonal regulalion*
    Antiandrogen therapy
    Estrogen therapy
    Melatonin

4. *Other miscellaneous treatments*
    Antihistamines

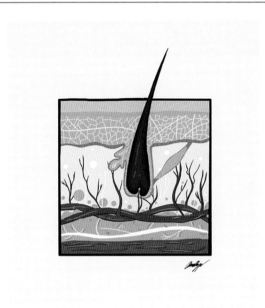

Fig. 16.1 Emerging treatments for androgenetic alopecia. (Image author: Amanda Nguyen)

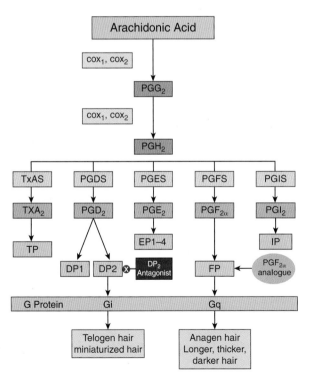

Fig. 16.2 Hair growth mechanistic pathways of prostaglandins and their associated therapies. (Image author: Amanda Nguyen)

synthase pathways (PGDS) (level of evidence: 4).[4,6] PGD_2 acts as a proinflammatory mediator when released from mast cells and T helper (Th2) lymphocytes and has been implicated in the inhibition of hair growth.[7] PGDS activity and PGD_2 levels increase prior to the catagen phase, suggesting their role in the cessation phase of the hair cycle. In murine models, elevated levels of PGD_2 induce follicle miniaturization, sebaceous gland hyperplasia, and alopecia (level of evidence: 5).[4,8] In human balding scalps, there are increased levels of PGD_2, potentially caused by the upregulation of PGDS in comparison to normal scalps.[4] PGD_2 stimulates the expression of androgen-receptor related genes in human dermal papilla cells (DPCs), such as transforming growth factor beta 1 (TGF-β1). New investigational medications targeting prostaglandin pathways are being explored for the treatment of AGA (Table 16.1).

Topical Prostaglandin Analogs

Topical prostaglandin analogs include latanoprost (PGF analog) and bimatoprost (synthetic prostamide F2 analog), which are eyedrops indicated for treatment of open-angle glaucoma.[8] The stimulating effects of PGs on hair growth were first observed as a side effect, prompting further studies and eventual FDA approval of bimatoprost

TABLE 16.1 Inflammatory Pathway Targets Prostaglandin for the Treatment of Androgenetic Alopecia

Medication	Mechanism of Action	Route	Dose	Adverse Effects	Treatment Regimen
Latanoprost	$PGF_{2\alpha}$ analog	Topical	0.1% solution	Eyelash hypertrichosis, malar vellus hair formation, erythema, folliculitis	Once daily
Bimatoprost	Synthetic PGE_2 analog	Topical	0.03% solution	Eyelash hypertrichosis, malar vellus hair formation	Once daily
Setipiprant	Selective PGD_2 receptor antagonist	Oral	500 mg	Gastrointestinal disorders, upper respiratory infection, liver enzyme abnormalities	Twice daily

0.03% solution for eyelash hypotrichosis. PG analogs interact with local receptors to extend the length of the anagen phase while simultaneously stimulating resting telogen-to-anagen hair follicles, with hair bulb and dermal papilla growth. The major reported side effects for both topical PG analogs include eyelash hypertrichosis and malar area vellus hair growth.[9-11]

Bimatoprost (0.03% ophthalmic solution, *Latisse*, Allergan Inc., Irvine, CA) is a synthetic PGE_2 analog that increases the time hair follicles spend in the anagen growth phase.[12-14] The initial excitement for its potential to grow scalp hair has thus far been supported by limited evidence, but clinical trials are still in progress at the time of publication. Studies suggest a concentration-dependent increase in the (a) number of anagen follicles and (b) follicular growth rates.[15] Two large clinical trials evaluated the effect of topical bimatoprost on mean change in hair growth (mm/cm^2) from baseline compared with vehicle-treated groups in men with mild-to-moderate AGA after 24 weeks of treatment. Scalp application of topical bimatoprost 0.03% solution once or twice a day produced a 0.92 mm/cm^2 and 0.76 mm/cm^2 mean change in hair growth, respectively (level of evidence: 1b).[17] However, another large clinical trial reported higher total hair counts with application of minoxidil 2% twice daily compared with once daily application of topical bimatoprost 0.03% among women with AGA after 6 months of treatment (level of evidence: 1b).[18] Common adverse effects included application site pruritis and upper respiratory tract infections.

Latanoprost (*Xalatan*, Pfizer, Inc.) is a PGF_2 analog currently approved by the FDA for the treatment of open-angle glaucoma and ocular hypertension. It acts as an inducer of the hair anagen phase, making it interesting for use in AGA. Evidence on the efficacy of compounded topical formulations, however, is lacking. A single clinical trial reported 16 men with mild AGA who were treated daily for 24 weeks with topical latanoprost 0.1% had a good clinical response and increased hair density compared with baseline ($p<0.001$) (level of evidence: 1b).[19] Common adverse effects included erythema and folliculitis.

Prostaglandin Antagonists

Setipiprant is a selective PG D2 receptor (PGD2R) antagonist that has been linked to the regulation of inflammatory pathways in asthma and allergies. At the time of publication, a clinical trial was underway to study the efficacy and safety of oral setipiprant 1000 mg twice daily relative to placebo in men with AGA (level of evidence: 1b).[20] Results are eagerly awaited, as setipiprant has been shown to be well-tolerated and with a favorable safety profile for other indications.[21]

Janus Kinase Inhibitors

JAK inhibitors are novel treatment options for alopecia area (AA) with therapeutic potential for other alopecia types. JAK inhibitors are a family of tyrosine kinases that mediate cytokine-receptor signaling through phosphorylation and activation of signal transducer and activator of transcription (STAT) nuclear proteins, which are critical for leukocyte activation and proliferation and play a major role in immune regulation.[22,23]

Oral JAK inhibitors (e.g., baricitinib, ruxolitinib, and tofacitinib) are emerging as a favorable treatment modality for a variety of inflammatory conditions, with current FDA approval for myelofibrosis, rheumatoid arthritis, polycythemia vera, psoriatic arthritis, ulcerative colitis, and graft-versus-host disease. JAK-STAT inhibitors play a major role in hair regrowth by regulating T-cell mediated responses at the level of the hair follicle, affecting hair follicle growth and promoting anagen progression.[24,25]

Topical JAK inhibitor preparations in AGA have resulted in anagen phase activation and rapid hair regrowth.[26] Investigational topical JAK 1/3 inhibitor (ATI-50002, applied twice daily to scalp) effectively treated both women and men with AGA, with an increase of 8.6 hairs/cm^2 in total nonvellus hair count over 26 weeks and without any serious adverse events (level of evidence: 1b).[27] However, oral JAK inhibitor treatments have not shown to be as effective for AGA thus far, as one study showed that, among men with AA with hair regrowth, the loss in AGA pattern was preserved.[28] Similarly, in a later small observational study, men with severe AA on an oral JAK 1/3 inhibitor for 24 to 50 weeks experienced significant hair regrowth, but the AGA-pattern loss remained (level of evidence: 4).[29]

Future studies are needed to address the conflicting results and determine the specific types of JAK inhibitors of use in AGA. As systemic JAK inhibition can have immunosuppressive properties, there is an inherent risk of increased infections (e.g., herpes zoster),[30-32] laboratory abnormalities (anemia, leukopenia, elevated cholesterol levels), and potential risk for malignancy and thrombosis.[33-35]

GROWTH REGULATORY PATHWAYS

Complex arrays of growth factors are integral paracrine signals that regulate the hair follicle growth cycle.[36] Induction of the anagen phase requires an elevation in Wnt signaling and stabilization of β-catenin within follicular bulge cells, allowing stem-cell differentiation and growth.[36] Also, fibroblast growth factor (FGF) is involved in β-catenin expression and stabilization, while also promoting angiogenesis and improved dermal fibroblast and hair follicle mitogenesis.[37] Maintenance of the anagen phase requires upregulation of three key growth factors: insulin-like growth factor- 1 (IGF-1), hepatocyte growth factor, and vascular endothelial growth factor (VEGF). IGF-1 promotes cellular proliferation and migration, while simultaneously inhibiting the onset of catagen.[38] Hepatocyte growth factor enhances hair follicle elongation and proliferation of follicular epithelial cells,[37] and VEGF is responsible for angiogenesis to support proper vasculature of the growing hair follicle.[38] Several additional paracrine growth factors are believed to play critical roles in the growth cycle, but the entire mechanism remains to be uncovered to further discern new targets in hopes of generating hair growth (Table 16.2).[36]

TABLE 16.2	Growth Regulation Pathways for Treatment of Androgenetic Alopecia				
Medication	Mechanism of Action	Route	Formulation / Dose	Adverse Effects	Treatment Regimen
Various Topical Growth Factor Combinations	Paracrine stimulation of hair follicles	Topical or Intradermal	Formulation: FGF (2.5μg/mL), IGF-1 (1 μg/mL), stem cell factor (2.5 μg/mL, VEGF (2.5 μg/mL), keratinocyte growth factor-2 (2.5 μg/mL), superoxide dismutase-1 (5 μg/mL), Noggin (2.5 μg/mL)	NR	Topical and intradermal preparations

(Continued)

TABLE 16.2	Growth Regulation Pathways for Treatment of Androgenetic Alopecia—cont'd				
Medication	**Mechanism of Action**	**Route**	**Formulation / Dose**	**Adverse Effects**	**Treatment Regimen**
Wnt Pathway Mediators					
Hair Stimulating Complex	Follistatin and Wnt proteins	Intradermal	Proprietary bioengineered Wnt proteins and growth factors, nondisclosed	NR	Single treatment
SM04554	Small molecule that stimulates the Wnt pathway	Topical	0.15% or 0.25% solution	Erythema, site burning or stinging, pruritus, skin exfoliation	Once daily
Adenosine	Upregulated expression of VEGF and FGF-7	Topical	0.75% adenosine lotion	Scaling, seborrhea, folliculitis, pruritus	Twice daily
Botulinum toxin	Stimulation of TGF-β1 in dermal papilla cells	Intradermal	5 to 150 units in at least 30 injection sites	Pain, edema, erythema at the injection site	One to four sessions
Caffeine	Phosphodiesterase inhibitor and IGF-1 stimulator	Topical	0.2 to 1% lotion	NR	Once daily

NR, Not reported.

Wnt Pathway Mediators

Wnt/β-catenin signaling is a well-described pathway that influences the inductive potential of dermal papilla cells and induces the differentiation of bulge stem cells into hair follicles.[39,40] Specifically, Wnt proteins activate the signal transduction pathways for hair germ formation during the next anagen phase and induce the transition from telogen to anagen.[39,41,42]

There are no currently approved alopecia medications targeting Wnt pathways; however, there are promising results from investigational small molecules that activate the Wnt pathway. Topical application of 0.15% SM04554 significantly increases hair follicle counts (average increase of 4.5 hairs/cm^2) and density (average increase of 217.9 μm) after 6 months compared with placebo, while also increasing hair bulb nuclear expression of Ki-67, a marker of cell proliferation (level of evidence: 1b).[43,44] Similarly, an investigational complex consisting of a proprietary concentration of bioengineered Wnt proteins (among other growth factors) increases hair thickness by 6.3%, hair density by 12.8%, and terminal hair density by 20.6% when assessed 52 weeks after a single session of intradermal injections (level of evidence: 1b).[41] The adverse events reported include erythema, site burning or stinging, pruritus, and skin exfoliation.[44]

Topical Growth Factors

Topical growth factors are increasingly popular components of cosmetic hair products, with very little evidence to substantiate their claims of promoting hair growth. Treatment with topical growth factors for hair loss is not FDA approved. Limited studies have examined the efficacy of topical nonautologous growth factor formulations in the treatment of AGA, and the existing preliminary results are positive but may have commercial bias. A topical growth factor solution (2.5 μg/ mL of FGF, IGF-1, VEGF, keratinocyte growth factor [KGF]-2, stem cell factor, Noggin, 5μg/mL superoxide dismutase-1) improved scalp hair-shaft density by greater than 10% when applied weekly with microneedling among 11 female patients (level of evidence: 2b).[45] Similarly, an investigational formulation of topical FGF (with microneedling) improved hair density and hair diameter among 40 men with AGA (level of evidence: 2b).[46] Intradermal injections every 3 weeks of investigational bioengineered, recombinant growth factor formulations (0.01 to 100 mg/L of FGF, VEGF, IGF, and KGF; 0.005 to 100mg/L thymosin β4; and, 0.1 to 500 mg/L copper tripeptide-1) were shown to increase the number of terminal hairs, increase the hair-shaft diameter (3μm), and reduce vellus hair counts after eight sessions of multiple scalp injections in 680 males and 320 females (level of evidence: 2b).[38] More studies are needed in this area to determine the growth factor ingredients and their optimal concentrations to improve AGA outcomes.

Adenosine

Adenosine is an extracellular purine nucleoside that has far-reaching effects across many organ systems, with systemic therapeutic use for cardiovascular regulation.[47] Adenosine regulates several growth factor transduction pathways within dermal papilla cells and is known to upregulate the expression of VEGF.[48,49] When bound to adenosine receptor A2b, production of FGF-7 increases and TGF-β levels decrease.[50] TGF-β is an inhibitory factor in DPCs, which can be induced by androgens.[51]

Several clinical trials show promising results for off-label use of topical adenosine in the treatment of AGA. Topical 0.75% adenosine lotion increases the quantity of thick hair (>60 μm) by 5.5 hairs/cm² after 6 months (level of evidence: 4),[52,53] with comparable clinical improvement to patients using topical minoxidil (relative recovery rate of 1.9% vs. 2.4%, respectively, p = 0.17) (level of evidence: 2b).[54] After 12 months, topical adenosine is reported to increase the ratio of thick hairs (>80 μm) and increase the anagen growth rate by at least 0.4 mm/day (level of evidence: 1b).[50] Adverse events are minimal, including scaling and seborrhea, folliculitis, and pruritus.[52,54]

Botulinum Toxin

Botulinum toxin (BTX) prevents the release of acetylcholine at the neuromuscular junction and is a treatment modality for various neurologic and dermatologic conditions.[55-57] It has gathered attention as an emerging therapy for AGA after several successful clinical studies. Though the mechanisms are not fully understood, botulinum toxin has potential as another future treatment for patients with AGA.

Its success in AGA has been speculative and attributed to increased oxygen delivery to tissue secondary to musculature relaxation. Higher concentrations of oxygen allow for greater quantities of testosterone to be converted to estradiol rather than dihydrotestosterone (DHT), with potential reduction of hair loss.[58] DHT is known to induce TGF-β1 in DPCs to inhibit follicular epithelial cell growth; therefore botulinum toxin type A (BTX) may indirectly inhibit TGF-β1 secretion within the hair bulb, similar to its action on scar tissue fibroblasts.[59]

Several open-label studies have evaluated the safety and efficacy of BTX injections, with varying dosages (5 to 150 units) injected into the muscles surrounding the scalp with over 30 injection sites and variable numbers of sessions (one to four). One study showed a statistically significant increase of mean hair counts between baseline and week 48 (p<0.0001) and visible hair growth in men with AGA after 60 weeks and three treatment cycles (level of evidence: 4).[58] Other studies report 70% of patients with good-to-excellent responses after 24 weeks (Fig. 16.3) (level of evidence: 4)[60] and hair regrowth in 36% of subjects 6 months after receiving one BTX treatment (level of evidence: 4).[61] The latest open-label study showed a superior therapeutic effect demonstrated by higher hair counts with the combination of BTX and oral finasteride compared with BTX alone after a total of four sessions (one BTX injection every 3 months) (level of evidence: 2b).[62] Commonly described transient side effects are pain, edema, or erythema at the injection site.[61,62] As there are also reports

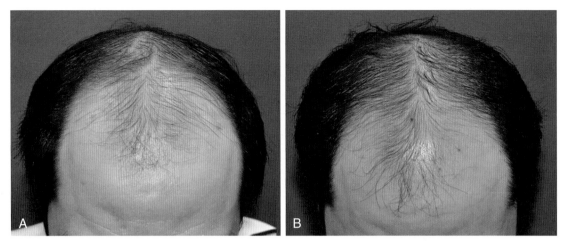

Fig. 16.3 Clinical photographs of a male patient with AGA at baseline (A) and at 6 months after treatment (B) with botulinum toxin. (Source: Shon U, Kim MH, Lee DY, Kim SH, Park BC. The effect of intradermal botulinum toxin on androgenetic alopecia and its possible mechanism. *J Am Acad Dermatol.* 2020;83(6):1838-1839. doi:10.1016/j.jaad.2020.04.082)

of facial and scalp hair loss secondary to botulinum toxin treatment for other indications, it is imperative that the details of its effects and mechanisms are well established and confirmed in larger, randomized trials.

Caffeine

Caffeine is a phosphodiesterase inhibitor that increases cell cyclic adenosine monophosphate levels, thereby promoting cellular proliferation and metabolism.[63] It is consumed in foods and beverages (2 to 200 mg of caffeine per 100 mL) and over-the-counter pain and weight-loss supplements, and it can cross the blood-brain barrier as a central nervous system stimulant.[64]

Although topical caffeine-containing products have not been FDA approved for hair loss, many investigational studies have focused on its use for the treatment of AGA. Topical caffeine easily crosses skin barriers, and *in vivo* studies demonstrated good follicular penetration and absorption (level of evidence: 5).[65] Several *in vitro* studies have noted that caffeine can promote hair growth [63] by (1) reversing the testosterone-inhibiting effect on keratinocyte proliferation[66]; (2) enhancing hair shaft elongation, prolonging anagen duration, and stimulating keratinocyte proliferation of the hair matrix[67]; (3) increasing IGF-1 expression (which promotes hair growth in both males and females)[67]; and (4) downregulating testosterone-induced TGF-β_1 expression (level of evidence: 5).[67]

Daily use of caffeine shampoo (unspecified concentration) results in reduced hair shedding, decreased hair loss intensity, and fewer hairs extracted during hair-pull test in both men and women with AGA (level of evidence: 1b).[68-70] Similarly, caffeine lotion (unspecified concentration) has shown decreases in hairs extracted during the hair-pull test with potential increase in hair tensile strength for men with AGA (level of evidence: 2b).[71] Topical caffeine has also been compared with other standard treatment modalities (topical minoxidil 5%, topical minoxidil 2.5%, azelaic acid 1.5%), with results showing improvements in anagen ratio (level of evidence: 1b),[72] increased patient satisfaction (level of evidence: 1b),[73] and decreased hair shedding (level of evidence: 1b).[74] No serious adverse events were reported.

HORMONAL REGULATION

Novel Antiandrogen Therapy

Classically, it is believed that 5α-reductase converts testosterone to DHT within DPCs and that DHT binds the androgen receptors resulting in the diminution of the number of terminal hairs.[75] Finasteride, a 5α-reductase inhibitor, is the only FDA approved antiandrogen treatment for AGA, but several additional antiandrogen medications are currently under review (Table 16.3).[76]

TABLE 16.3 Emerging Hormonal Targets for Treatment of Androgenetic Alopecia

Medication	Mechanism of Action	Route	Dose	Adverse Effects	Treatment Regimen
Anti-Androgen Therapies					
Clascoterone	Direct androgen receptor inhibitor	Topical	2.5%, 5%, or 7.5% solution	NR	Once daily
Pyrilutamide	Androgen receptor antagonist	Oral	2.5-5 mg	NR	Once to twice daily
Fluridil	Competitive androgen receptor antagonist	Topical	2% solution	Scalp yellowing, reactivation of seborrheic dermatitis, allergic reaction	Once daily
Flutamide	Selective nonsteroidal androgen receptor antagonist	Oral	62.5-250 mg	Liver toxicity, depressed plasma androgen levels, headaches, respiratory tract disorders, nausea and/or vomiting, diarrhea, dry skin, reduced libido	Once daily, increasing the dose as tolerated
Estrogen Therapies					
17α-estradiol	Inhibition of 5α-reductase	Topical	0.025% solution	Irritation, mild pruritus, erythema, scaling	Once daily
Estradiol valerate	Inhibition of 5α-reductase	Topical	0.03% lotion	Irritation, mild pruritus, erythema, scaling, postmenopausal uterine bleeding	Once daily
Melatonin Therapy					
Melatonin	Antioxidant and prolactin stimulator	Topical	0.0033% solution	Headache, gastrointestinal distress, pruritus, erythema	Once daily

NR, Not reported.

Topical Anti-Androgens

Clascoterone is an ester derivative of cortexolone and is a potent direct androgen receptor inhibitor.[77] When applied topically, the drug penetrates the skin and binds to androgen receptors within sebaceous glands and hair follicles and inhibits DHT-stimulated signaling. At the time of publication, clascoterone was approved for acne vulgaris treatment and under investigation for treatment of AGA. A clinical trial with 400 men with AGA reported increased hair counts (growth of additional 10 to 14 hairs per 1-cm^2 area, on average) with use of a 2.5%, 5%, or 7.5% clascoterone solution for 12 months, without any reported adverse events (level of evidence: 1b).[77]

Fluridil is an investigational topical nonsteroidal antiandrogen that competitively binds to androgen receptors in the dermal papilla. A clinical trial of 43 men with AGA receiving topical fluridil 2% reported increases in anagen counts and decreases in telogen counts compared with placebo (level of evidence: 1b).[78] Minimal adverse reactions were reported, including yellowing of the scalp, reactivation of seborrheic dermatitis by sun exposure, and allergic reaction after concurrent application of topical deodorant.

Oral Anti-Androgens

Flutamide is a pure selective nonsteroidal antiandrogen and acts peripherally to competitively block the binding of androgens to cytoplasmic and/or nuclear androgen receptors, and is currently approved for oral administration (250 mg thrice daily) solely for the treatment of metastatic prostate cancer.[79,80] Few studies have examined the efficacy of off label use of flutamide for AGA, but preliminary results note improvements in Ludwig scores with daily oral 62.5 to 250 mg flutamide (level of evidence: 2b).[79,81] Reported adverse reactions include depressed plasma androgen levels, elevated transaminase levels, headaches, respiratory tract disorders, nausea and vomiting, diarrhea, dry skin, and reduced libido.[79]

Pyrilutamide is an oral androgen receptor antagonist currently investigated for AGA. A randomized, double-blind, placebo-controlled clinical trial is in progress, using oral pyrilutamide 2.5 to 5 mg daily in 120 men with AGA (level of evidence: 1b).[82] There are no known serious side effects.

Estrogen Therapies

The mechanism delineating how estrogen may benefit AGA-affected hair follicles remains unclear despite prolific scientific efforts. At the level of the hair follicle, 17 α-estradiol can suppress the function of 5α-reductase and diminish the quantity of DHT formed.[83] Moreover, by stimulating P-450 aromatase, it may upregulate the conversion of testosterone to 17β-estradiol and the conversion of androstenedione to estrone, further decreasing pathologic levels of DHT.[83,84]

Topical estrogen therapy is currently FDA approved for treatment of postmenopausal symptoms and for hormone replacement therapy.[85] In terms of AGA, evidence for estradiol off label use has predominantly shown promising results. Postmenopausal women (ages 48 to 71 years) applying estradiol valerate 0.03% lotion to the scalp for 12 weeks experienced an anagen-to-telogen ratio increase from 1.57 to 2.27, indicating a decreased telogen rate and/or increased anagen rate (level of evidence: 1b).[84] Female patients applying topical

0.025% 17 α-estradiol solution experienced increases in total hair counts by an average of 60.08 hairs/cm^2 and hair caliber from 0.058 ± 0.016 μm to 0.073 ± 0.015 μm ($p < 0.05$) after 12 months of therapy (level of evidence: 2b).[86] Another study concurred that topical 0.025% 17 α-estradiol increases total hair counts by an average of 31.57 hairs/cm^2 and hair diameter by an average of 10.39 μm after 8 months of therapy (level of evidence: 2b).[83] However, one clinical trial using topical 0.025% alfatradiol therapy among 51 women for 6 months demonstrated no significant difference in hair thickness or absolute hair density from baseline (level of evidence: 1b).[87] Similarly, oral cyproterone acetate therapy was found to be inferior to topical minoxidil therapy among 66 women after 12 months of treatment (level of evidence: 1b).[88] Reported adverse events include irritation, mild pruritus, erythema, and/or scaling from the topical formulations. A case of breast adenocarcinoma was reported in a patient who used estradiol valerate topical therapy, but no direct causation was established.[84]

Fulvestrant

Fulvestrant is an estrogen receptor antagonist without any known agonist properties, originally formulated for intramuscular administration (250 mg/mL) in the treatment of breast cancer.[89,90] When bound to the estrogen receptor, the complex is destabilized and internalized within the cell for degradation.[91] Interestingly, topical formulations have demonstrated preclinical murine success in the treatment of hair loss by causing hair follicles to transition from the telogen to anagen phase (level of evidence: 5).[92] Despite this preclinical success, to date, clinical trials using topical 30 μL/cm^2 of fulvestrant 70 mg/mL solution reported no improvement in men and women over the age of 18 with Hamilton-Norwood grades III to Va or Ludwig I to II after 16 weeks of use (level of evidence: 1b).[92]

Melatonin

Melatonin (5-methoxy-N-acetyltryptamine) is a lipophilic hormone synthesized and secreted by the pineal gland from a pathway that includes both tryptophan and serotonin.[93] The well-established function of melatonin is its involvement in circadian rhythm and sleep cycle control and its strong antioxidant properties.[93,94] Human skin is known to have its own melatoninergic antioxidative system, which includes melatonin receptors within hair follicle keratinocytes and dermal papilla fibroblasts.[95] Keratinocytes, fibroblasts, and melano-cytes have functional melatonin receptors located in the hair root sheath, which are thought to assist in hair growth regulation and hair shaft stabilization.[96] *In vitro* studies demonstrated that low doses of melatonin enhance human follicle proliferation, while melatonin antagonists suppress follicular stimulation. Thus, it is theorized that melatonin has a specific receptor-mediated effect on follicular oxidative stress and growth, making it a possible candidate to counteract the oxidative stress associated with AGA.[97]

Several trials have evaluated the safety and efficacy of topical melatonin 0.0033% application in women and men with AGA, but it is currently not FDA approved. Various open-label and observational studies indicate topical melatonin 0.0033% cosmetic hair solution is highly tolerable with positive effects on hair growth. Specifically, daily application of 0.003% topical melatonin therapy did not increase serum melatonin levels (level of evidence: 1b),[98] but showed significantly reduced hair loss severity (level of evidence: 2b)[99] and increased hair density and hair count (level of evidence: 2b).[100] One large clinical trial evaluating men with stage I or II AGA (Hamilton scale) and women with stage I or II AGA (Ludwig scale) reported fewer patients with a positive hair-pull test and significant new hair growth (p<0.001) after 6 months of daily 0.0033% topical melatonin application (level of evidence: 1a).[101] Interestingly, one study noted only women with AGA experienced hair-loss reduction in comparison to men after a 6 month treatment period of daily topical melatonin 0.0033% solution (level of evidence: 2b).[102] Common side effects include headache,[100] pruritis,[101] burning, itching, erythema, and sensitivity.[102]

OTHER MISCELLANEOUS TREATMENTS

Antihistamines

There has been an increased interest in the role of histamine in various types of alopecias, as it is involved in modulating both innate and adaptive immune responses.[103,104] Two antihistamines, cimetidine and cetirizine, are theorized to help treat AGA based on limited evidence of inherent antiinflammatory properties independent of their blockade of histamine receptors.[105]

Cimetidine is a selective histamine receptor 2 (H2) antagonist, originally FDA approved to reduce gastric acid secretion. Evidence from a small study in the 1980s in women with AGA (n = 10) recorded clinical improvement at a dose of 300 mg five times daily for up to 9 months of therapy.[103,106] However, no further relevant studies have been conducted, and interest surrounding its use for AGA has faded, mostly as a result of its side effect profile (dizziness, somnolence).[103]

Cetirizine, a second-generation selective histamine receptor 1 (H1) antagonist, functions by blocking eosinophil activation and mast cell degranulation. Cetirizine is approved for the treatment of allergic rhinitis and chronic urticaria, administered in oral doses between 5 mg and 10 mg, and is generally well tolerated with minimal side effects such somnolence, fatigue, and dry mouth.[107] Interestingly, cetirizine has antiinflammatory and PGD2 suppressive properties.[104] These newly uncovered PGD2 suppressive properties sparked interest in using cetirizine in hair loss, as PGD2 production is implicated in the pathogenesis of AGA.[4] Investigational topical cetirizine 1% increased new hair growth (based on dermatoscopic exam) in 43.3% of patients after 6 months of daily scalp application (level of evidence: 3b).[108] Similarly, it increases total hair density by 11% and terminal hair density by 18% while reducing vellus hair density by 15% after 6 months (level of evidence: 2b).[105] There have been no reports of adverse reactions to topical cetirizine therapy.

EVIDENCE SUMMARY

- Prostaglandin analog topical therapies show significant evidence of efficacy in the treatment of androgenetic alopecia (strength of recommendation: C).
- Janus kinase inhibitors are greatly beneficial in the treatment of alopecia areata (strength of recommendation: A). Comparable results in the treatment of AGA remain to be seen.
- Growth factor therapy stimulates hair follicle growth at the cellular level, and both topical and intradermal preparations have shown success (strength of recommendation: D).
- Wnt pathway mediators are therapeutic options that may emerge as efficacious in the treatment of androgenetic alopecia, based on preliminary results (strength of recommendation: D).
- Topical adenosine, caffeine, and melatonin may improve hair regrowth by reducing hair loss severity and increasing hair density and hair count in

patients with androgenetic alopecia (strength of recommendation: D).

- Botulinum toxin injections have unclear effects on hair growth in patients with androgenetic alopecia and thus are last-line therapies in refractory cases (strength of recommendation: D).
- Novel antiandrogen therapy encompasses several drugs that have shown moderate success in increasing terminal hair growth (strength of recommendation: D).
- Estrogen therapy has shown inconsistent efficacy in the treatment of androgenetic alopecia and is associated with serious adverse reactions that require careful deliberation of treatment options before use (strength of recommendation: D).

REFERENCES

1. Jain R, De-Eknamkul W. Potential targets in the discovery of new hair growth promoters for androgenic alopecia. *Expert Opin Ther Targets.* 2014;18(7):787-806. doi:10.1517/14728222.2014.922956.
2. Ricciotti E, FitzGerald GA. Prostaglandins and inflammation. *Arterioscler Thromb Vasc Biol.* 2011;31(5):986-1000. doi:10.1161/ATVBAHA.110.207449.
3. Johnstone MA, Albert DM. Prostaglandin-induced hair growth. *Surv Ophthalmol.* 2002;47(suppl 1):S185-S202. doi:10.1016/s0039-6257(02)00307-7.
4. Garza LA, Liu Y, Yang Z, et al. Prostaglandin D2 inhibits hair growth and is elevated in bald scalp of men with androgenetic alopecia. *Sci Transl Med.* 2012;4(126):126ra34. doi:10.1126/scitranslmed.3003122.
5. Sasaki S, Hozumi Y, Kondo S. Influence of prostaglandin F2alpha and its analogues on hair regrowth and follicular melanogenesis in a murine model. *Exp Dermatol.* 2005;14(5):323-328. doi:10.1111/j.0906-6705.2005.00270.x.
6. Urade Y, Watanabe K, Hayaishi O. Prostaglandin D, E, and F synthases. *J Lipid Mediat Cell Signal.* 1995;12(2-3):257-273. doi:10.1016/0929-7855(95)00032-l.
7. Tanaka K, Ogawa K, Sugamura K, Nakamura M, Takano S, Nagata K. Cutting edge: differential production of prostaglandin D2 by human helper T cell subsets. *J Immunol.* 2000;164(5):2277-2280. doi:10.4049/jimmunol.164.5.2277.
8. Alkhalifah A. Topical and intralesional therapies for alopecia areata. *Dermatol Ther.* 2011;24(3):355-363. doi:10.1111/j.1529-8019.2011.01419.x.
9. Hart J, Shafranov G. Hypertrichosis of vellus hairs of the malar region after unilateral treatment with bimatoprost. *Am J Ophthalmol.* 2004;137(4):756-757. doi:10.1016/j.ajo.2003.09.002.
10. Tosti A, Pazzaglia M, Voudouris S, Tosti G. Hypertrichosis of the eyelashes caused by bimatoprost. *J Am Acad Dermatol.* 2004;51(suppl 5):S149-S150. doi:10.1016/j.jaad.2004.05.002.
11. Herane MI, Urbina F. Acquired trichomegaly of the eyelashes and hypertrichosis induced by bimatoprost. *J Eur Acad Dermatol Venereol.* 2004;18(5):644-645. doi:10.1111/j.1468-3083.2004.01020.x.
12. Cohen JL. Enhancing the growth of natural eyelashes: the mechanism of bimatoprost-induced eyelash growth. *Dermatol Surg.* 2010;36(9):1361-1371. doi:10.1111/j.1524-4725.2010.01522.x.
13. Barrón-Hernández YL, Tosti A. Bimatoprost for the treatment of eyelash, eyebrow and scalp alopecia. *Expert Opin Investig Drugs.* 2017;26(4):515-522. doi:10.1080/13543784.2017.1303480.
14. Emer JJ, Stevenson ML, Markowitz O. Novel treatment of female-pattern androgenetic alopecia with injected bimatoprost 0.03% solution. *J Drugs Dermatol.* 2011;10(7):795-798.
15. Khidhir KG, Woodward DF, Farjo NP, et al. The prostamide-related glaucoma therapy, bimatoprost, offers a novel approach for treating scalp alopecias. *FASEB J.* 013;27(2):557-567. doi:10.1096/fj.12-218156.
16. A Safety and Efficacy Study of Bimatoprost in Men with Androgenic Alopecia (AGA). Full Text View - ClinicalTrials.gov. Available at: https://clinicaltrials.gov/ct2/show/NCT01904721. Accessed July 22, 2013.
17. Safety and Efficacy Study of Bimatoprost in the Treatment of Men with Androgenic Alopecia. Full Text View - ClinicalTrials.gov. Available at: https://clinicaltrials.gov/ct2/show/NCT01325337. Accessed March 29, 2011.
18. Safety and Efficacy Study of Bimatoprost in the Treatment of Women with Female Pattern Hair Loss. Full Text View - ClinicalTrials.gov. Available at: https://clinicaltrials.gov/ct2/show/NCT01325350. Accessed March 29, 2011.
19. Blume-Peytavi U, Lönnfors S, Hillmann K, Garcia Bartels N. A randomized double-blind placebo-controlled pilot study to assess the efficacy of a 24-week topical treatment by latanoprost 0.1% on hair growth and pigmentation in healthy volunteers with androgenetic alopecia. *J Am Acad Dermatol.* 2012;66(5):794-800. doi:10.1016/j.jaad.2011.05.026.
20. Allergan. *Multicenter, Randomized, Double-Blind, Placebo-Controlled, Phase 2A Study of Setipiprant Tablets in Androgenetic Alopecia in Males.* clinicaltrials.gov; 2019. Available at: https://clinicaltrials.gov/ct2/show/results/NCT02781311. Accessed April 12, 2021.
21. Ratner P, Andrews CP, Hampel FC, et al. Efficacy and safety of setipiprant in seasonal allergic rhinitis: results from Phase 2 and Phase 3 randomized, double-blind, placebo- and active-referenced studies. *Allergy Asthma*

Clin Immunol. 2017;13:18. doi:10.1186/s13223-017-0183-z.

22. Murray PJ. The JAK-STAT signaling pathway: input and output integration. *J Immunol.* 2007;178(5):2623-2629. doi:10.4049/jimmunol.178.5.2623.

23. Clark JD, Flanagan ME, Telliez JB. Discovery and development of Janus kinase (JAK) inhibitors for inflammatory diseases. *J Med Chem.* 2014;57(12):5023-5038. doi:10.1021/jm401490p.

24. Ito T, Tokura Y. The role of cytokines and chemokines in the T-cell-mediated autoimmune process in alopecia areata. *Exp Dermatol.* 2014;23(11):787-791. doi:10.1111/exd.12489.

25. Strazzulla LC, Wang EHC, Avila L, et al. Alopecia areata: An appraisal of new treatment approaches and overview of current therapies. *J Am Acad Dermatol.* 2018;78(1):15-24. doi:10.1016/j.jaad.2017.04.1142.

26. Harel S, Higgins CA, Cerise JE, et al. Pharmacologic inhibition of JAK-STAT signaling promotes hair growth. *Sci Adv.* 2015;1(9):e1500973. doi:10.1126/sciadv.1500973.

27. *Aclaris Therapeutics Announces Positive 6-Month Results from a Phase 2 Open-Label Clinical Trial of ATI-502 Topical in Patients with Androgenetic Alopecia (Male/Female Pattern-Baldness).* BioSpace. Available at: https://www.biospace.com/article/aclaris-therapeutics-announces-positive-6-month-results-from-a-phase-2-open-label-clinical-trial-of-ati-502-topical-in-patients-with-androgenetic-alopecia-male-female-pattern-baldness-/. Accessed June 17, 2019.

28. Liu LY, Craiglow BG, Dai F, King BA. Tofacitinib for the treatment of severe alopecia areata and variants: a study of 90 patients. *J Am Acad Dermatol.* 2017;76(1):22-28. doi:10.1016/j.jaad.2016.09.007.

29. Yale K, Pourang A, Plikus MV, Mesinkovska NA. At the crossroads of 2 alopecias: androgenetic alopecia pattern of hair regrowth in patients with alopecia areata treated with oral Janus kinase inhibitors. *JAAD Case Rep.* 2020;6(5):444-446. doi:10.1016/j.jdcr.2020.02.026.

30. Verstovsek S, Mesa RA, Gotlib J, et al. Efficacy, safety, and survival with ruxolitinib in patients with myelofibrosis: results of a median 3-year follow-up of COMFORT-I. *Haematologica.* 2015;100(4):479-488. doi:10.3324/haematol.2014.115840.

31. O'Sullivan JM, McLornan DP, Harrison CN. Safety considerations when treating myelofibrosis. *Expert Opin Drug Saf.* 2016;15(9):1185-1192. doi:10.1080/14740338.2016.1185414.

32. Arana Yi C, Tam CS, Verstovsek S. Efficacy and safety of ruxolitinib in the treatment of patients with myelofibrosis. *Future Oncol.* 2015;11(5):719-733. doi:10.2217/fon.14.272.

33. Verden A, Dimbil M, Kyle R, Overstreet B, Hoffman KB. Analysis of spontaneous postmarket case reports submitted to the FDA regarding thromboembolic adverse events and JAK inhibitors. *Drug Saf.* 2018;41(4):357-361. doi:10.1007/s40264-017-0622-2.

34. Wollenhaupt J, Silverfield J, Lee EB, et al. Safety and efficacy of tofacitinib, an oral janus kinase inhibitor, for the treatment of rheumatoid arthritis in open-label, long-term extension studies. *J Rheumatol.* 2014;41(5):837-852. doi:10.3899/jrheum.130683.

35. Papp KA, Krueger JG, Feldman SR, et al. Tofacitinib, an oral Janus kinase inhibitor, for the treatment of chronic plaque psoriasis: long-term efficacy and safety results from 2 randomized phase-III studies and 1 open-label long-term extension study. *J Am Acad Dermatol.* 2016;74(5):841-850. doi:10.1016/j.jaad.2016.01.013.

36. Houschyar KS, Borrelli MR, Tapking C, et al. Molecular mechanisms of hair growth and regeneration: current understanding and novel paradigms. *Dermatology.* 2020;236(4):271-280. doi:10.1159/000506155.

37. Gentile P, Garcovich S. Systematic review of platelet-rich plasma use in androgenetic alopecia compared with Minoxidil, Finasteride, and adult stem cell-based therapy. *Int J Mol Sci.* 2020;21(8):2702. doi: 10.3390/ijms21082702.

38. Kapoor R, Shome D. Intradermal injections of a hair growth factor formulation for enhancement of human hair regrowth - safety and efficacy evaluation in a first-in-man pilot clinical study. *J Cosmet Laser Ther.* 2018;20(6):369-379. doi:10.1080/14764172.2018.1439965.

39. Shimizu H, Morgan BA. Wnt signaling through the beta-catenin pathway is sufficient to maintain, but not restore, anagen-phase characteristics of dermal papilla cells. *J Invest Dermatol.* 2004;122(2):239-245. doi:10.1046/j.0022-202X.2004.22224.x.

40. Millar SE. Molecular mechanisms regulating hair follicle development. *J Invest Dermatol.* 2002;118(2):216-225. doi:10.1046/j.0022-202x.2001.01670.x.

41. Zimber MP, Ziering C, Zeigler F, et al. Hair regrowth following a Wnt- and follistatin containing treatment: safety and efficacy in a first-in-man phase 1 clinical trial. *J Drugs Dermatol.* 2011;10(11):1308-1312.

42. Gentile P, Garcovich S. Advances in regenerative stem cell therapy in androgenic alopecia and hair loss: Wnt pathway, growth-factor, and mesenchymal stem cell signaling impact analysis on cell growth and hair follicle development. *Cells.* 2019;8(5):466. doi:10.3390/cells8050466.

43. Yazici Y, Swearingen C, Simsek I, et al. *Safety, tolerability and efficacy of a topical treatment (sm04554) for androgenic alopecia (AGA): results from a phase 2 trial.* Poster Session presented at the: American Academy of Dermatology (AAD); March 4, 2016; Washington, DC.

44. Seykora J, Simsek I, DiFrancesco A, et al. *Safety and biopsy outcomes of a topical treatment (sm04554) for male*

androgenic alopecia (AGA): results from a phase 2, multi-center, randomized, double-blind, vehicle-controlled trial. Poster Session presented at the: American Academy of Dermatology (AAD); March 3, 2017; Orlando, FL.

45. Lee YB, Eun YS, Lee JH, et al. Effects of topical application of growth factors followed by microneedle therapy in women with female pattern hair loss: a pilot study. *J Dermatol.* 2013;40(1):81-83. doi:10.1111/j.1346-8138.2012.01680.x.

46. Yu CQ, Zhang H, Guo ME, et al. Combination therapy with topical minoxidil and nano-microneedle-assisted fibroblast growth factor for male androgenetic alopecia: a randomized controlled trial in Chinese patients. *Chin Med J (Engl).* 2020;134(7):851-853. doi:10.1097/CM9.0000000000001195.

47. Layland J, Carrick D, Lee M, Oldroyd K, Berry C. Adenosine: physiology, pharmacology, and clinical applications. *JACC Cardiovasc Interv.* 2014;7(6):581-591. doi:10.1016/j.jcin.2014.02.009.

48. Iino M, Ehama R, Nakazawa Y, et al. Adenosine stimulates fibroblast growth factor-7 gene expression via adenosine A2b receptor signaling in dermal papilla cells. *J Invest Dermatol.* 2007;127(6):1318-1325. doi:10.1038/sj.jid.5700728.

49. Li M, Marubayashi A, Nakaya Y, Fukui K, Arase S. Minoxidil-induced hair growth is mediated by adenosine in cultured dermal papilla cells: possible involvement of sulfonylurea receptor 2B as a target of minoxidil. *J Invest Dermatol.* 2001;117(6):1594-1600. doi:10.1046/j.0022-202x.2001.01570.x.

50. Oura H, Iino M, Nakazawa Y, et al. Adenosine increases anagen hair growth and thick hairs in Japanese women with female pattern hair loss: a pilot, double-blind, randomized, placebo-controlled trial. *J Dermatol.* 2008;35(12):763-767. doi:10.1111/j.1346-8138.2008.00564.x.

51. Inui S, Fukuzato Y, Nakajima T, Yoshikawa K, Itami S. Androgen-inducible TGF-beta1 from balding dermal papilla cells inhibits epithelial cell growth: a clue to understand paradoxical effects of androgen on human hair growth. *FASEB J.* 2002;16(14):1967-1969. doi:10.1096/fj.02-0043fje.

52. Watanabe Y, Nagashima T, Hanzawa N, et al. Topical adenosine increases thick hair ratio in Japanese men with androgenetic alopecia. *Int J Cosmet Sci.* 2015;37(6):579-587. doi:10.1111/ics.12235.

53. Iwabuchi T, Ideta R, Ehama R, et al. Topical adenosine increases the proportion of thick hair in Caucasian men with androgenetic alopecia. *J Dermatol.* 2016;43(5):567-570. doi:10.1111/1346-8138.13159.

54. Faghihi G, Iraji F, Rajaee Harandi M, Nilforoushzadeh M-A, Askari G. Comparison of the efficacy of topical minoxidil 5% and adenosine 0.75% solutions on male

androgenetic alopecia and measuring patient satisfaction rate. *Acta Dermatovenerol Croat.* 2013;21(3):155-159.

55. Başar E, Arıcı C. Use of botulinum neurotoxin in ophthalmology. *Turk J Ophthalmol.* 2016;46(6):282-290. doi:10.4274/tjo.57701.

56. Scott AB, Rosenbaum A, Collins CC. Pharmacologic weakening of extraocular muscles. *Invest Ophthalmol.* 1973;12(12):924-927.

57. Carruthers JD, Carruthers JA. Treatment of glabellar frown lines with C. botulinum-A exotoxin. *J Dermatol Surg Oncol.* 1992;18(1):17-21. doi:10.1111/j.1524-4725.1992.tb03295.x.

58. Freund BJ, Schwartz M. Treatment of male pattern baldness with botulinum toxin: a pilot study. *Plast Reconstr Surg.* 2010;126(5):246e-248e. doi:10.1097/PRS.0b013e3181ef816d.

59. Shon U, Kim MH, Lee DY, Kim SH, Park BC. The effect of intradermal botulinum toxin on androgenetic alopecia and its possible mechanism. *J Am Acad Dermatol.* 2020;83(6):1838-1839. doi:10.1016/j.jaad.2020.04.082.

60. Singh S, Neema S, Vasudevan B. A pilot study to evaluate effectiveness of botulinum toxin in treatment of androgenetic alopecia in males. *J Cutan Aesthet Surg.* 2017;10(3):163-167. doi:10.4103/JCAS.JCAS_77_17.

61. Zhang L, Yu Q, Wang Y, Ma Y, Shi Y, Li X. A small dose of botulinum toxin A is effective for treating androgenetic alopecia in Chinese patients. *Dermatol Ther.* 2019;32(4):e12785. doi:10.1111/dth.12785.

62. Zhou Y, Yu S, Zhao J, Feng X, Zhang M, Zhao Z. Effectiveness and safety of botulinum toxin type A in the treatment of androgenetic alopecia. *Biomed Res Int.* 2020;2020:1501893. doi:10.1155/2020/1501893.

63. Fischer TW, Hipler UC, Elsner P. Effect of caffeine and testosterone on the proliferation of human hair follicles in vitro. *Int J Dermatol.* 2007;46(1):27-35. doi:10.1111/j.1365-4632.2007.03119.x.

64. Völker JM, Koch N, Becker M, Klenk A. Caffeine and its pharmacological benefits in the management of androgenetic alopecia: a review. *Skin Pharmacol Physiol.* 2020;33(3):93-109. doi:10.1159/000508228.

65. Trauer S, Lademann J, Knorr F, et al. Development of an in vitro modified skin absorption test for the investigation of the follicular penetration pathway of caffeine. *Skin Pharmacol Physiol.* 2010;23(6):320-327. doi:10.1159/000313514.

66. Tsianakas A, Hüsing B, Moll I. An ex vivo model of male skin - caffeine counteracts testosterone effects. *Arch Dermatol Res.* 2005;296:450.

67. Fischer TW, Herczeg-Lisztes E, Funk W, Zillikens D, Bíró T, Paus R. Differential effects of caffeine on hair shaft elongation, matrix and outer root sheath keratinocyte proliferation, and transforming growth factor-β2/

insulin-like growth factor-1-mediated regulation of the hair cycle in male and female human hair follicles in vitro. *Br J Dermatol.* 2014;171(5):1031-1043. doi:10.1111/bjd.13114.

68. Sisto T, Bussoletti C, Celleno L. Efficacy of a cosmetic caffeine shampoo in androgenetic alopecia management. *J Appl Cosmetol.* 2012;31:57-66.

69. Bussoletti C, Mastropietro F, Tolani M. Use of a caffeine shampoo for the treatment of male androgenetic alopecia. *J Appl Cosmetol.* 2011;29:167-180.

70. Bussoletti C, Tolaini MV, Celleno L. Efficacy of a cosmetic phyto-caffeine shampoo in female androgenetic alopecia. *G Ital Dermatol Venereol.* 2020;155(4):492-499. doi:10.23736/S0392-0488.18.05499-8.

71. Bussoletti C, Mastropietro F, Tolaini M, Celleno L. Use of a cosmetic caffeine lotion in the treatment of male androgenetic alopecia. *J Appl Cosmetol.* 2011;29:167-180.

72. Dhurat R, Chitallia J, May TW, et al. An open-label randomized multicenter study assessing the noninferiority of a caffeine-based topical liquid 0.2% versus Minoxidil 5% solution in male androgenetic alopecia. *Skin Pharmacol Physiol.* 2017;30(6):298-305. doi:10.1159/000481141.

73. Golpour M, Rabbani H, Farzin D, Azizi F. Comparing the effectiveness of local solution of minoxidil and caffeine 2.5% with local solution of Minoxidil 2.5% in treatment of androgenetic alopecia. *J Mazandaran Univ Med Sci.* 2013;23(106):30-36.

74. Pazoki-Toroudi H, Moghadam R, Ajami M, Nassiri-Kashani M, Ehsani A, Tabatabaie H. The efficacy and safety of minoxidil 5% combination with azelaic acid 1/5% and caffeine 1% solution on male pattern hair loss. *J Invest Dermatol.* 2013;133:S84.

75. Sun HY, Sebaratnam DF. Clascoterone as a novel treatment for androgenetic alopecia. *Clin Exp Dermatol.* 2020;45(7):913-914. Available at: https://doi.org/10.1111/ced.14292.

76. Zito PM, Bistas KG, Syed K. Finasteride. In: *StatPearls.* StatPearls Publishing; 2021. Available at: http://www.ncbi.nlm.nih.gov/books/NBK513329/. Accessed May 4, 2021.

77. *Cassiopea Announces Very Positive Phase II Twelve Months Results for Breezula (Clascoterone) in Treating Androgenetic Alopecia.* Cassiopea. Published April 16, 2019. Available at: https://www.bloomberg.com/press-releases/2019-04-16/cassiopea-announces-very-positive-phase-ii-twelve-monthsresults- for-breezula-clascoterone-in-treating-androgenetic. Accessed March 28, 2021.

78. Sovak M, Seligson AL, Kucerova R, Bienova M, Hajduch M, Bucek M. Fluridil, a rationally designed topical agent for androgenetic alopecia: first clinical experience. *Dermatol Surg.* 2002;28(8):678-685. doi:10.1046/j.1524-4725.2002.02017.x.

79. Paradisi R, Porcu E, Fabbri R, Seracchioli R, Battaglia C, Venturoli S. Prospective cohort study on the effects and tolerability of flutamide in patients with female pattern hair loss. *Ann Pharmacother.* 2011;45(4):469-475. doi:10.1345/aph.1P600.

80. Johnson DB, Sonthalia S. Flutamide. In: *StatPearls.* Florida: StatPearls Publishing; 2021. Available at: http://www.ncbi.nlm.nih.gov/books/NBK482215/. Accessed May 4, 2021.

81. Carmina E, Lobo RA. Treatment of hyperandrogenic alopecia in women. *Fertil Steril.* 2003;79(1):91-95. doi:10.1016/s0015-0282(02)04551-x.

82. *Kintor Pharmaceutical's Completion of Patients Enrolment for Pyrilutamide's Phase II Clinical Trial for Treatment of Androgenetic Alopecia.* Kintor Pharmaceutical Limited. Available at: https://en.kintor.com.cn/news/155.html. Accessed Dec. 30, 2020.

83. Kim JH, Lee SY, Lee HJ, Yoon NY, Lee WS. The efficacy and safety of 17α-estradiol (Ell-Cranell alpha 0.025%) solution on female pattern hair loss: single center, open-label, non-comparative, phase IV study. *Ann Dermatol.* 2012;24(3):295-305. doi:10.5021/ad.2012.24.3.295.

84. Georgala S, Katoulis AC, Georgala C, Moussatou V, Bozi E, Stavrianeas NG. Topical estrogen therapy for androgenetic alopecia in menopausal females. *Dermatology.* 2004;208(2):178-179. doi:10.1159/000076497.

85. Hariri L, Rehman A. Estradiol. In: *StatPearls.* StatPearls Publishing; 2021. Available at: http://www.ncbi.nlm.nih.gov/books/NBK549797/. Accessed May 4, 2021.

86. Choe SJ, Lee S, Choi J, Lee WS. Therapeutic efficacy of a combination therapy of topical 17α-estradiol and topical minoxidil on female pattern hair loss: a noncomparative, retrospective evaluation. *Ann Dermatol.* 2017;29(3):276-282. doi:10.5021/ad.2017.29.3.276.

87. Blume-Peytavi U, Kunte C, Krisp A, Garcia Bartels N, Ellwanger U, Hoffmann R. Comparison of the efficacy and safety of topical minoxidil and topical alfatradiol in the treatment of androgenetic alopecia in women. *J Dtsch Dermatol Ges.* 2007;5(5):391-395. doi:10.1111/j.1610-0387.2007.06295.x.

88. Vexiau P, Chaspoux C, Boudou P, et al. Effects of minoxidil 2% vs. cyproterone acetate treatment on female androgenetic alopecia: a controlled, 12-month randomized trial. *Br J Dermatol.* 2002;146(6):992-999. doi:10.1046/j.1365-2133.2002.04798.x.

89. Frank LA. OEstrogen receptor antagonist and hair regrowth in dogs with hair cycle arrest (alopecia X). *Vet Dermatol.* 2007;18(1):63-66. Available at: https://doi.org/10.1111/j.1365-3164.2007.00559.x.

90. Farooq M, Patel SP. Fulvestrant. In: StatPearls. *StatPearls* Publishing; 2021. Available at: http://www.ncbi.nlm.nih.gov/books/NBK560854/. Accessed May 4, 2021.

91. Lai AC, Crews CM. Induced protein degradation: an emerging drug discovery paradigm. *Nat Rev Drug Discov.* 2017;16(2):101-114. doi:10.1038/nrd.2016.211.

92. Gassmueller J, Hoffmann R, Webster A. Topical fulvestrant solution has no effect on male and postmenopausal female androgenetic alopecia: results from two randomized, proof-of-concept studies. *Br J Dermatol.* 2008;158(1):109-115. doi:10.1111/j.1365-2133.2007.08276.x.

93. Ekmekcioglu C. Melatonin receptors in humans: biological role and clinical relevance. *Biomed Pharmacother.* 2006;60(3):97-108. doi:10.1016/j.biopha.2006.01.002.

94. Tan D, Chen L, Poeggeler B, Manchester L, Reiter R. Melatonin: a potent, endogenous hydroxyl radical scavenger. *Endocr J.* 1993;1:57-60.

95. Fischer TW, Sweatman TW, Semak I, Sayre RM, Wortsman J, Slominski A. Constitutive and UV-induced metabolism of melatonin in keratinocytes and cell-free systems. *FASEB J.* 2006;20(9):1564-1566. doi:10.1096/fj.05-5227fje.

96. Fischer TW, Slominski A, Tobin DJ, Paus R. Melatonin and the hair follicle. *J Pineal Res.* 2008;44(1):1-15. doi:10.1111/j.1600-079X.2007.00512.x.

97. Fischer TW, Trüeb RM, Hänggi G, Innocenti M, Elsner P. Topical melatonin for treatment of androgenetic alopecia. *Int J Trichology.* 2012;4(4):236-245. doi:10.4103/0974-7753.111199.

98. Macher JP. Pharmacokinetics and clinical and biological tolerability of repeated topical application of a melatonin-containing cosmetic hair solution in healthy female volunteers. A double-blind, placebo-controlled, crossover design study. Clinical Study Report. MEL-COS-1. Data on file. Asatona AG, Switzerland.

99. Lorenzi S, Caputo R. Melatonin cosmetic hair solution: Open study of the efficacy and the safety on hair loss (telogen) control and hair growth (anagen) stimulation. MEL-COS-AS01. Data on file. Asatona AG, Switzerland.

100. Lorenzi S, Barbareschi M, Caputo R. Efficacy and safety of a melatonin-containing cosmetic hair solution in the treatment of early stages of male androgenic alopecia.

Open study with Trichoscan evaluation. Report/Protocol. MEL-COS-AS03. Data on file. Asatona AG, Switzerland.

101. Innocenti M, Barbareschi M. Open-label, non comparative, multicenter clinical study on efficacy and safety of a melatonin-containing cosmetic hair solution in the treatment of hair loss (telogen) and in the stimulation of hair re-growth (anagen) Report. MEL-COS-AS05. Data on file. Asatona AG, Switzerland.

102. Schmid HW. Use Test with of a melatonin-containing cosmetic hair solution to determine the change of the appearance and texture of thinning and fine hair following the application. Statistical Report. MEL-COS-AS04. Data on file. Asatona AG, Switzerland.

103. Jafarzadeh A, Nemati M, Khorramdelazad H, Hassan ZM. Immunomodulatory properties of cimetidine: its therapeutic potentials for treatment of immune-related diseases. *Int Immunopharmacol.* 2019;70:156-166. doi:10.1016/j.intimp.2019.02.026.

104. Charlesworth EN, Kagey-Sobotka A, Norman PS, Lichtenstein LM. Effect of cetirizine on mast cell-mediator release and cellular traffic during the cutaneous late-phase reaction. *J Allergy Clin Immunol.* 1989;83(5):905-912. doi:10.1016/0091-6749(89)90104-8.

105. Rossi A, Campo D, Fortuna MC, et al. A preliminary study on topical cetirizine in the therapeutic management of androgenetic alopecia. *J Dermatolog Treat.* 2018;29(2):149-151. doi:10.1080/09546634.2017.1341610.

106. Aram H. Treatment of female androgenetic alopecia with cimetidine. *Int J Dermatol.* 1987;26(2):128-130. doi:10.1111/j.1365-4362.1987.tb00546.x.

107. Naqvi A, Gerriets V. Cetirizine. In: *StatPearls.* StatPearls Publishing; 2021. Available at: http://www.ncbi.nlm.nih.gov/books/NBK549776/. Accessed May 4, 2021.

108. Zaky MS, Abo Khodeir H, Ahmed HA, Elsaie ML. Therapeutic implications of topical cetirizine 1% in treatment of male androgenetic alopecia: a case-controlled study. *J Cosmet Dermatol.* 2021;20(4):1154-1159. doi:10.1111/jocd.13940.

17

Devices and Genomic Therapies

Alana Kurtti and Jared Jagdeo

KEY POINTS

- Using clustered, regularly interspaced, short palindromic repeats-CRISPR associated protein 9, hair follicles with high steroid type II 5α-reductase enzyme activity can be genetically altered into follicles with suppressed SRD5A2 enzyme activity, theoretically allowing hair follicles to grow new hairs for a lifetime, without side effects.
- High-efficiency delivery of therapeutic proteins and genetic elements to target cells in the hair follicle is achieved with cutting-edge nanoparticle carrier systems.
- Small interfering RNA and microRNA regulate gene expression at the posttranscriptional level and can be used to reduce the production of proteins involved in androgenetic alopecia pathogenesis.

INTRODUCTION

Androgenetic alopecia (AGA) is an arduous disease for both providers and patients. Over the last few decades, numerous topical, intralesional, oral, and surgical therapies have been developed.[1] However, many of these therapies offer incomplete or temporary improvement and are associated with serious adverse effects, leaving patients frustrated and dissatisfied with disease management.[1,2]

There is an unmet medical need for tolerable and effective AGA therapies. Currently, there are several innovative therapies being investigated to overcome the aforementioned limitations. Additionally, the cellular pathways involved in the pathogenesis of AGA are being elucidated to uncover new potential therapeutic targets and treatment strategies.[3] This chapter explores several emerging hair-loss therapies including CRISPR-Cas9 (clustered, regularly interspaced, short palindromic repeats-CRISPR associated protein 9) gene editing, small interfering RNA (siRNA), microRNA (miRNA), and tissue engineering.

GENE THERAPIES

AGA is classified as an inherited genetic condition.[4,5] It is thus a promising candidate for gene therapy, which is defined as the manipulation of gene expression to alter the biological properties of living cells for therapeutic use.[6] In the twenty-first century, there has been a surge of interest in gene-based therapies targeting hair follicles for the management of hair disease.[1] This new generation of advanced medical therapies including CRISPR-Cas9 gene editing, siRNAs, and miRNA-based therapies shows great promise for AGA because of the suitability and easy accessibility of the target hair follicles.[1,7]

CRISPR-Cas9

Designing DNA-modifying gene therapies necessitates several challenging steps: gene identification, gene modification, and implementation in living humans. In gene identification, researchers must determine which of tens of thousands of genes promote disease pathogenesis. The next step is determining how these target genes must be modified to achieve the desired therapeutic effect. The final step is safely and efficiently implementing these changes in target cells in humans. Although gene identification and modification have been successfully carried out in preclinical studies, there are still many unknowns regarding application in human studies. In this section, we explore CRISPR-Cas9, a promising DNA-modifying therapy in development for the treatment of AGA.

CRISPR-Cas9, originally discovered in in the *Escherichia coli* genome, allows for the addition, removal, and alteration of sections of the DNA sequence.[8] There are two major molecules in the CRISPR-Cas9 system: the guide RNA (gRNA) and Cas9 enzyme (Fig. 17.1).[9] The gRNA is a short strand of preconstructed RNA within a longer RNA scaffold, designed to locate and bind a complimentary target DNA sequence in the genome.[9] The gRNA "guides" the Cas9 enzyme to the target site in the DNA sequence. The enzyme subsequently cuts across both DNA strands. At this time, the cell recognizes the Cas-mediated double-strand break and initiates repair via the high-fidelity homology-directed repair (HDR) pathway or the error-prone nonhomologous end joining (NHEJ) pathway.[10] NHEJ can be used to produce insertions and deletions that knockout the target gene, while HDR can be used for precise nucleotide sequence modifications, such as point mutation correction.[11-13] HDR requires the delivery of a DNA repair template with the gRNA and Cas9 enzyme.[14] The repair template must contain the desired edit flanked by homologous arms directly upstream and downstream of the target sequence.[15] Using CRISPR-Cas9, genes involved in AGA pathogenesis can be suppressed, to potentially prevent and treat AGA.

The steroid type II 5α-reductase (*SRD5A2*) gene has been identified as a major target for gene editing (level of evidence: 5).[16] The SRD5A2 enzyme is responsible for converting testosterone to dihydrotestosterone (DHT).[17] DHT is the key androgen involved in the pathogenesis of male AGA as it mediates follicular miniaturization, a process that shortens the anagen phase of hair follicles, leading to shorter, thinner vellus hair shafts.[18] In theory, gene editing technologies can treat AGA by suppressing the *SRD5A2* gene. This notion is supported by the absence of male pattern hair loss in males with genetic deficiency of *SRD5A2*.[19]

Many current clinical therapies target SRD5A2 enzyme activity, but not without efficacy and tolerability issues. Systemic oral therapies such as finasteride yield

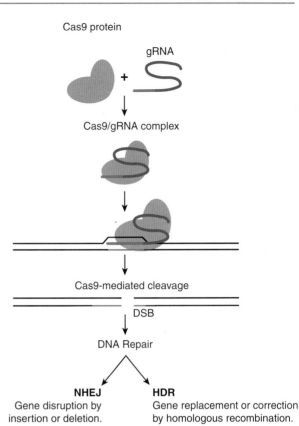

Cas9 protein

gRNA

Cas9/gRNA complex

Cas9-mediated cleavage

DSB

DNA Repair

NHEJ
Gene disruption by insertion or deletion.

HDR
Gene replacement or correction by homologous recombination.

Fig. 17.1 Schematic of CRIPSR-Cas9 (clustered, regularly interspaced, short palindromic repeats-CRISPR associated protein 9) gene editing. The Cas9 enzyme follows the guide RNA (gRNA) to the target site in the DNA sequence. The enzyme cuts across both DNA strands, creating a double-strand break (DSB). The cell recognizes the Cas-mediated DSB and initiates repair via the high-fidelity homology-directed repair (HDR) pathway or the error-prone nonhomologous end joining (NHEJ) pathway.[10] NHEJ can be used to produce insertions and deletions that knockout the target gene, while HDR can be used for precise nucleotide sequence modifications, such as point mutation correction.[11-13]

various side effects, including sexual dysfunction, anxiety, depression, and skin rash.[2,20,21] Contrarily, topical agents such as minoxidil face low transfer efficiency, which restricts efficacy.[2] A genetic approach to AGA therapy may overcome such limitations by accurately and efficiently targeting the causative gene in target cells while leaving nontarget cells unaffected. Hair follicles with high SRD5A2 enzyme activity could be genetically altered into follicles with suppressed SRD5A2 enzyme activity, allowing hair follicles to grow new hairs for a lifetime, without side effects (Pearl 17.1).

PEARL 17.1: Using CRISPR-Cas9 (clustered, regularly interspaced, short palindromic repeats-CRISPR associated protein 9), hair follicles with high SRD5A2 enzyme activity can be genetically altered into follicles with suppressed SRD5A2 enzyme activity, theoretically allowing hair follicles to grow new hairs for a lifetime, without side effects.

PEARL 17.2: High efficiency delivery of therapeutic proteins and genetic elements to target cells in the hair follicle may be achieved with cutting-edge nanoparticle carrier systems.

Designing a delivery system that efficiently transports CRISPR-Cas9 molecules to the intracellular spaces of target dermal papilla cells (DPCs) in the stratum corneum has been challenging.[16] When administered into serum, unprotected Cas9 proteins can be neutralized by binding to serum proteins and bloods cells, suffer from serum instability, and undergo rapid degradation or inactivation by proteases.[16,22] To overcome these hurdles, researchers have designed several nanoparticle systems to protect and facilitate the transport of protein complexes, with some systems showing excellent efficiency (Fig. 17.2, Pearl 17.2).[23,24] Among the more successful designs is the cutting-edge microbubble conjugated nanoliposome (MB-NL) delivery system (level of evidence: 5).[16] In this model, nanoliposomes encapsulate the Cas9 protein and gRNA (Fig. 17.3). The nanoliposomes are conjugated to microbubbles.

Determining the proper route of administration of the MB-NL carrier system has presented additional challenges. Systemic administration of genetic elements has been reported to produce severe side effects as a result of nontarget organs being affected.[25,26] Contrarily, when genetic elements are applied topically in an attempt to bypass off-target effects, there is insufficient penetration of nanoparticles, especially in the skin.[16] To resolve these issues, researchers created an ultrasound

(US)-activated topical MB-NL solution.[16] After the topical solution is applied to skin containing hair follicles, US is administered and causes the microbubbles to burst. This creates transient cavities in the surface of the skin to transport the nanoliposomes through the epidermis and into the DPCs (Fig. 17.4).[16] The topical administration keeps the therapeutic effects localized, while the US provides the external force necessary to efficiently transport the MB-NL into the target DPCs.

In a 2020 study, this novel method was tested on mouse models.[16] Male mice underwent hair removal

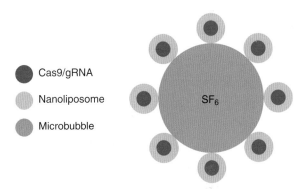

Cas9/gRNA

Nanoliposome

Microbubble

SF$_6$

Fig. 17.3 Schematic of the microbubble conjugated nanoliposome (MB-NL) system. The nanoliposomes (NLs), which encapsulate the Cas9/guide RNA (gRNA) gene editing molecules, are conjugated onto the microbubble (MB) particle surface.[16]

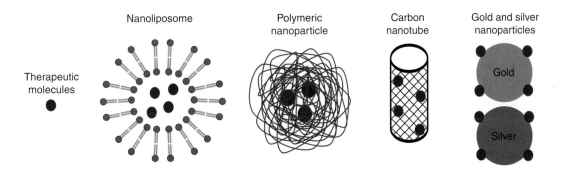

Therapeutic molecules   Nanoliposome   Polymeric nanoparticle   Carbon nanotube   Gold and silver nanoparticles

Gold

Silver

Fig. 17.2 Example nanoparticle carrier systems for delivery of therapeutic molecules.

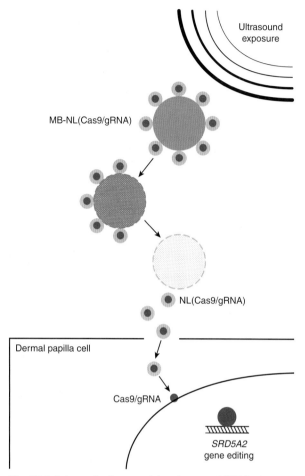

Ultrasound exposure

MB-NL(Cas9/gRNA)

NL(Cas9/gRNA)

Dermal papilla cell

Cas9/gRNA

SRD5A2
gene editing

Fig. 17.4 Schematic diagram of the ultrasound (US) flash exposure and enhancement of nanoliposome (NL) particle penetration to the dermal papilla cell (DPC) cytosol. US administration causes the microbubbles (MBs) to burst, creating momentary cavities in the surface of the skin to transport the NLs through the epidermis and into the DPCs.[16]

using hair clippers at 7 weeks of age, so that hair follicles were synchronized in the telogen phase. Topical testosterone was applied to the depilated skin of mice in all noncontrol groups daily for 7 weeks. Daily topical MB-NL solution was applied and US performed on mice in the treatment group for 5 days. The novel US-activated MB-NL system exhibited remarkable gene editing efficiency (71.6%), and SRD5A2 mRNA showed approximately 70% reduction from the control.[16] Additionally, the topical administration did not affect SRD5A2 function in other organs. Regarding hair growth, mice that were subject to US-activated MB-NL showed initiation of hair generation on the third week; by the seventh week, hair follicle density was similar to the non-testosterone-treated control mouse. By contrast, testosterone-treated mice without US-activated MB-NL treatment maintained their telogen hair cycle for 7 weeks. Mice treated with naked Cas9/sgRNA complexes with US and NL (Cas9/gRNA) with the US showed a similar pattern to the testosterone-treated mice, suggesting that these methods are insufficient for penetration of the complexes to regenerate hair.[16] Researchers appear to have identified a functional topical technique to achieve adequate penetration and high gene editing efficiency for hair regeneration while avoiding systemic side effects.

Although CRISPR-Cas9 has great promise as a simple, efficient, accurate gene editing tool, research is largely being conducted in animal models and cultured human cells, with the goal of using the system routinely in humans in the future (Pearl 17.3). The US-activated MB-NL system has shown great success in preliminary mouse studies and should be further investigated as a potential therapy for AGA in humans.

Small interfering RNA

RNA interference (RNAi) has been touted as one of the newest and most innovative approaches in gene therapy (Pearl 17.4). Small interfering RNAs (siRNAs) are double-stranded RNA molecules approximately 21 to 23 nucleotides in length that "interfere" with the expression of genes of complementary nucleotide sequence.[27,28] In the RNAi pathway, siRNAs are incorporated into the effector complex RNA-induced silencing complex (RISC), a multiprotein complex (Fig. 17.5). During RISC assembly, the siRNA is unwound and the single-stranded RNA binds with the complementary target

> **PEARL 17.3:** Gene therapy research is largely being conducted in animal models and cultured human cells, with the goal of eventually using gene-based modalities routinely in humans.

> **PEARL 17.4:** Small interfering RNAs and microRNAs regulate gene expression at the posttranscriptional level and can be used to reduce the production of proteins involved in androgenetic alopecia pathogenesis.

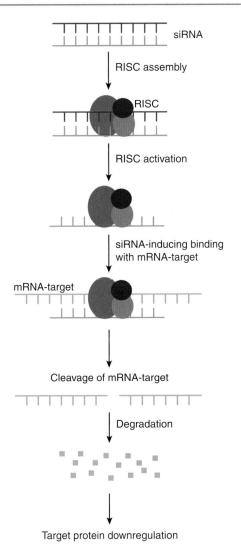

siRNA

RISC assembly

RISC

RISC activation

siRNA-inducing binding with mRNA-target

mRNA-target

Cleavage of mRNA-target

Degradation

Target protein downregulation

Fig. 17.5 Schematic of the small interfering RNA (siRNA) pathway. Small interfering RNAs (siRNAs) are incorporated into the effector complex RNA-induced silencing complex (RISC), a multiprotein complex. During RISC assembly, the siRNA is unwound and the single-stranded RNA binds with the complementary microRNA (mRNA) target sequence. The activated RISC then cleaves the mRNA target, leaving it subject to degradation by proteases, thereby preventing translation.[28]

mRNA sequence.[28] The activated RISC then cleaves the mRNA target, leaving it subject to degradation by proteases, thereby preventing translation. siRNAs share many functional properties with miRNAs, as they are both able to repress the expression of target mRNAs by either inhibiting their translation or promoting their

degradation.[28] In other fields, such as oncology, researchers have capitalized this newfound knowledge by constructing siRNAs that can inactivate cancer-causing gene mutations in oncogenes and tumor suppressor genes.[29] At this time, three FDA-approved siRNA-based therapies are on the market, with none in the field of dermatology.[30] However, the potential of siRNA-based therapies for the treatment of dermatologic disease, particularly hair disease, has not been overlooked and is currently being extensively researched.

Several features of siRNAs make it an attractive option for AGA therapy. For one, siRNAs can downregulate target gene expression with high specificity and thus be used to suppress causative AGA genes.[30] *SRD5A2* and androgen receptor (AR) mRNA have been identified as promising targets, as their protein products are crucial to AGA pathogenesis. Compared with CRISPR-Cas9, siRNA has the appealing feature of not being integrated into DNA.[29] Therefore, the genome is not permanently altered. This provides the option to halt and modify the siRNA therapy at any time, an important regulatory and safety consideration.[29,31]

There is a paucity of published studies investigating siRNA therapies for AGA. However, in a published conference abstract, topical application of liposome-formulated siRNA targeting ARs on human scalp skin explants yielded a significant dose-dependent decrease of AR mRNA and protein levels (level of evidence: 5).[32,33] The topical solution reduced AR levels only at the site of application and did not show evidence of absorption in systemic circulation both *in vivo* in mice and *ex vivo* in Franz diffusing cells containing human skin. The efficacy of topical siRNA for hair loss treatment was further demonstrated in the mouse model of chemotherapy-induced alopecia using p53 targeted siRNA. Translation of p53 mRNA produces a protein in matrix keratinocytes that, when exposed to chemotherapy, results in their apoptosis. The results of this model showed that p53 siRNA-treated mice were partly rescued from hair loss and demonstrated significantly accelerated hair regrowth in the affected area compared with control.[32,33]

Despite its exciting potential, siRNA application faces several challenges, many of which are shared by CRISPR-Cas9. For one, naked siRNA suffers a short half-life in the bloodstream as a result of degradation by enzymes and rapid renal clearance.[34] When applied topically, siRNA faces low permeability through the epidermis because of its large size, negative charge, and susceptibility to degradation by enzymes.[35-37] Further, siRNAs are unable to enter cells by passive diffusion mechanisms.[27] As a result, topical siRNA delivery efforts are centered around constructing carrier molecules that mask siRNA-negative charges, compress the siRNA molecule to make it smaller, and protect siRNA from degradation.[1,38]

Several carrier molecules have been scrutinized for siRNA applications.[39,40] Nakamura et al. demonstrated the safe and effective delivery of siRNA using biodegradable cationized gelatin microspheres in a murine model of alopecia areata (AA) and demonstrated high-specificity inhibition of target gene expression, resulting in the restoration of hair shaft elongation (level of evidence: 5).[1,39] This carrier system may also be suitable for siRNA-based AGA therapies. Nanocarriers have been shown to effectively encapsulate siRNA, helping prevent degradation and increasing delivery efficiency.[40] Further research comparing the safety and efficacy of these transport methods will help determine the ideal system for AGA therapy.

Among the different categories of RNA therapeutics, siRNA has seemingly generated the most anticipation. Successful therapeutic application of siRNA requires further research on achieving efficient delivery to the desired cells. Moreover, extensive preclinical testing is required before siRNA therapy can be implemented in AGA human studies.

Micro RNA

Micro RNAs are small single-stranded RNA molecules approximately 22 nucleotides in length that regulate gene expression at the posttranscriptional level (Fig. 17.6).[41,42]

These noncoding RNA strands regulate the expression of nearly one-third of genes in humans by targeting mRNAs based on sequence complimentarity.[43,44] The exact mechanisms of miRNA silencing are still being elucidated, but based on our current knowledge, it is believed that, after extensive processing, miRNA binds the RISC.[45] The complex then associates with a target mRNA with two to eight bases of sequence complementarity. The target mRNA then encounters translational blockage or degradation subsequent to cleavage or adenylation and decapping.[46-48]

Almost every aspect of cellular processes is affected by miRNAs, including cell cycle control, apoptosis, developmental staging, differentiation, and metabolic pathways, and deregulation of their expression has been noted in many human diseases.[51,52] This can be used as a potential therapeutic by miRNA replacement therapy using miRNA mimics or inhibition of miRNA activity by anti-miRNAs.[49] In the replacement approach, synthetic miRNA mimics are used to mimic the function of the endogenous miRNAs, leading to mRNA inhibition and thus a gene silencing effect.[50] The anti-miRNA approach is similar to antisense therapy, in which constructed anti-miRNA strands act as antagonists to inhibit the activity of endogenous miRNAs.[50] Several preclinical studies using a variety of disease models have assessed miRNA-based therapeutics, with several progressing into clinical studies.[49]

There are documented roles of miRNAs in hair follicle formation and hair growth.[53,54] It is well known that hair follicles are derived from hair follicle stem cells, and that miRNAs affect the formation of hair follicles by regulating the proliferation, differentiation, and

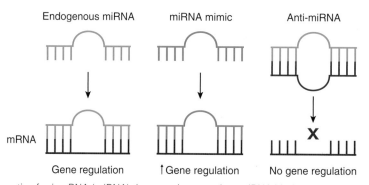

Fig. 17.6 Schematic of microRNA (miRNA) therapeutic strategies. miRNA binds to a complementary mRNA sequence, regulating its expression. The miRNA mimic promotes miRNA activity, while the anti-miRNA strand inhibits endogenous miRNA action.[49,50]

apoptosis of hair follicle stem cells.[54,55] Further, changes in miRNA expression levels appear to affect the hair follicle growth cycle, and AGA is associated with abnormal expression of various miRNAs.[44,56] Studying the abnormal expression of miRNAs in regions affected by AGA can reveal the pathogenesis of AGA at the genetic level and is expected to be useful for identifying potential new therapeutic targets for AGA.

Herein, we discuss several miRNA molecules that may function in AGA pathogenesis. Several studies have identified abnormal expression of miRNAs in the Wnt/β-Catenin pathway, a significant regulatory pathway in hair follicle growth.[57-59] Wnt/β-Catenin signaling plays an important role in promoting hair morphogenesis and DPC proliferation and maintaining the cycle of long hair growth.[57,60] In a study by Deng et al, miRNA microarray profiling identified 43 miRNAs that were significantly differentially expressed in AGA patients (21 upregulated and 22 downregulated), and qRT-PCR verified that 8 miRNAs were significantly differentially expressed (level of evidence: 5).[56]

Among the abnormally expressed miRNAs, miR-133b was of particular interest to researchers, as further analysis revealed overexpression of miR-133b inhibited the proliferation and induction ability of DPCs via the Wnt/β-catenin pathway.[56] As researchers speculate that miR-133b may inactivate the Wnt/β-catenin pathway and ultimately regulate hair growth, inhibiting miR-133b using anti-miRNAs may be a promising strategy to treat AGA.

Several other studies have identified miRNAs that appear to regulate the Wnt/β-catenin pathway and thus may be responsible for hair follicle growth.[58] For example, miR-218-5p positively regulates the Wnt/β-catenin pathway, thereby promoting growth of hair shafts, while miR-195-5p inhibits Wnt/β-catenin to regulate hair follicle inductivity.[58,61] Additionally, Ge et al. found that miR-29a/b1 inhibits hair follicle stem cell lineage progression by spatiotemporally suppressing Wnt and bone morphogenetic protein signaling (level of evidence: 5).[59] Several miRNA activators and inhibitors of the Wnt/β-catenin pathway have been identified and can serve as the basis for future studies. Developing miRNA mimics to activate the Wnt/β-catenin and anti-miRNAs to suppress inhibitors of the Wnt/β-catenin are promising strategies to promote hair follicle growth.

Other studies have identified promising miRNA targets involved in the mitogen-activated protein kinase (MAPK) and transforming growth factor (TGF)-β signaling pathways.[62]

DHT has been shown to stimulate synthesis of TGF-β, resulting in premature entry of hair follicles into the catagen phase and inducing male pattern baldness.[63] Further, TGF-β antagonists have been reported to prevent catagen-like morphologic changes and promote elongation of hair follicles in vivo and in vitro.[63] Previous studies have shown that the MAPK cascade is implicated in keratinocyte terminal differentiation.[64] Mohammadi et al. generated miRNA signatures for normal and AGA follicular stem and progenitor cells (level of evidence: 3b).[62] The study revealed that miR-324-3p was depleted in AGA patient stem cells compared with normal stem and progenitor cells and that miR-324-3p promotes differentiation and migration of cultured keratinocytes, likely through the regulation of MAPK and TGF-β signaling.[62] The data indicates that miR-324-3p is a probable candidate to regulate human hair keratinocyte differentiation.[62] Topical application of an miR-324-3p mimic therefore may be a promising new therapeutic for hair loss.

Substantial progress has been made in clarifying the roles of miRNAs in hair follicle development and hair cycle-associated tissue remodeling. However, miRNA studies largely remain in the therapeutic target identification phase. Researchers are still diligently working to define the "microRNome" of AGA patients. As miRNA therapy progresses toward clinical application, researchers will have to overcome several design challenges. Like siRNAs, miRNA therapies face significant delivery challenges. Unprotected RNA molecules are subject to instability, degradation, and rapid clearance in the bloodstream, and their hydrophilic nature, negative charge, and high molecular weight make penetration into target cells extremely difficult.[50] As siRNAs and miRNAs share many physicochemical properties and have the same intracellular site of action, similar delivery technologies can likely be used for both types of RNA molecules.[50] Nonetheless, extensive development and preclinical testing is required before implementing miRNA therapy in AGA human studies.

TISSUE ENGINEERING

Tissue engineering is defined as the practice of assembling scaffolds, cells, and biologically active molecules into functional tissues.[65] Scaffolds are three-dimensional

(3D) structures, typically made of polymeric biomaterials, that provide the physical support for cell attachment and growth.[66] The scaffold and cells are exposed to growth factors and other regulatory signals to direct cell behavior and differentiation into specific cell types, with the aim of producing fully functional tissue suitable for implantation (Fig. 17.7).[67] Bioengineered human skin constructs (HSCs) do exist, but they are limited by poor long-term viability and lack of appendages, including hair follicles, sebaceous glands, and sweat glands.[1,68] In theory, the ability to create a transplantable, fully functional hair organ via tissue engineering could cure hair loss without adverse side effects (Pearl 17.5).[69,70]

Various hair-producing HSCs are in development, with some showing great promise.[68,71] Abaci et al. regenerated fully functional, hair-bearing skin from cultured human cells in an entirely *ex vivo* environment (level of evidence: 5).[68] To achieve this, researchers used 3D-printing technology to recreate the physiologic conformation of cells in the hair follicle microenvironment. This 3D model guided the arrangement of genetically

> **PEARL 17.5:** In theory, the ability to create a transplantable, fully functional hair organ via tissue engineering would cure hair loss without adverse side effects.

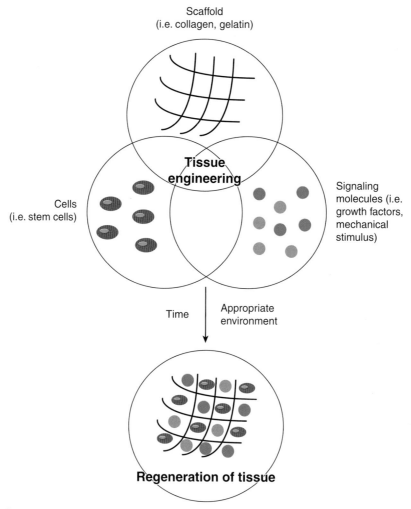

Fig. 17.7 Schematic of the tissue engineering triad. Combing appropriate scaffolds, cells, and signaling molecules produces functioning tissue.

reprogrammed cells into physiologically relevant conformations with proper epithelial-mesenchymal and cell-extracellular matrix interactions, enabling the formation of functional hair follicle units capable of hair neogenesis. When these in vitro-conditioned structures were transplanted onto rodent skin, they induced formation of hundreds of hair follicles starting from just a single strip of donor tissue, a feat that was not possible with previous techniques.[68] This biomimetic method presents an innovative, feasible approach for producing hair-bearing HSCs from cultured human cells in an entirely *ex vivo* context.

There has been a surge of interest and substantial progress in the field of hair follicle bioengineering. However, there are uncertainties about whether these methods can be safely and effectively applied in humans, as studies have yet to expand beyond mouse models. A regenerative medicine therapy for human hair loss will only be successfully achieved when hair follicles constructed *in vitro* enable de novo hair follicle formation after transplantation of the bioengineered structures into the human patient's bald scalp.[69]

EVIDENCE SUMMARY

There is an unmet medical need for safe and effective androgenetic alopecia therapy. In the twenty-first century, there have been tremendous advancements in our understanding of androgenetic alopecia pathogenesis, permitting the development of novel therapeutic strategies. Gene-based therapies and tissue engineering represent cutting-edge technologies that may potentially be harnessed to treat androgenetic alopecia. Both the US-activated microbubble conjugated nanoliposome and liposome-formulated small interfering RNA systems have shown great success in preliminary mouse studies and should be further investigated as potential therapies for androgenetic alopecia in humans (strength of recommendation: D). However, extensive research investigating the safety and efficacy of these modalities is required before they can be employed in human studies.

REFERENCES

1. Martinez-Lopez A, Montero-Vilchez T, Sierra-Sánchez Á, Molina-Leyva A, Arias-Santiago S. Advanced medical therapies in the management of non-scarring alopecia: areata and androgenic alopecia. *Int J Mol Sci.* 2020; 21(21):8390.
2. Khandpur S, Suman M, Reddy BS. Comparative efficacy of various treatment regimens for androgenetic alopecia in men. *J Dermatol.* 2002;29(8):489-498.
3. Falto-Aizpurua L, Choudhary S, Tosti A. Emerging treatments in alopecia. *Expert Opin Emerg Drugs.* 2014;19(4): 545-556.
4. Birch MP, Messenger AG. Genetic factors predispose to balding and non-balding in men. *Eur J Dermatol.* 2001; 11(4):309-314.
5. Nyholt DR, Gillespie NA, Heath AC, Martin NG. Genetic basis of male pattern baldness. *J Invest Dermatol.* 2003; 121(6):1561-1564.
6. FDA U. Long Term Follow-up After Administration of Human Gene Therapy Products. Guidance for Industry. 2020.
7. Mistriotis P, Andreadis ST. Hair follicle: a novel source of stem cells for cell and gene therapy. In: Danquah MK, Mahato RI, eds. *Emerging Trends in Cell and Gene Therapy.* Totowa, NJ: Humana Press; 2013:97-118.
8. Ishino Y, Krupovic M, Forterre P. History of CRISPR-Cas from encounter with a mysterious repeated sequence to genome editing technology. *J Bacteriol.* 2018;200(7): e00580-00517.
9. Cui Y, Xu J, Cheng M, Liao X, Peng S. Review of CRISPR/ Cas9 sgRNA design tools. *Interdiscip Sci.* 2018;10(2): 455-465.
10. Wu SS, Li QC, Yin CQ, Xue W, Song CQ. Advances in CRISPR/Cas-based gene therapy in human genetic diseases. *Theranostics.* 2020;10(10):4374-4382.
11. Gaj T, Gersbach CA, Barbas CF III. ZFN, TALEN, and CRISPR/Cas-based methods for genome engineering. *Trends Biotechnol.* 2013;31(7):397-405.
12. Lieber MR. The mechanism of double-strand DNA break repair by the nonhomologous DNA end-joining pathway. *Annu Rev Biochem.* 2010;79:181-211.
13. Chiruvella KK, Liang Z, Wilson TE. Repair of double-strand breaks by end joining. *Cold Spring Harb Perspect Biol.* 2013;5(5):a012757.
14. Hsu PD, Lander ES, Zhang F. Development and applications of CRISPR-Cas9 for genome engineering. *Cell.* 2014; 157(6):1262-1278.
15. Sansbury BM, Hewes AM, Kmiec EB. Understanding the diversity of genetic outcomes from CRISPR-Cas generated homology-directed repair. *Commun Biol.* 2019;2:458.
16. Ryu JY, Won EJ, Lee HAR, et al. Ultrasound-activated particles as CRISPR/Cas9 delivery system for androgenic alopecia therapy. *Biomaterials.* 2020;232:119736.
17. Ellis JA, Stebbing M, Harrap SB. Genetic analysis of male pattern baldness and the 5α-reductase genes. *J Invest Dermatol.* 1998;110(6):849-853.

18. Kaufman KD. Androgens and alopecia. *Mol Cell Endocrinol.* 2002;198(1-2):89-95.

19. Wilson JD, Griffin JE, Russell DW. Steroid 5α-reductase 2 deficiency. *Endocr Rev.* 1993;14(5):577-593.

20. Di Loreto C, La Marra F, Mazzon G, Belgrano E, Trombetta C, Cauci S. Immunohistochemical evaluation of androgen receptor and nerve structure density in human prepuce from patients with persistent sexual side effects after finasteride use for androgenetic alopecia. *PLoS One.* 2014;9(6):e100237.

21. Motofei IG, Rowland DL, Georgescu SR, et al. Finasteride adverse effects in subjects with androgenic alopecia: a possible therapeutic approach according to the lateralization process of the brain. *J Dermatolog Treat.* 2016; 27(6):495-497.

22. Gu Z, Biswas A, Zhao M, Tang Y. Tailoring nanocarriers for intracellular protein delivery. *Chem Soc Rev.* 2011;40(7): 3638-3655.

23. Staahl BT, Benekareddy M, Coulon-Bainier C, et al. Efficient genome editing in the mouse brain by local delivery of engineered Cas9 ribonucleoprotein complexes. *Nat Biotechnol.* 2017;35(5):431-434.

24. Zuris JA, Thompson DB, Shu Y, et al. Cationic lipid-mediated delivery of proteins enables efficient protein-based genome editing in vitro and in vivo. *Nat Biotechnol.* 2015;33(1):73-80.

25. Gilbert LA, Horlbeck MA, Adamson B, et al. Genome-scale CRISPR-mediated control of gene repression and activation. *Cell.* 2014;159(3):647-661.

26. Kim H, Kim ST, Ryu J, Kang BC, Kim JS, Kim SG. CRISPR/Cpf1-mediated DNA-free plant genome editing. *Nat Commun.* 2017;8(1):1-7.

27. Kesharwani P, Gajbhiye V, Jain NK. A review of nanocarriers for the delivery of small interfering RNA. *Biomaterials.* 2012;33(29):7138-7150.

28. Laganà A, Veneziano D, Russo F, et al. Computational design of artificial RNA molecules for gene regulation. *Methods Mol Biol.* 2015;1269:393-412. doi:10.1007/978-1-4939-2291-8_25.

29. Tatiparti K, Sau S, Kashaw SK, Iyer AK. siRNA delivery strategies: a comprehensive review of recent developments. *Nanomaterials.* 2017;7(4):77.

30. Zhang MM, Bahal R, Rasmussen TP, Manautou JE, Zhong XB. The growth of siRNA-based therapeutics: updated clinical studies. *Biochem Pharmacol.* 2021:114432.

31. Resnier P, Montier T, Mathieu V, Benoit JP, Passirani C. A review of the current status of siRNA nanomedicines in the treatment of cancer. *Biomaterials.* 2013;34(27):6429-6443.

32. Feinstein E. Topical application of siRNA against androgen receptor for treatment of androgenic alopecia and female pattern hair loss. Oral presentation at: 10th World Congress for Hair Research; October, 2017; Kyoto, Japan.

33. Feinstein E, Gao S, Avkin S, Kalinski H, Spivak I, Brafman A, Huang J, Luo N, Zhang H, Ashush H. Topical application of siRNA for treatment of hair follicle pathologies. Joint Conference on 9th Clinical Dermatology Congress & 2nd International Conference on Psoriasis, Psoriatic arthritis & Skin infections; October, 2017; New York, NY.

34. Soutschek J, Akinc A, Bramlage B, et al. Therapeutic silencing of an endogenous gene by systemic administration of modified siRNAs. *Nature.* 2004;432(7014):173-178.

35. Ruan R, Chen M, Sun S, et al. Topical and targeted delivery of siRNAs to melanoma cells using a fusion peptide carrier. *Sci Rep.* 2016;6(1):29159.

36. Baroli B. Penetration of nanoparticles and nanomaterials in the skin: fiction or reality? *J Pharm Sci.* 2010;99(1):21-50.

37. Lenn JD, Neil J, Donahue C, et al. RNA aptamer delivery through intact human skin. *J Invest Dermatol.* 2018;138(2): 282-290.

38. Singhal M, Lapteva M, Kalia YN. Formulation challenges for 21st century topical and transdermal delivery systems. *Expert Opin Drug Deliv.* 2017;14(6):705-708.

39. Nakamura M, Jo J, Tabata Y, Ishikawa O. Controlled delivery of T-box21 small interfering RNA ameliorates autoimmune alopecia (Alopecia Areata) in a C3H/HeJ mouse model. *Am J Pathol.* 2008;172(3):650-658.

40. Haigh O, Depelsenaire AC, Meliga SC, et al. CXCL1 gene silencing in skin using liposome-encapsulated siRNA delivered by microprojection array. *J Control Release.* 2014;194:148-156.

41. Goodarzi HR, Abbasi A, Saffari M, Tabei MB, Daloii MRN. MicroRNAs take part in pathophysiology and pathogenesis of male pattern baldness. *Mol Biol Rep.* 2010;37(6):2959-2965.

42. de Planell-Saguer M, Rodicio MC. Analytical aspects of microRNA in diagnostics: a review. *Anal Chim Acta.* 2011;699(2):134-152.

43. Lewis BP, Burge CB, Bartel DP. Conserved seed pairing, often flanked by adenosines, indicates that thousands of human genes are microRNA targets. *Cell.* 2005;120(1): 15-20.

44. Mardaryev AN, Ahmed MI, Vlahov NV, et al. Micro-RNA-31 controls hair cycle-associated changes in gene expression programs of the skin and hair follicle. *FASEB J.* 2010;24(10):3869-3881.

45. Ryan B, Joilin G, Williams JM. Plasticity-related microRNA and their potential contribution to the maintenance of long-term potentiation. *Front Mol Neurosci.* 2015;8:4.

46. Eulalio A, Huntzinger E, Nishihara T, Rehwinkel J, Fauser M, Izaurralde E. Deadenylation is a widespread effect of miRNA regulation. *RNA.* 2009;15(1):21-32.

47. O'Brien J, Hayder H, Zayed Y, Peng C. Overview of MicroRNA biogenesis, mechanisms of actions, and circulation. *Front Endocrinol (Lausanne).* 2018;9:402.

48. Shah MY, Ferrajoli A, Sood AK, Lopez-Berestein G, Calin GA. microRNA therapeutics in cancer—an emerging concept. *EBioMedicine.* 2016;12:34-42.

49. Rupaimoole R, Slack FJ. MicroRNA therapeutics: towards a new era for the management of cancer and other diseases. *Nat Rev Drug Discov.* 2017;16(3):203-222.

50. Lam JKW, Chow MYT, Zhang Y, Leung SWS. siRNA Versus miRNA as therapeutics for gene silencing. *Mol Ther Nucleic Acids.* 2015;4(9):e252.

51. Erson A, Petty E. MicroRNAs in development and disease. *Clin Genet.* 2008;74(4):296-306.

52. Medina PP, Slack FJ. microRNAs and cancer: an overview. *Cell Cycle.* 2008;7(16):2485-2492.

53. Goodarzi H, Abbasi A, Saffari M, Fazelzadeh Haghighi M, Tabei M, Noori Daloii M. Differential expression analysis of balding and nonbalding dermal papilla microRNAs in male pattern baldness with a microRNA amplification profiling method. *Br J Dermatol.* 2012;166(5):1010-1016.

54. Yi R, O'Carroll D, Pasolli HA, et al. Morphogenesis in skin is governed by discrete sets of differentially expressed microRNAs. *Nat Genet.* 2006;38(3):356-362.

55. Liu G, Li S, Liu H, et al. The functions of ocu-miR-205 in regulating hair follicle development in Rex rabbits. *BMC Dev Biol.* 2020;20(1):8.

56. Deng W, Hu T, Han L, et al. miRNA microarray profiling in patients with androgenic alopecia and the effects of miR-133b on hair growth. *Exp Mol Pathol.* 2021;118:104589.

57. Chen X, Liu B, Li Y, et al. Dihydrotestosterone regulates hair growth through the Wnt/β-catenin pathway in C57BL/6 mice and in vitro organ culture. *Front Pharmacol.* 2020;10:1528.

58. Zhu N, Huang K, Liu Y, et al. miR-195-5p regulates hair follicle inductivity of dermal papilla cells by suppressing Wnt/β-catenin activation. *BioMed Res Int.* 2018;2018:4924356.

59. Ge M, Liu C, Li L, et al. miR-29a/b1 inhibits hair follicle stem cell lineage progression by spatiotemporally suppressing WNT and BMP signaling. *Cell Rep.* 2019;29(8):2489-2504.e4.

60. Shimizu H, Morgan BA. Wnt signaling through the β-catenin pathway is sufficient to maintain, but not restore, anagen-phase characteristics of dermal papilla cells. *J Invest Dermatol.* 2004;122(2):239-245.

61. Zhao B, Chen Y, Yang N, et al. miR-218-5p regulates skin and hair follicle development through Wnt/β-catenin signaling pathway by targeting SFRP2. *J Cell Physiol.* 2019;234(11):20329-20341.

62. Mohammadi P, Nilforoushzadeh MA, Youssef KK, et al. Defining microRNA signatures of hair follicular stem and progenitor cells in healthy and androgenic alopecia patients. *J Dermatol Sci.* 2021;101(1):49-57.

63. Hibino T, Nishiyama T. Role of TGF-β2 in the human hair cycle. *J Dermatol Sci.* 2004;35(1):9-18.

64. Haase I, Hobbs RM, Romero MR, Broad S, Watt FM. A role for mitogen-activated protein kinase activation by integrins in the pathogenesis of psoriasis. *J Clin Invest.* 2001;108(4):527-536.

65. National Institutes of Health. *Tissue Engineering and Regenerative Medicine.* Accessed March 28, 2021 https://www.nibib.nih.gov/science-education/science-topics/tissue-engineering-and-regenerative-medicine.

66. Chan B, Leong K. Scaffolding in tissue engineering: general approaches and tissue-specific considerations. *Eur Spine J.* 2008;17(4):467-479.

67. Hasan A, Morshed M, Memic A, Hassan S, Webster TJ, Marei HE-S. Nanoparticles in tissue engineering: applications, challenges and prospects. *Int J Nanomedicine.* 2018;13:5637-5655.

68. Abaci HE, Coffman A, Doucet Y, et al. Tissue engineering of human hair follicles using a biomimetic developmental approach. *Nat Commun.* 2018;9(1):5301.

69. Castro AR, Logarinho E. Tissue engineering strategies for human hair follicle regeneration: how far from a hairy goal? *Stem Cells Transl Med.* 2020;9(3):342-350.

70. Toyoshima KE, Asakawa K, Ishibashi N, et al. Fully functional hair follicle regeneration through the rearrangement of stem cells and their niches. *Nat Commun.* 2012;3:784.

71. Zhang L, Wang WH, Jin JY, et al. Induction of hair follicle neogenesis with cultured mouse dermal papilla cells in de novo regenerated skin tissues. *J Tissue Eng Regen Med.* 2019;13(9):1641-1650.

INDEX

Page numbers followed by '*f*' indicate figures, those followed by '*t*' indicate tables.